Medicine for Disasters

Edited by
PETER BASKETT BA MBBCH BAO FFARCS
ROBIN WELLER MB BS FFARCS
Department of Anaesthetics, Frenchay Hospital, Bristol

with a foreword by
John S. M. Zorab

WRIGHT
London Boston Singapore Sydney Toronto Wellington

John Wright
is an imprint of Butterworth Scientific

First published 1988

© **Butterworth & Co. (Publishers) Ltd, 1988**

British Library Cataloguing in Publication Data
Medicine for disasters.
    1. Disaster medicine
    I. Baskett, Peter J. F.   II. Weller,
    Robin M.
616'.025   RC86.7

ISBN 0-7236-0949-7

Photoset by BC Typesetting, Exeter EX2 8PN
Printed and bound in Great Britain by Butler and Tanner, Frome, Somerset

FOREWORD

John S. M. Zorab FFARCS
Consultant Anaesthetist, Frenchay Hospital, Bristol
Secretary, World Federation of Societies of Anaesthesiologists

It is our first duty to serve society . . .

Samuel Johnson, 1709–1784

The late Professor Rudolf Frey (Mainz, FRG) devoted much of his professional life to serving society and, in particular, created an awareness of the responsibilities of the medical profession towards those suffering from the effects of both natural and man-made disasters. In 1977, he formed the 'Club of Mainz on Emergency and Disaster Medicine Worldwide' which has now developed into the 'World Association for Emergency and Disaster Medicine'.

In the preface to the *Proceedings of the International Congress on Disaster Medicine* (Mainz 1977), Professor Frey wrote, 'The missions and roles of the medical profession include the prevention, diagnosis and treatment, not only of individual patients' health problems but also of disasters which strike communities or nations and result in mass casualties.'

Disasters continue to occur with distressing regularity and the medical involvement in disaster management is now sufficiently important to have generated many conferences, innumerable published papers, a journal devoted to the subject* and, at last, an authoritative textbook.

This book is long overdue. It is likely to become the standard work in the field providing, as it does, an introduction to all types of disasters with a generous list of references to allow deeper penetration into specific fields.

Much of its value arises from the international nature of the contributors, and the editors are to be congratulated on having drawn together a group who have personal experience on which to draw and the literary ability with which to express themselves.

I believe this book forms a basic text on all aspects of disaster medicine and, as such, will be of great value to all who may find themselves working in this field, as well as being fascinating reading. Rudolf Frey would be proud and gratified to see his own field of interest being advanced in this way.

---

* 'Emergency and Disaster Medicine', later to become *Journal of the World Association of Emergency Disaster Medicine*.

This book is dedicated to the members of the
World Association for Emergency and Disaster Medicine.

PREFACE

Most doctors, nurses and other health workers look forward to a life pursuing their chosen career in relative order, peace and tranquility. However, the unexpected, by its very nature, may strike anywhere, at any time, and involve anybody or everybody, including those who are unprepared.

Some of these same professional people by chance, by inclination, through their special training or skills, or even determined by such a mundane fact as where they live, develop an interest in or involvement with the disasters that strike mankind.

This book is an attempt not only to provide an opportunity for this small second group to share their experiences amongst each other, but also, and more importantly, for them to bring their experience and wisdom to the attention of the much larger first group. For surely it is the duty of all health care workers, and doctors in particular, to react professionally and efficiently, rationally and effectively when disaster strikes. To do so, they need some fundamental principles and knowledge on which to base their activities.

Disasters come in all shapes and sizes. If you, or a member of your family, happen to be personally involved in a car accident, even if only one or two are hurt, it will rank as a disaster. At the other end of the scale, earthquakes and famines can kill and maim hundreds of thousands, or even millions of people. In each case, and in the many disasters of greater or lesser scale in between, what can be expected to happen? What planning might help alleviate their effects? What can be done to help afterwards?

The earlier chapters in this book cover the general management of disasters. They can be applied in a wide range of circumstances. Many, obviously, contain the condensed wisdom of the authors. Whole books have been written on nearly all the subjects, so none can be considered or are intended to be fully comprehensive. The later chapters deal with specific disasters; firstly, those that are natural and, secondly, those that are man-made. Many of those include descriptions of specific disasters with which the authors are personally familiar.

Editors do not write books. This one could not have been produced without the willing co-operation of its many authors. The experience of many of them is unique. The bodies and organizations for whom they work cover the range of disasters that strike this world. The editors owe an enormous debt of gratitude to them all for their unstinting efforts. It would be invidious to pick out any in particular, but Dr S. W. A. Gunn, having produced three chapters, has the experience and knowledge to have written the book on his own. Compared with his work in disaster medicine, and that of many others, the editors are mere novices, and have really done little more than gather up the pearls of wisdom from what they believe is a well and widely chosen field of genuine experts.

Lastly, but certainly not least, the editors wish to acknowledge a few people without whom this volume would never have seen the light of day. First, there are Mr Roy Baker and Mrs Merilyn Chambers from John Wright who provided us, respectively, with the initial encouragement and the guidance to keep us on the straight and narrow. But, especially, our thanks are due to two of the smartest, quickest, most efficient ladies we know, Mrs Barbara Burgess and Mrs Lynne Scott, our secretaries in the Anaesthetics Department at Frenchay.

P. J. F. B.
R. M. W.

CONTENTS

THE CONTINUING PHASE

SPECIFIC SECTION

CONTRIBUTORS

Jakov Adler MD

Peter J. F. Baskett BA MBBCH BAO FFARCS

Nicholas G. Bircher BS MD

Howard R. Champion FRCS FACS

Claude de Ville de Goyet MD

Morgan Fahey OBE FRNZCGP MRCGP

Judith Fisher MBBS MRCGP

Patricia S. Gainer MPA

Frank Golden OBE PhD Dip Av Md

S. William A. Gunn MD MS FRCS(C)

Jessie Hackes MA

Ian Haywood MBBS FRCS

Ken Hines MB BS

Richard J. Knight MB BS(London) MRCS LRCP FFARCSI

Timothy Lusty MB BCh

Ellen G. McDaniel MD

Sergio Magalini MD

Corrado Manni MD

Marshall Midda BDS FDSRCS FFDRCSI

Marjorie A. Moreau RN CEN

James P. Orlowski MD

Ernesto A. Pretto MD

Rudolph Proietti MD

John Restall MBBS FFARCS

Brian Robertson MRCS LRCP

Peter Safar MD

Patricia H. Sanner MD

Peter E. A. Savage MS FRCS

Martin E. Silverstein MD

Roberta E. Steadman RN MN

Michael Tarry

Robin M. Weller MB BS FFARCS

José L. Zeballos MD

BIOGRAPHIES

Jakov Adler was born in Czechoslovakia, qualifying from the Hebrew University, Hadassah Medical School in 1961. He is now Chief Surgeon of the Civil Defence in Israel, and Director of the Emergency Medical Services, Shaare Zedek Medical Centre, Jerusalem. He organizes the Israel Medical Teams assisting Cambodian refugees in Thailand, leading the first team in 1979. He has been Chief Medical Officer of the Ministry of Health Assistance Team to South Lebanon. He has always been actively involved with the training and teaching of resuscitation and the organization of services in natural disasters and mass casualty situations.

Peter Baskett is a consultant anaesthetist at Frenchay Hospital and the Royal Infirmary, Bristol, and a teacher in anaesthetics at the University of Bristol. He has been Honorary Secretary/Treasurer of the World Association for Emergency and Disaster Medicine since 1980 and is a past chairman of the British Association for Immediate Care.

He is currently Chairman of the WFSA CPR Committee, President of the European Regional Section of the WFSA and President of the Anaesthetic Monospecialist Committee for the European Community.

He is Vice-President of the Association of Anaesthetists of Great Britain and Ireland and a member of the Board of Faculty of Anaesthetists of the Royal College of Surgeons in England.

He is a Founder Member of the Resuscitation Council UK and a member of the Royal Automobile Club Motor Sport Association's Medical Panel, and an officer in the Territorial Army.

He is the author of several books, chapters and articles on immediate care and disaster medicine, cardiopulmonary resuscitation, training and organization of paramedic ambulancemen and the relief of acute pain in emergency situations.

Nicholas G. Bircher, born in 1954, is a graduate of Harvard University (BS) and the University of Pittsburgh (MD and Anesthesiology Residency). In 1978, while still a medical student, he became the first research fellow and later became co-ordinator of research on cardiopulmonary resuscitation methods at the International Resuscitation Research Center of the University of Pittsburgh. He is the author of about 100 scientific publications and has participated in the writing of national and international guidelines for cardiopulmonary resuscitation and emergency cardiac care. During 1984–8, he is serving as a Lieutenant Commander in the Medical Corps of the US Navy, as a staff anesthesiologist of the US Naval Hospital, and as Assistant Professor of Anesthesiology of the Uniformed Services University of the Health Sciences, Bethesda, Maryland. Dr Bircher is an Assistant Professor of Anesthesiology at the University of Pittsburgh and a member of the Cardiopulmonary Resuscitation Committee of the World Federation of Societies of Anesthesiologists.

Howard R. Champion is Chief of the Trauma Service and the Director of Surgical Critical Care at the Washington Hospital Center, Washington DC, USA. Dr Champion established the MedSTAR trauma service in Washington DC, and has been involved in national and international efforts to improve trauma assessment and care and disaster medicine since 1972.

Claude de Ville de Goyet has been extensively involved with disaster medicine throughout his medical career and has had vast experience of disasters in Central and Southern America. He is Medical Adviser to the Emergency Preparedness and Disaster Relief Co-ordination Program of the Pan-American Health Organization and has been associated with many relief missions involving communicable diseases.

He is a past Member of the Executive Council of the World Association for Emergency and Disaster Medicine.

Morgan Fahey is a family practitioner in Christchurch, New Zealand. He has devoted a very considerable part of his professional life to immediate care and disaster medicine and has been the leading pioneer in these specialties in his country. His particular interest has been in traffic medicine on land, at sea and in the air. He is adviser to Air New Zealand, the International Civil Aviation Organization and the World Health Organization. He is currently the President of the World Association for Emergency and Disaster Medicine.

Judith Fisher is a general practitioner in East London and a member of the North East Metropolitan Accident Unit. She qualified as gold medallist in surgery from the Royal Free Hospital, University of London in 1963. After qualifying she accompanied her husband on tour with the Royal Army Medical Corps and was enticed into becoming a locally employed medical officer to the Royal Scots Greys. She also became an amateur SCUBA diver and then a training officer for amateur divers. Returning to the United Kingdom she entered general practice where she retained her interests in teaching and pre-hospital care. She became founder Chairman of the Resuscitation Council (UK) and is currently Honorary Secretary of the British Association for Immediate Care. She is a trainer in general practice and a member of the Royal Free Hospital General Practice Teaching Group.

Patricia S. Gainer is the Administrative Director for Surgical Critical Care at the Washington Hospital Center. Ms Gainer has been involved in emergency medical and trauma systems development and administration since 1978.

Frank Golden qualified in medicine in Cork, Ireland, in 1960. Following his intern residencies and a period as a general practitioner in London, he joined the Royal Navy where subsequently an interest in applied physiology grew out of his involvement with aviation medicine and air-sea rescue in particular. He took his Diploma in Aviation Medicine in 1969 and PhD in physiology at Leeds University in 1979.

In the 1970s he chaired the working party on cold water survival for the International Maritime Organization and was made an Honorary Fellow of the Nautical Institute in 1982 for his services to safety at sea. For many years he worked at the Institute of Naval Medicine, latterly as Director of Research. Currently in a staff job but retaining an interest in physiology, particularly in relation to immersion in cold water.

William Gunn is a senior international health official with particular involvement in disaster management. For many years head of global emergency operations of the World Health Organization, he took part in the WHO study on the Effects of Nuclear War on Health and Health Services. He is now Special Adviser to the Red Cross League. Author of over 150 scientific papers, he is co-editor of the book *Refugee Community Health Care,* compiler of the *WHO Emergency Health Kit* and author of the *Dictionary of Emergency Relief and Disasters.* As GLAWARS Commissioner, his latest task has been the report *London Under Attack.*

A forerunner in establishing disaster medicine as a discipline, he is on the Executive Committee of the World Association for Emergency and Disaster Medicine, and the Board of the Société Internationale de Médecine des Catastrophes, and the Council of Europe's Disaster Medicine Centre in San Marino.

Jessie Hackes is the Director for Program Assessment of the US Department of Health and Human Services.

Ian Haywood is a serving officer in the Royal Army Medical Corps. He is a graduate of St Thomas's Hospital and the University of London and a Fellow of the Royal College of Surgeons of England. He has received a surgical training in military and civilian hospitals in the United Kingdom and in the past held appointments in teaching hospitals in London and Edinburgh, which have included being a Lecturer in Surgery to the Westminster Hospital Medical School and the Medical College of St Bartholomew's Hospital. He has served as a consultant surgeon in several military hospitals and until recently was the Consultant in Charge of the Trauma Unit of the Cambridge Military Hospital, Aldershot. At present he is the Joint Professor of Military Surgery to the Royal

College of Surgeons of England and the Royal Army Medical College, London.
Military service on several occasions in Northern Ireland and in the Middle East has brought him into contact with the clinical management of the victims of terrorism.

Kenneth Hines is a family practitioner in London, UK. He has had a lifelong interest and involvement in immediate care and has been particularly interested in the co-ordination of medical and rescue services in pre-hospital care.

He has had extensive experience of rescue and emergency medical care in London, including road and rail accidents, chemical accidents, terrorist activities and incidents at major crowd events and has participated in many of the activities of the British Association for Immediate Care.

Richard Knight was Consultant Anaesthetist to the Royal Army Medical Corps. In addition to serving in military hospitals worldwide, he obtained civilian experience as a registrar in Southampton, as senior registrar at Reading and the Westminster, and as supernumerary consultant at Frenchay Hospital, Bristol, UK. His expertise in the anaesthesia of gunshot wounds was gained in Northern Ireland, Cyprus, Oman and the Falkland Islands Campaign, for which latter he shared a Pask Certificate of Honour. His publications cover equipment for field anaesthesia, beta blockers in obstetric anaesthesia and aspects of the Falklands War. He is currently working in a 500 bed multispeciality hospital in Saudi Arabia, but intends to return to UK anaesthetic practice.

Timothy Lusty has worked for many years in the field of medical relief for the developing world, particularly in the African Continent. He is Senior Health Adviser to the Health Unit of Oxfam, one of the major voluntary relief agencies. He is an expert on famine relief and has travelled extensively to stricken areas to direct famine relief programmes.

He is a past Member of the Executive Council of the World Association for Emergency and Disaster Medicine.

Ellen McDaniel attended Carnegie-Mellon University and received her medical degree from the University of Michigan in 1966. Postgraduate training included an internship at the Wilmington Medical Center, a psychiatric residency at Ohio State University and the University of Maryland, and psychoanalytic training at the Baltimore-DC Institute for Psychoanalysis. She is currently an Associate Professor in Psychiatry at the University of Maryland School of Medicine in Baltimore, where she serves as an Associate Dean for Admissions and as Training Director of the Forensic Fellowship Program, in addition to having a private practice in psychiatry, both general and forensic.

Sergio Magalini is the Associate Professor of Clinical Toxicology at the Catholic University of the Sacred Heart, Rome, and Director of the Antipoison Centre,

Rome. He is a member of the World Association for Emergency and Disaster Medicine, and European Secretary of the World Federation of Associations of Antipoison Centres.

Corrado Manni is the President of the Society of International Disaster Medicine, and a member of the Executive Committee of both the European Academy of Anaesthesiology and the World Federation of Anaesthesiologists. He holds the Chair of Anaesthesia and Resuscitation at the Medical School of the Catholic University of the Sacred Heart, Rome.

Marshall Midda is a consultant dental surgeon at the University of Bristol Dental Hospital and School and Director of the School of Dental Hygiene. He is a member of the Working Party on Forensic Odontology of the British Dental Association and Adviser in Forensic Dentistry to Her Majesty's Government. He is a lecturer in forensic dentistry to the Home Office and a past member of the Aviation Pathology Team of the Royal Air Force. He has lectured and published extensively on the subject of dental identification in mass disasters and other aspects of forensic odontology.

Marjorie A. Moreau is the Training Co-ordinator for Surgical Critical Care at the Washington Hospital Center. Ms Moreau is a board-certified Emergency Nurse with 10 years' experience in pre-hospital education, trauma education and international emergency medicine.

James Orlowski is Director of Paediatric Intensive Care and Assistant Director of the Surgical Intensive Care Unit at the Cleveland Clinic Foundation. He received his medical degree from Case Western Reserve University School of Medicine and his postgraduate training included a residency in Paediatrics at the Cleveland Clinic, a residency year in Anaesthesia at University Hospitals of Cleveland, and a fellowship in Paediatric Intensive Care at Rainbow Babies' and Children's Hospital. He was the recipient of an International Travelling Fellowship Award from the International Center for Specialty Studies. He is a member of Team I of the International Medical Disaster Teams of The Southern Baptist Convention and his experience with hurricane disaster medicine relief came in response to Hurricanes David and Frederick which struck the Dominican Republic in September of 1979. He is also a member of the World Association of Emergency and Disaster Medicine.

Ernesto A. Pretto, born in 1952, received his MD degree from the University of Panama and trained in anesthesiology at the Albert Einstein College of Medicine, New York. He trained in critical care medicine at the Presbyterian University Hospital and was Chief Research Fellow at the International Resuscitation Research Center, both of the University of Pittsburgh. His research interests include use of the isolated perfused rat heart preparation, and emergency cardiopulmonary bypass. During 1985–7 he served as a Lieutenant Commander in the Medical Corps of the US Navy, as Staff Intensivist and Anesthesiologist of the US Naval Hospital, and as Assistant Professor of Anesthesiology of the Uniformed Services University of Health Sciences, Bethesda, Maryland. He is a member of the Education and Public Information Task Force of the National Disaster Medical System (NDMS). He is an Assistant Professor of Anesthesiology/Critical Care Medicine and Resuscitation Research Center Investigator at the University of Pittsburgh.

Rudolf Proietti works in the Anaesthetic and ITU Departments of the Policlinico A. Gemelli, Rome, and is an Associate Professor in special techniques for resuscitation. He is a member of the editorial board of *Medicina Informatica*.

John Restall qualified in 1958 at St Thomas's Hospital, London. He held junior anaesthetic posts at St Thomas's Hospital and the Southampton Group Hospitals. He joined the Royal Army Medical Corps in 1960, and obtained the FFARCS in 1967. He has served in Brunei, Malaya, Singapore, Belize, Northern Ireland and West Germany. He was Senior Consultant Anaesthetist for BAOR during 1981–4, Senior Lecturer at the Royal Army Medical College, London, 1984–6, and is currently Consultant Adviser in Anaesthetics and Resuscitation to the Director General AMS.

Brian Robertson is a general practitioner in Aldershot, Hampshire and Secretary of the Hampshire, Berkshire and Surrey Immediate Care Scheme. He has had vast experience of trauma associated with road and rail accidents and lectures extensively on the subject of pre-hospital care. He is a member of the Executive Council of BASICS and is Editor of the *BASICS Journal* and other publications associated with emergency and disaster medicine.

Peter Safar, born in 1924, is a graduate of the University of Vienna (MD 1948), and gained postgraduate experience in pathology, surgery and anesthesiology at the Universities of Vienna, Yale, Pennsylvania and Joh n Hopkins. He developed and chaired new academic departments and anesthesiology and resuscitation in Lima (Peru), Baltimore (Maryland) and Pittsburgh (Pennsylvania). He was one of the initiating researchers of modern cardio-pulmonary resuscitation in the 1950s and 1960s. He developed the first intensive care unit in the USA and the first critical care medicine physician training programme in the world. In the 1970s he extended cardiopulmonary resuscitation to cardiopulmonary-cerebral resuscitation. He is presently Distinguished Service Professor of Resuscitation Medicine and Director of the International Resuscitation Research Center of the University of Pittsburgh. He is the author of over 500 scientific publications. He was a founding member and past president of the Society of Critical Care Medicine (USA) and the World Association for Emergency and Disaster Medicine (Club of Mainz).

Patricia Sanner qualified at the Baylor College of Medicine, Houston, in 1976, and is now a major in the US Air Force Medical Corps. She has supervised courses on battlefield medicine and battlefield nursing, and has been involved with disaster planning and management courses developed by the American College of Emergency Physicians for the Federal Emergency Management Agency. She has published work on the stress reactions in mass casualty simulations.

Peter Savage qualified from St Mary's Hospital Medical School in 1960 and since 1974 has been consultant general surgeon with an interest in peripheral vascular surgery at Queen Mary's Hospital, Sidcup, Kent.

Throughout his career he has had a particular interest in resuscitation and the management of the severely injured casualty. While surgical registrar at Worthing Hospital he set up the hospital's cardiac arrest team, and equipped a resuscitation bay in the casualty department.

As senior registrar at Wexham Park Hospital, Slough, he first became involved in disaster planning, and since then has maintained a close interest in the organizational aspects of mass casualty management and hospital disaster planning. A regular speaker at disaster conferences, Peter Savage has written a number of papers on the subject, and in 1979 published a book: *Disasters – Hospital Planning*.

Martin Silverstein is a Senior Fellow in Science and Technology (Disaster) at Georgetown University's Center for Strategic and International Studies and Clinical Professor of Surgery and of Military Medicine at the F. Edward Hebert School of Medicine, Uniformed Services University of the Health Sciences. He is the Chairman of the Board of Emergency Systems International, a disaster research and service organization with offices in Washington DC and Tucson, Arizona.

Roberta Steadman holds Bachelor's and Master's degrees in nursing, and is currently a doctoral candidate in education. She is an Assistant Professor of Nursing at the Intercollegiate Center for Nursing Education, Spokane, Washington, USA. She is also a staff nurse in the Intensive Care Unit at Deaconess Medical Center in the same city. She has been interested in disaster nursing since the early 1970s and has been a Red Cross disaster nurse volunteer since that time. She has lectured to nursing students and critical care nurses, and previously published on the subject.

Michael Tarry is the Chief Ambulance Officer for the County of Northampton, UK. He has been a strong supporter of integration between the ambulance service and pre-hospital medical care by doctors and directs his local immediate care scheme. He has developed an excellent communications network within his own ambulance authority, which has integrated the ambulance and medical services with the other rescue services.

He is currently a member of the Executive Council of the British Association for Immediate Care representing the ambulance service.

Robin Weller is a consultant anaesthetist at Frenchay Hospital, Bristol. He qualified at St Bartholomew's Hospital in 1966 and trained at Whipps Cross Hospital, London, and the Radcliffe Infirmary, Oxford, before moving to Bristol. He spent one year as Assistant Visiting Professor at the University of Virginia, Charlottesville. He is an officer in the Territorial Army, serving with the 308 Evacuation Hospital. He is interested in acute and disaster medicine, acting as medical officer at several sporting events. He has also been actively involved with aeromedical evacuation and is a member of the Council of the British Aeromedical Practitioners Association as well as a member of the British Association for Immediate Care (BASICS). He has served on the Council of the Anaesthetic Section of the Royal Society of Medicine and is joint editor of *Lectures in Anaesthesiology* produced twice-yearly for the WFSA. Lastly, he is founder, editor and sole producer of *Today's Anaesthetist.*

José Zeballos, a native of Bolivia, obtained his MD degree at the Universidad Mayor de San Andres, La Paz, Bolivia and his MPH at the School of Public Health, University of Puerto Rico. Further, he completed postgraduate studies in Argentina and Japan. Most of his professional experience is related to epidemiology. He was Chief of the Department of Epidemiology, Ministry of Public Health in Bolivia, at national level.

Dr Zeballos joined the Pan-American Health Organization in 1981 where he is presently working as Adviser on Emergency Preparedness and Disaster Relief Co-ordination. His most relevant experience in the disaster field was acquired during the Mexico earthquake in 1985 by providing technical assistance and expertise at top decision-making level.

GENERAL SECTION

M. Fahey

1

A History of Disaster Medicine

INTRODUCTION

Throughout history, disasters have had an impact on the development of medicine world-wide and, particularly in recent centuries, their management has been influenced by discoveries in medicine. Historical reports record a range of important disasters, both natural and man-made, which illustrate the problems of disaster management which were beyond the local or national organizations, and the technical resources available. Naturally-occurring phenomena in the past, such as earthquakes, floods, avalanches, whirlwinds and famine, together with man-made calamities including war, fire and explosion have resulted in fatalities, many of which could have been prevented if the disaster had occurred in this century, and if the victims could have been rescued and treated in time.

What follows is an account of a few of these disasters which best illustrate the problems of disaster management in the past and the consequences of their management and mismanagement.

NATURALLY-OCCURRING DISASTERS

Where in modern times we are exposed to an increasing degree to potential disasters resulting from technological advances, especially in transportation, our ancestors were tested more in coping with naturally-occurring disasters.

The Volcano

Perhaps the most spectacular and instantly terrifying of these is the volcano. Historically, volcanic activity has been limited to well defined areas. Sixty-two per cent have occurred along the boundaries of the Pacific Ocean. While it is recorded that volcanic eruptions caused the death of approximately 190 000 people from the years 1500 to 1914, the mortality figures before this are unknown. It is also recorded[1] that nearly 1000 deaths a year result from volcanic eruption. The first recorded death from a volcano, that of Pliny the Elder, occurred in the Vesuvius eruption of 19 AD. Sixty years later the ancient cities of Pompeii and Herculaneum, situated south-east of Naples, were destroyed by an eruption from the same mountain. Pliny the Younger recorded that Pompeii was covered with volcanic debris and ashes to a depth of seven metres. While it was felt by young Pliny that noxious gases were the main cause of death, later

3

research[2] suggests that the dominant cause of death in both Pompeii and Herculaneum was asphyxia caused by the avalanche of mud, metres deep.

Vulcan, the god of fire, has always been associated with volcanic death by fire from red hot lava. However, this is a rare cause of death in a volcanic eruption, as most of the lava flows are slow moving and some can be diverted.[3] Volcanoes are also often accompanied by earthquake—another factor contributing to the death tolls.

More recent evidence, particularly from the Mount St Helens eruption in 1980,[4] has shown that most volcanic deaths were due to suffocation which took only a few minutes and, to a lesser extent, from burns or blunt injuries. Of interest is the fact that deaths occurred between 7·2 and 28·2 km from the centre of that volcano. From a study of both early and recent volcanic disasters, it has been concluded[1] that modern resuscitation and primary care, even if available at the time, would have been too late to save the asphyxiated victims of Pompeii and Herculaneum. If such disasters had occurred today, all that could possibly be done to save life would be by prevention of exposure and evacuation of the population, aided by early volcanic monitoring. For those who died of burns, there would of course have been a greater chance of survival with modern treatments.

The Earthquake

Of all the natural disasters, the earthquake stands alone for its power to cause the immediate destruction of cities, land and thousands of people. Lives lost as a result of a single earthquake range up to hundreds of thousands. While crushing injuries have always been known to be the dominant cause of death in earthquakes, recent research[5] has identified the specific types of injuries involved and the causes of death from modern earthquake disasters.

Studies show the following breakdown of injuries with the expected proportions of patients receiving them: soft tissue injuries (wounds and contusions) 32–68 per cent, limb fractures 16–44 per cent, head injuries 4–37 per cent, injuries to the thorax 3–15 per cent, and spinal injuries 3–9 per cent. The proportion of victims with multiple injuries varies from 3 to 66 per cent or more. It has also been shown that neurogenic shock commonly occurs in earthquake disasters.

New research[6] shows that the 5–9 year age group and those over 60 are most vulnerable. It has been assumed that the rate of mortality to morbidity will be approximately 1:3 in earthquakes, and that this ratio is most likely to coincide with a Richter magnitude in the range 6·5–7·4.

The Infections

With the exception of sporadic outbreaks of cholera in developing countries, infections today are seldom regarded as an aspect of disaster medicine. Before the advent of disease control and treatment, however, epidemics which swept across nations unchecked, untreated and escalating, were disasters of great magnitude.

In *The Black Death*, historian Robert Gottfried traced the uncontrolled rampage of this legendary disease across Europe. Historians using tax records and church documents have recorded this epidemic which struck Europe in 1347, lasted over 300 years, ruptured the bonds of feudalism and dislodged accepted medical practice. In four early years of the epidemic, between 17 and 28 million people died and this should be compared to the 8·5 million casualties during World War I. In cities where sanitation was primitive and vermin rampant, mortality reached 60 per cent. Deaths in London, whose medieval population was no more than 50 000, averaged 290 per day during the summer of 1549 alone. The Black Death of the 14th century was a typical example of what can happen when an unfamiliar infection attacks a population for the first time— with no resistance, no cure and little relief from suffering. The cholera epidemics of the 19th century constitute a second but far less destructive example.

Imperfect records make it impossible to begin to appreciate the scale of earlier diseases and historians have often failed to appreciate the enormous difference between an outbreak of a familiar disease amid an experienced population and the effects of the same disease on a community which lacks immunity.

It is well known that outbreaks of disease could determine the outcome of military campaigns and change the course of history. Disease liability has also been influenced by the development of new skills to transform the balance of nature. Weapons were made to kill large-bodied herbivores that abounded in the grasslands of the African Savannah and on similar landscapes in Asia as much as 4 million years ago. New diseases were met as evolution developed. For example, sleeping sickness was and remains so devastating to human beings, that the ungulate herds of the African Savannah have survived to the present. Without modern prophylaxis humans cannot live in regions where the tsetse fly exists.

Agricultural development, with clearing of rain forest environments, multi- plied breeding places for a kind of mosquito that feeds by preference on human blood.

In the Yemen, for example, ablution pools attached to a mosque were found to harbour snails infected with schistosomiasis, and in India it is well known that the propagation of cholera was, and is, largely a sequel of religious pilgrimage.

Patterns of communication were slowly developed that allowed increasingly effective mutual support in moments of crisis and hunting efficiency improved human survival chances. However, the rise of cities meant that the concentration of large populations in communities offered potential disease organisms a rich and readily accessible food supply. Even the ceremonial bathing shared by thousands of pilgrims gathered to celebrate a holy festival offered human parasites an opportunity to adopt new hosts.

Biblical Diseases
The plagues of Egypt are described in the Book of Exodus where it is recorded that Moses brought down plagues upon Egypt—'sores that break into pustules on man and beast'. An epidemic suffered by the Philistines as punishment for their seizure of the Ark is also cited; so is the pestilence that killed 70 000 out of 1 300 000 able-bodied men in Israel and Judah, and the fatal visitation that 'slew in the camp of the Assyrians 185 000' overnight and caused the Assyrian King Sennacherib to withdraw from Judah without capturing Jerusalem. The writers of the Old Testament, when they put the text into the present form between

1000 and 500 BC, were quite familiar with the possibility of a sudden outbreak of death from disease and these epidemics were interpreted as acts of God.

By 500 BC, new diseases had begun to manifest themselves in many major civilized centres. Among the disasters mentioned in the Babylonian Epic of Gilgamesh, as preferable to death from the flood, was visitation from the god of pestilence.

Modern translation used the term 'plague' for disastrous events, since the principal disease that continued to erupt in Europe until the 18th century was bubonic plague. However, there is no reason to suppose that these ancient outbreaks of disease were in fact bubonic plague. Any of the now familiar diseases such as influenza, measles, smallpox, typhoid or dysentery, could have provided the type of sudden outbreak of epidemic deaths recorded in the Bible. The conclusion is that such diseases were familiar to ancient middle eastern populations well before 520 BC and played a significant role in reducing populations, though not to a level below that necessary for empire building. Otherwise, the Assyrian and Persian Empires could not have flourished as they did between the 9th and 5th centuries BC.

Fevers, including regularly recurring fevers (probably malaria), figure very prominently in ancient Chinese medical writings, and it is now clear that the Chinese had considerable success in combating early disease. Hippocrates, the father of Greek medicine (460–377 BC) recorded case histories with enough precision and detail to prove the existence of a great variety of infections in ancient Greece such as tuberculosis, influenza, diphtheria and malaria.

The Christian Era

It is known that by the beginning of the Christian era there were four divergent civilized disease pools that had come into existence (India, China, Western Eurasia and the Mediterranean) each sustaining infection that could be lethal if let loose among populations lacking any prior exposure or immunity. In the first two centuries of the Christian era, regular trade between these four areas implied exchange of infections as well as goods. It was still not appreciated that disease travelled less easily overland than by sea. By the 2nd century AD a great number of epidemics had arrived in Europe. One striking in 165 AD, which was initially brought to the Mediterranean by troops who had been campaigning in Mesopotamia, was probably smallpox and remained epidemic for 15 years killing up to one third of the affected population, at the rate of 5000 a day between 251 and 266 AD.

From the 3rd century the diseases that ravaged the Roman population were probably measles and smallpox. One great advantage that the Christians had over their pagan contemporaries was that the care of the sick, even in times of pestilence, was for them a recognized religious duty. Simple provision of adequate food, water and good nursing was all that could be offered to help. The effect of these disasters was to strengthen Christian churches at a time when other institutions were being discredited. For the Christians the support of their faith helped considerably in their disaster management and made life meaningful amid sudden death.

The Plague

By far the most important epidemic with long reaching influences on future disasters of infection was the Plague.

Daniel Defoe wrote in 1721 *A Journal of the Plague Year*. It was to be recognized not only for the quality of his descriptive brilliance but for its message of a disaster so frightening in devastation that few could believe that they were not reading fiction. Defoe recognized the 'Black Death' as the greatest environmental event in history and one of the major turning points in western civilization.

The epidemic which lasted over 300 years from its initial impact on Europe in the 14th century swept across the continent in 1665. By 1721, when the Plague reached Marseilles, it was recorded that men and children began to die like flies. The effects on human suffering, on social and anti-social behaviour, on governments so anxious to seek its control and elimination, were meticulously researched by Defoe and recorded for posterity. He spoke of the problem, still dominant in modern disasters, that those most affected are always the poor, the undernourished and the underprivileged. He spoke of the preying of the rich on the poor, of the looting, of the selling of remedies, of the superstition of foreigners and the lack of communication—still a dominant problem in 20th century disasters.

Defoe's account of the Plague was an excellent example of public health education based on sound observation. He wrote of the flight of the poor to the woods and forests; of the ability of the rich to buy isolation by chartering boats (up to 10 000 lived on ships); of the isolation of houses thought to be contagious by marking with a red cross; and of the greater increase in the spread of the disease in hot weather. He observed that the infections came into homes by way of servants sent into the streets to buy food, and that people were careful not to touch money. Breath, sweat and the stench of sores were regarded as a major means of spread of the disease. Defoe wrote that John Haywood, a gravedigger, and his wife, a nurse to infected people, never caught Plague. And when this was put down to the use of garlic, tobacco and vinegar, it was yet to be realized that many were building up immunity to this and other infections.

As with modern disasters, secondary causes of death became evident. For example, because so many midwives were dead, more babies died at birth or were stillborn. While it was clear that infection was usually spread by people who had been well, but who had been in contact with the sick, there was always doubt as to how well people could harbour the disease. The sick could not be easily distinguished from the sound because the 'incubation' period was not recognized.

It was not until 1894 that the bacillus of Plague (*Pasteurella pestis*) was discovered. After the Great Plague of London in 1665, the bacillus withdrew from north-western Europe, though it remained active in the Eastern Mediterranean and Russia throughout the 18th and 19th centuries.

There was, of course, no cure for the disaster of Plague, only relief of symptoms with nursing, adequate food and water, bleeding for fevers and the application of a wide variety of substances to the erupting wounds. Infection was minimized by quarantine, even in the 14th century, stemming from a biblical passage prescribing the ostracism of lepers, and by treating Plague sufferers as if they were temporary lepers. Other public health measures included the construction of houses in stone or brick, rather than wood, and the replacement of thatched roofs with tiles, all measures limiting rodents. In Italy, especially, local governments responded quickly to the Plague by efficient organization of burials, by safeguarding food supplies and deliveries, by setting up quarantine and by hiring Plague doctors—especially between 1350 and 1550.

By the 16th century, throughout Europe, there were emerging standard rules of quarantine and other prophylactic measures against the spread of Plague. Three centuries later the containment of Plague through international medical communication and co-operation marks one of the most dramatic triumphs of modern medicine.

Cholera

As a world disease, the rise and fall of cholera belongs to the history of a single century—the 19th. Before 1817 it was largely a local disease of India, but within 6 years it had spread to Japan and Europe. In India alone, cholera killed more than 7 million people in 20 years of the present century.

Until the development of the vaccines to increase resistance to cholera, the prevention of cholera focused largely on hygiene—cleaning up the privies, drinking water, hog pens, rag and bone shops and garbage stores. Again, like modern disasters, it affected those most at risk—the poor, hungry and under-privileged. The first outbreak of cholera in Britain promoted the establishment of local boards of health with specific functions to improve public sanitation and sewage disposal. International medical co-operation was especially generated over the disease cholera, and from 1850, when medical conferences became common in many countries, there was greater communication on all aspects of control. It became apparent that cholera seemed capable of by-passing any man-made obstacle and any quarantine.

In 1883 Koch found the bacillus responsible for cholera after a London doctor, John Snow, showed cases of cholera could be traced to a single source of drinking water in 1855. In 1913 compulsory innoculation against cholera was first established.

In terms of disaster management of cholera outbreaks, the most important primary care function was to replace lost body fluid, and then to improve water supplies and sanitation. The serious effects of dehydration from diarrhoea were often not appreciated by those caring for the victims, and it was not until recently that the value of simple, cheap, oral electrolyte powders and solutions was appreciated for their value in mass disaster management of cholera.

Influenza

The influenza of 1918 and 1919, known as the 'Spanish Influenza', killed more victims in a few months than all the armies in 4 years. In the United States alone, 500 000 died.

In India, 6 months of influenza accounted for nearly as many deaths as 20 years of cholera. This pandemic of 1918–1919 ranks with the Plague of Justinian and the Black Death as one of the most destructive outbreaks of disease known to man. However, the chance of surviving influenza was good. While the Black

Death killed 9 out of 10 when it attacked, cholera sometimes 4 out of 5, influenza in 1918 killed only 2 or 3 out of 100. Treatment relied mainly on good nursing care and nutrition with, occasionally, vaccines. Crowd contacts were limited, schools were closed, wearing of masks became compulsory, e.g. in San Francisco.

Plague, cholera and influenza have been discussed because they represent a range of disasters occurring over some five centuries. Many others, including smallpox, typhus, typhoid and yellow fever, could have been mentioned but their history and control is well documented, and their influence on disaster management less than the three diseases discussed.

Water

There has been little reliable information recorded of the numbers who have perished in historical flood disasters. Historians have recorded the major floods of Paris (1658 and 1910), of Warsaw (1861), of Frankfurt am Main (1854 and 1930) and of Rome (1530 and 1557), but the mortality from these is unknown.

Floods may occur from ice jams during the spring rise, from tsunamis, or from the result of summer thunderstorms in mountains—the so-called flashflood— probably the most dangerous of all floods. With floods, the common cause of death is from drowning or blunt injury of the body against rocks or debris. With disasters at sea a further hazard is of course hypothermia, when the body is immersed in freezing water.

While primitive means of resuscitation were used involving gravity, removal of inhaled water from the lungs, the recognition of hypothermia and its treatment and the efficient techniques of resuscitation appropriate for the near-drowned victims, were all triumphs of this century, especially of the past 25 years. They were largely developed through a world-wide improvement in surf life-saving and the teaching of resuscitation techniques to surf life-savers and first-aiders.

MAN-MADE DISASTERS

Wars

War is understood to be an armed conflict involving more than 50 000 combatants and it is beyond the scope of this paper to outline a history of wars, but rather to concentrate on those historical issues and landmarks which most influenced morbidity and mortality in the mass casualties created by them.

Of all the types of disasters that have most influenced modern disaster preparedness and management, war would have to dominate all other disasters, whether natural or man-made.

The Weapons

Injury types have changed progressively with the development of weaponry. Clubbing, spearing, slinging, shooting arrows and trampling from horses dominated the warfare tactics used in the ancient world of the Greeks and Romans. Death resulted largely from haemorrhage or blunt injury to the head for which there was no effective treatment.

Explosives possibly originated in China in the 10th century, but certainly were used by the Arabs in the 14th century, when the first real gun was developed which fired an arrow from a bamboo tube. Firearms were probably the invention of a 14th century German monk, named Berthold Schwarz. Explosive injury from firearms or black powder changed the pattern of injury to include not only internal and external haemorrhage, but also untreatable destruction of vital internal organs including the heart, lungs, liver, spleen and bowel. Death, if not immediate, soon came with the infection and chemical imbalance from shock, which was unrecognized and beyond any healing skills. With the discovery of the physiology of the circulation of the blood by William Harvey in 1628, greater understanding developed of the importance of controlling haemorrhage, for there was no replacement therapy. Thomas Spencer Wells gained first hand experience of the nature of gun shot wounds when he served in the Crimean War in 1854, and from this experience he invented the haemostatic artery forceps, which bear his name and which replaced the traditional use of the fingers of an assistant used to control bleeding during an operation.

Shells were first used extensively in the Swedish Thirty Years War of the 17th century, and created their own types of injury, with infection from metallic fragments and large soft tissue wounds which soon became contaminated.

Chemical warfare using poison gas brought to World War I major problems of injury to the respiratory tract, which was often permanent.

As the means of transportation in war developed, with a great number of men confined within narrow static areas such as trenches, or in tanks and ships, their vulnerability to shellfire increased. Thermal injuries rose dramatically from World War I to World War II, and this was compounded by the fires arising from air battles and blitzkrieg, which affected not only military personnel but also large numbers of civilians.

The Tactics and the Strategies

A study of wars, both ancient and recent, shows how tactics, independent of physical combat, greatly influenced survival chances. Napoleon has a pre-eminent place in the history of strategy. Deception, surprise and fear of numbers were part of a psychological warfare. The tactic of keeping the enemy constantly moving, without rest or adequate food, lowered their resistance to both disease and injury and made them more vulnerable when the conflict became physical. One of the most destructive forms of war disaster was that of hypothermia when thousands of troops could perish in a few hours following exposure to freezing temperatures. This state was also influenced by, and often resulted from, strategies designed to move the enemy away from shelter. This was just one sequel of the 'strategy of exhaustion' and one which Napoleon's Grand Army suffered itself on its retreat from Moscow in 1812.

The Hazard of Numbers

Wars added another series of risks to survival because soldiers were confined, often in thousands in one area, vulnerable to lack of sufficient food, to severe exposure and to disease. It was well recorded how the Plague destroyed more soldiers than were killed by armed combat. There was another risk with wound cross-infections so easily spread where hygiene was poor, and the means to cleanse wounds absent or inadequate. It was much harder too for immediate aid to be given to some hundreds of soldiers or sailors, victims of explosive warfare, with lack of ability to escape readily from the area under attack, let alone sort out their dead from their injured. The hazard of numbers was particularly evident in water accidents during many wars where the number of lifeboats was inadequate to cope with many soldiers and sailors suddenly exposed to freezing water.

TREATMENT

With all disasters, ancient or modern, the most common causes of death were: massive haemorrhage; multiple injuries; crushing; airway obstruction; infections; dehydration and starvation. The essentials of immediate care are now recognized simply as airway and ventilation control, restoration of good circulation and pain relief. In any disaster this immediate care cannot be competently delivered without a system of disaster preparedness, disaster management, good communication, triage, casualty management and appropriate transportation. Even small disasters could not be managed without communication, transportation and other support, and could soon develop into major disasters.

Bacteriology

The history of the bacteriological advances with the discovery of the causes of epidemics is well documented in numerous publications, and has been referred to briefly earlier in this chapter.

The Circulation

John Hunter, the brilliant Scottish physician of the 18th century, contributed most to the understanding of the circulation of the blood—and particularly noted that venous blood was dark and arterial blood florid. His observation contributed much to the early understanding of the nature of gunshot wounds and stabbings.

Previously, William Harvey (1578–1657) had shown that blood continuously circulated, and Michael Servetus (1511–53) had shown that blood had a separate path through the lungs. Harvey demonstrated that blood was changed from venous to arterial in the lungs with 'respiration' exchanging gases between air and blood and this was identified as the key to understanding the reason for blood circulation some time later.

The suggestion that blood could be given back into veins was first made as early as the 17th century, notably by Johann Daniel Major of Padua, but the major step of replacing lost blood did not develop until the 1920s and 1930s, following the brilliant work of Landsteiner in describing the major red blood cell types. The necessity for urgent transfusion after blood loss resulted from not only experience of warfare, but also the increasing trauma resulting from road accidents.

The Surgeon

Biblical information on medicine is limited, though there was reference to surgery for circumcision. In the 2nd to 6th centuries AD, Jewish writers had discussed means of reducing dislocations and the management of injuries to many organs.

It was not until the 18th century, after following the scientific study of anatomy, that surgical developments progressed rapidly. In 1743 a Royal decree in France forbade barbers from practising all except minor procedures in surgery. A half a century later the Royal College of Surgeons of England was granted a charter, and surgery became a skilled and controlled specialty.

The surgeon soldiers became the first group to bring disaster medicine delivery to the front line of battles. In World War I, particularly with the development of antiseptic techniques and front line surgery, soldiers who previously would have died survived through early surgical skills. This was disaster medicine in action—early triage to separate the casualties and decide who required immediate care, with field hospitals well equipped to cope with an influx of many casualties.

The finest and best researched account of early war medicine is to be seen in *Medical and Surgical History of the War of the Rebellion (1861–1865)*—better known as the American Civil War. This work documented for the first time treatment protocols for mass disaster problems based on well kept statistics. Of those within the Union Army who died in this war, 44238 were killed in action, 49205 died of fatal battle wounds, 186298 died from disease or disease-related causes, and 24103 died from unknown causes. Within the Confederate Army documentation was not accurate, though it is recorded that some 200000 died and that three-quarters of the deaths were due to disease. Chest and abdominal wounds were nearly always fatal. Immediate first aid in the battle field was primitive, transportation of the wounded unplanned, and only available when a vehicle was not needed to haul military supplies. The injured were treated in makeshift hospitals located far to the rear of the battle zones in abandoned schools and churches.

However, within two years of the outbreak of this war there had been a significant improvement in disaster medicine. This was brought about by a number of factors, both organizational and medical. The first was the improved efficiency of the military medical departments with better training of doctors, ambulance corps and nurses who were able to cope with the greater demands of front line care, and the improved efficiency of medical supply delivery. The second was related to the medical advances occurring about this time which improved survival rates of the injured. These included Pasteur's discovery of the role of bacteria in 1863, and by 1867 Lister had recognized the organisms' relation to wound infection and proposed his method of antisepsis.

Records showed that other medical advances developed at this time included improved dressing materials, surgical instruments and syringes, as well as recognition of good nutrition as being important to survival under such unsanitary conditions. New drugs, including purgatives, opiates, mercurials, drying agents and emetics, were used in the military hospitals, and a number of fermentations and poultices developed to relieve pain. While general anaesthesia, especially chloroform, was widely used, local anaesthesia was still not to be available for another four decades. Blood transfusion was used on two occasions in the Civil War, involving transfusions of 2 oz and 16 oz, with no hazard recorded.

By 1863, front line care had developed markedly, with a recognition of the need to administer immediate first aid and start resuscitation on the battlefield. This marks a most important development in disaster medicine—the recognition of basic life support within minutes of the accident. The regimental surgeons would apply dressings of lint or linen to a wound, perform minor surgical procedures and sort out priorities of transportation and care. Serious cases were transported in so-called 'ambulances' to the nearby field hospital, where wounds were explored and metal and other foreign bodies removed. Because the legs were so often injured with resultant damage to blood vessels and bone, amputation was common as there was little splinting suitable for serious fractures. There was a mortality rate of 26 per cent with leg amputation, and over 90 per cent died following fracture of the femur. There was a total of 29 980 amputations performed in this Civil War involving fingers, hands and limbs. Haemorrhage on the battle front was controlled by tourniquets or by the local application of styptics, including silver nitrate, tannic acid and iron solutions. If surgical ligation of blood vessels failed, amputation was undertaken to save life. Other causes of death, with close to 100 per cent mortality listed in the official war history, included tetanus (505 reported cases), gangrene (2642 cases), erysipelas (1097 cases) and septicaemia (2818 cases).

The Civil War of 1861–5 has been considered in this chapter in some depth because of its significant impact on improving many aspects of the delivery of disaster medicine. These included particularly the development and training of the front line ambulance corps, rudimentary triage, front line surgical care of severe haemorrhage, improved pain relief and surgical care. These facts were well recorded by the military historians and the lessons of management and mismanagement were remembered 50 years later in World War I.

The Anaesthetist

Pain is as old as mankind and is perhaps the most constant and most feared sequelae of any major accident. It is a symptom never neglected by the disaster historians who recorded that Napoleon's painful piles are reputed to have sealed his fate at the battle of Waterloo, and that Magellan was tortured with war wounds. Early remedies for pain were often in the hands of priests who relied on prayers, together with what natural remedies were available at the time. Hippocrates wrote that, 'divine is the work to subdue pain', and knew of the value of cold in causing pain relief, but it was not until the middle of the 19th century that this was used as a skilled tool in regional anaesthesia. In 1807 Napoleon's Surgeon-General Baron Dominique Jean Larrey observed that amputation could be painlessly performed on soldiers who had been lying for some time in the snow.

While many ancient writings refer to a state similar to anaesthesia as we know it, pain-relieving drugs are of recent origin. Alcohol, opiates and plants containing hyoscyamus had been known for their pain-relieving properties for thousands of years before inhalation anaesthesia was discovered in the 19th century. It was known that some amputations were carried out under the sedative powers of alcohol.

In 1792 in Bristol, England, Thomas Beddoes set up a small hospital laboratory and later developed techniques to adminster medications by inhalation. Humphry Davy, appointed by Beddoes as superintendent of the Pneumatic Institution about this time, demonstrated the pain-relieving properties of nitrous oxide (previously discovered by Joseph Priestley in 1772)—an agent which to this day has a most valuable place in disaster medicine. It was not, however, until 1842 that Dr Crawford Long applied its use to surgery.

The value of ether and chloroform in bringing pain relief and improving surgical efficiency is now well recorded in the history of disaster medicine. These two, together with nitrous oxide, have been widely used in the wars and other disasters since the 1860s. While the popularity of both ether and chloroform has now been surpassed by other safer anaesthetics, nitrous oxide is still widely used. Since their maturation as a specialty world-wide, anaesthetists have played a significant role in disaster management through their skills of resuscitation and pain relief.

The Moving of the Sick

Almost every means of transportation has been used over the centuries to shift the sick and wounded—from mules, camels and horse-drawn ambulances to trains and ships. The Civil War raged for two years in the 1860s before effective ambulance and hospital systems evolved. It took about another century for medical science to agree that an ambulance was not so much a transport vehicle as a treatment vehicle and that the severely injured should never be transported until their shock is mollified.

In dealing with disasters of such magnitude as earthquake and flooding, which may occur in remote and underdeveloped areas, normal transportation for the carriage of the victims may, of course, be non-existent as it was with many early disasters before the development of aero-medical evacuation. Essential in the efficient use of any transport system involved in a disaster is effective communication, which was lacking until this century.

CONCLUSION

In his reading as a background to this work, the writer concluded that the history of medicine is inexorably linked with the history of disasters; for almost every major discovery in medicine became necessary as a result of a disaster which was beyond the existing range of treatment.

Modern disaster medicine has developed only through wise observation of many crippling disasters. It will continue to develop only if we are prepared to remember the mistakes of the past.

REFERENCES

1. Editorial (24 Feb 1982) *New Zealand Medical Journal*, p. 115.
2. Bullard F. M. (1976) *Volcanoes of the Earth* (Revised ed.) Austin, University of Texas.
3. Waltham A. C. (1978) *Catastrophe, the Violent Earth*. London, MacMillan.

4. Decker R. (1981) Eruption of Mount St. Helens. *Sci. Am.* **244**, 52–64.
5. Alexander D. (1985) Death and injury in earthquakes. *Disasters* **9** (1).
6. Gueri M. and Alzate H. (1984) The Popayan earthquake. *Disasters* **8** (1).

FURTHER READING

Bailey H. (1959) *Notable Names in Surgery*. 3rd ed. London, H. K. Lewis.

Cartwright F. F. (1978) *A Social History of Medicine*. London and New York, Longman.

Crosby A. W. (1976) *Epidemic and Peace 1918*. Westport, Greenwood Press.

Defoe D. (1963) *Journal of the Plague Year*. Signet Classics.

50 Years of Medicine 1900–1949. (1950) A symposium from the *Br. Med. J.*

Glover M. (1979) *The Napoleonic Wars*. London, Batsford.

Gottfried R. S. (1983) *The Black Death*. New York, Free Press.

Haggard H. W. (1929) *Devils, Drugs and Doctors*. London, Heinemann.

Harbottle's Dictionary of Battle, 2nd ed. (1979) London, Granada.

Hare R. (1954) *Pomp and Pestilence*. London, Victor Gollancz.

Keen H. (ed.) (1976) *Triumphs of Medicine*. London, Paul Elek.

King H. S. (ed.) (1971) *A History of Medicine*. Harmondsworth, Penguin.

King L. *The Medical World of the 18th Century*. The University of Chicago Committee on Publication in Biology and Medicine (Cat. no. 58-7332).

Lyons A. S. and Petrinelli R. J. (1979) *Medicine: An Illustrated History*. Bentveld, Abrams.

McNeill W. H. (1976) *Plagues and Peoples*. New York, Anchor Press/Doubleday.

Medical and Surgical History of the War of the Rebellion (1861–1865) (1900) US Acts of Congress publications under the direction of Surgeon General Joseph Barnes.

Rubin S. (1974) *Mediaeval English Medicine*. Newton Abbott, David & Charles.

Savitt T. (1978) *Medicine and Slavery*. Chicago, University of Illinois Press.

Smith A. (1943) *Plague on Us*. New York, The Commonwealth Fund; London, Oxford University Press.

THE IMMEDIATE PHASE

Medical Skills

H. R. Champion, Marjorie M. Moreau and Patricia S. Gainer

2

Assessment and Triage

Early resuscitation and critical care life support are crucial to minimizing the potential morbidity and mortality that follow a disaster. Providing effective care to disaster victims, however, is often impeded by the nature of the disaster, the number of victims affected, the availability of medical care and the co-ordination of rescue efforts among personnel at the disaster site, the existence of modes of rapid evacuation and the availability of post-evacuation tertiary care. Once in the throes of a disaster, existing resources will be taxed and a logical and flexible disaster response must be implemented in order to achieve maximum results. The goal in multiple or mass casualty scenarios is to minimize mortality and morbidity. Consequently, the most basic disaster response must include, at its core, a method for assessing the disaster and the extent of injury to victims, as well as methods for determining which victims will receive treatment first and what types of treatment will be given during the various stages of the disaster. This basic need exists regardless of the environment in which the disaster occurs, whether large or small numbers of victims are involved, or whether the disaster occurs in a 'developing' or 'developed' country.

THE STAGES OF DISASTER RESPONSE

Generally, disasters have discrete stages, during each of which specific responses should occur.[1] For the purposes of this chapter, five temporal stages are presented:

1. *Within seconds/minutes*—Initial emergency treatment provided by

19

bystanders and victims with minor injuries. Initial determination of disaster magnitude.

2. *Within minutes to 1 hour*—Detailed assessment of the disaster scene. Mobilization of disaster response. Resuscitative interventions.
3. *Within 4 to 6 hours*—Definitive wound care and vascular surgery to preserve limbs and tissues and prevent subsequent sepsis.
4. *Within 1 to 5 days*—Intensive care for critically injured; combined care for the less critically injured. Treatment of early complications and sequelae.
5. *Within 2 to 7 days and beyond*—Public health issues associated with the disaster are identified and addressed.

This chapter will discuss the assessment and triage techniques necessary to respond to the first three stages of a disaster, namely: (1) the response needed within seconds/minutes; (2) the response needed within minutes to 1 hour; and (3) the response needed within 4 to 6 hours.

Assessment of the Disaster Scene

Initial notice that a disaster has occurred is usually provided by bystanders or victims with minor injuries, whose ability to communicate details about the nature of the disaster and the extent of damage is often affected by their reaction to the frightening scene unfolding before them. These individuals will normally notify local authorities, whose actions will determine the subsequent pace, level and intensity of the initial medical and rescue responses.

Generally, two types of information are necessary to provide local authorities with a reasonable basis from which to determine the initial rescue and medical responses.[2] The first type of information is *general* in nature and includes the extent of the damage, the geographical area of the disaster, the population affected, the extent of actual damage to existing structures, such as highways, roads and land, as well as apparent damage to the availability of water, power and telecommunications. The second type of information is *medical*, which, as specifically as possible, estimates the number of dead and injured and characterizes the general nature of the injuries, e.g. 'burns'.

The disaster site may be physically remote from essential resources, access to the site may be hampered because of the damage from the disaster itself, and prompt mobilization of rescue and medical personnel may be precluded. Consequently, bystanders or victims with minor injuries are realistically the only persons available to provide first aid in the critical minutes following the disaster. It is probable that the effort of these individuals will be less than effective, since it is likely that few of these persons will have received prior training in first aid techniques. Ultimately, it usually falls to rescue and medical personnel to provide initial effective medical care to the injured.

Arrival of the first cohorts of rescue and medical personnel should occur within one hour following the disaster.

The rescue personnel are responsible for:

1. Accurately assessing the nature and extent of the disaster.
2. Securing the disaster scene, while enabling other rescue and medical personnel to have unrestricted access and egress.
3. Assessing the risks associated with rescue of disaster victims.

4. Performing necessary manoeuvres to remove hazards created by the disaster, e.g. extinguishing fires.

In developed countries, fire department and police personnel will assume the rescue responsibilities, augmented by state or national military personnel as needed. In developing countries, rescue responsibilities may be performed primarily by members of the military, since municipal services may not be available.

The medical personnel are responsible for:

1. Estimating the number of casualties.
2. Determining the nature and severity of the injuries suffered.
3. Specifying the resources needed to treat the injured initially at the disaster site and the hospital resources needed for subsequent, definitive care.
4. Assessing and triaging disaster victims.
5. Providing initial treatment and resuscitation, where necessary.

Medical Organization and Deployment

If not specifically controlled and directed, the medical response will not necessarily match the needs of the disaster. Over-response to the disaster may dangerously deplete valuable resources, while under-response may increase mortality. Clear identification of the most experienced medical authority at the disaster scene will lay the groundwork for appropriate medical organization and deployment. This individual should define the medical response required and direct the actual deployment of the triage treatment teams. It is axiomatic that a physician should be deployed to the disaster site to perform this role. Additional physicians should be dispatched to the disaster site if it appears that transport of victims to hospitals will be delayed or prolonged, or if on-site surgical intervention is necessary, e.g. for trapped victims.

Members of the medical triage treatment teams, working under physician direction, identify the medical needs of the victims, perform lifesaving therapeutics, remove the victims from the disaster site, and make primary and secondary patient assessments.[3] Teams should be assigned to specific physical areas of disaster, which will provide a mechanism for ensuring that all disaster victims are eventually assessed and treated, as well as enabling better communication among team members.

Patient Assessment

In a mass casualty circumstance, the number of injured victims will exceed that which may be cared for by the health system operating under normal conditions. There may be a high proportion of individuals with multiple injuries to vital organs, suffering from internal and external haemorrhage, shock, depressed consciousness or burns. Ideally, patient assessment at the disaster site is conducted by emergency medical personnel, trained and certified to perform specific procedures without physician supervision. Realistically, the initial response to a disaster will almost always be lacking in adequately trained medical personnel, medical materials and rapid transport to tertiary care to provide optimal immediate care for the victims. Nonetheless, the goal of the disaster response is to minimize mortality and morbidity, and effective care must be rendered as best as possible no matter how difficult the conditions. Therefore, it is necessary to simplify the assessment process to the point where it may be adequately performed by personnel with minimal medical training functioning within the disaster environment. For this reason, the patient assessment techniques presented here are equally useful in developing and developed countries. Initial resuscitation and treatment techniques are discussed elsewhere in this text. (*See* Chapter 3.)

Individual patient assessment in the disaster setting is divided into two distinct phases—primary and secondary surveys.

The Primary Survey

The primary survey deals with life-threatening or evolving life-threatening illness or injuries. In this phase, special attention is given to a basic assessment and physical examination of the airway, breathing and circulation (the 'ABCs'). Airway patency should be assured by either chin lift or jaw thrust, since hyper-extension of the head and neck may aggravate any cervical spine injuries present. Once an airway has been established, the respiratory system is checked by the 'look, listen and feel' method: *look* for respiratory effort by watching for movement of the chest wall, *listen* for breathing by placing one's ear close enough to the victim's mouth and nose to hear air exchange, and, at the same time, *feel* for air movement against one's face. Respiratory rate is a sensitive measure of respiratory distress and should be counted for 15 seconds and multiplied by 4 to give the rate per minute.

Circulation is checked by feeling for a carotid pulse in adults and the brachial pulse in infants. Pulse rate and blood pressure should be obtained and recorded. While assessing for airway, breathing and circulation, a rapid inspection of the total body should be made to determine the presence of major haemorrhage. During the initial assessment, the chest should be bared so that obvious life-threatening anterior chest injuries may be seen (*see Table* 2.1.). The level of consciousness should be recorded with the other vital signs and the time on the patient's skin or tag.

The primary survey is used to separate out those individuals whose life-threatening injuries are treatable by swift intervention. It identifies those persons who will surely die if not treated immediately. Resuscitative manoeuvres and immobilization of important areas (e.g. spine) should ideally take place before moving the patient. The secondary survey is performed after life-threatening injuries have been identified and further danger to the victim has been minimized. The purpose of the secondary survey is to identify any other less significant injuries which the victim may have suffered.

The Secondary Survey

The secondary survey is a systematic head-to-toe physical examination utilizing the usual inspection, palpation, auscultation and percussion techniques. A brief history of mechanism of injury and symptoms may be obtained. The secondary survey is particularly important for the unconscious, paediatric, or deaf victim,

Table 2.1. Primary survey algorithm

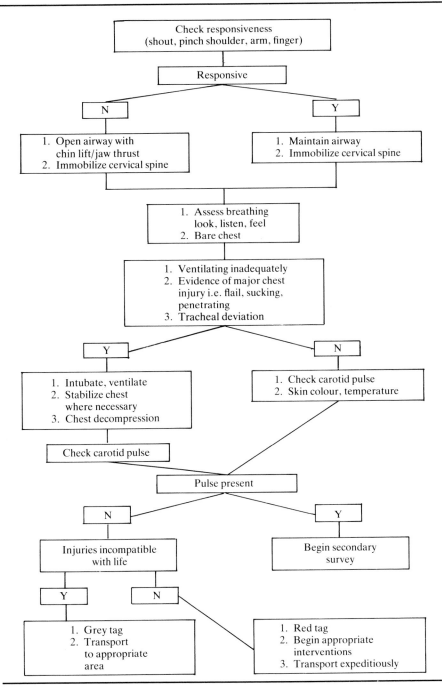

$$Y = Yes \qquad N = No$$

where normal communication between examiner and victim is impaired or impossible.

Ideally, the secondary survey is completed at the staging area, well away from the actual disaster site. The information derived from this evaluation will serve to re-allocate victims into the appropriate triage and transport category. When done correctly, no area of the body is left unassessed, and since the examination is not interrupted for treatment, it can be accomplished in one to two minutes. Upon completion of the secondary survey, therapy may be instituted on the basis of the injuries found, coupled with the vital signs or the Trauma Score (*see below*), derived from the combination of information from the primary and secondary surveys.

The secondary survey is completed in the following manner. Start with the head and palpate the back and top of the head, as well as the facial bones, to look for lacerations, abrasions, contusions and deformity. Check the ears and the nose for blood and cerebrospinal fluid. Open the mouth and check for blood, lacerations and foreign bodies, such as broken teeth and/or dentures. Check the pupils for size and reaction to light. Assess the neck for deformity of the cervical spine and the position of the trachea. While positioned to one side of the victim, rapidly palpate the clavicle, scapula, humerus, elbow, ulna, radius and hand to determine if deformity, tenderness or swelling is present. Upon reaching the hand, a neurovascular assessment is completed by checking capillary refill and squeezing the finger. After excluding injury to this extremity, take the pulse and blood pressure. Should there be an injury to this particular upper extremity, the examiner should move rapidly around the patient (i.e. not step over the patient), and repeat the examination to the other upper extremity before taking vital signs. Once the blood pressure and pulse have been ascertained, auscultation of the heart and lungs can be completed. Afterwards, the sternum and ribs are palpated to check for deformity and/or tenderness and the entire chest inspected for lacerations, abrasions and contusions. Next, paying careful attention to any contusion, abrasion or laceration, the abdomen should be palpated in all four quadrants to assess for rigidity, tenderness and distension. The pelvis is then gently rocked to elicit the integrity of the pelvic girdle. Moving down to the lower extremity closest to the assessor, the femur, patella, tibia and fibula are palpated for deformity, swelling, and/or tenderness. After removing the shoe and sock, where necessary, the foot is inspected and palpated. A neurovascular assessment is again completed by checking capillary refill and squeezing the toe. Moving to the other foot, the examination of the lower extremity is repeated from foot to hip. After inspection and palpation of the remaining upper extremity, if not previously done, a second set of vital signs is taken. The victim is then log-rolled onto the side toward the assessor, to inspect and palpate the back and buttocks. Should there be the need to immobilize the victim or apply pneumatic anti-shock trousers, this can easily be accomplished by rolling the victim back onto the appropriate equipment.

PATIENT TRIAGE

Triage refers to the classification and allocation of priority for the injured. The technique of triage was first used by Baron Dominique Jean Larrey, Napoleon's chief medical officer, who developed the principle of sorting patients for treatment based on medical need. Larrey used triage sorting techniques to identify soldiers who were dangerously wounded in battle. These soldiers at risk of dying from their injuries received surgery first. Care of the less severely injured occurred after the gravely wounded were treated.[4]

Modern triage is based on the assessment of the patient that is completed at the accident site, and a judgement of the actual or possible severity of the victim's injuries. Triage of disaster victims gives priority to those patients who will derive the most medical benefit from immediate treatment. Unlike Larrey's triage scheme, however, where treatment was given first to those with the gravest injuries, modern disaster triage gives highest priority to victims who will live only if treated. Victims who will live without treatment and victims who will die despite treatment receive lower priority.[3,4]

In a disaster with mass casualties, the process of triage must facilitate the application of lifesaving maneouvres.[5] If large numbers of victims have been injured in the disaster and health resources are insufficient to care for all the injured simultaneously, the process of determining which patients should receive treatment first will often be the key to minimizing mortality. Further, application of a strategic triage system to identify those who need immediate treatment will optimize the use of available medical personnel and resources, which are generally in short supply during catastrophic events.

Completion of the primary and secondary surveys will provide an assessment of the injuries suffered by each victim. It is often difficult to use this 'raw' information as a basis for determining which victims are to be treated first because the sheer volume of injured victims may preclude effective use of the mass of injury information obtained. For this reason, physiological severity scores, which quantify the information, have been found to be useful in the triage of mass casualty victims.[6,7] For a severity score to be used effectively for disaster triage, however, the score must meet several prerequisites. First, the score must be correlated with mortality so that each level of severity represented within the score has a specific probability of survival or death associated with that level. Second, the score must have a high degree of consistency so that when applied by different personnel with varying degrees of training, similar results will be obtained. Third, the score must be simple enough for application in the difficult physical and emotional environment of a disaster.

Vital signs (pulse, blood pressure, respiration and level of consciousness) are initially assessed during the primary survey, and then again during the secondary survey. The Trauma Score[8] is a physiologic measure of injury severity that mathematically combines into one number which is pertinent to the vital sign information; specifically the Glasgow Coma Scale[9] and cardiovascular and respiratory system variables. (See Table 2.2.) Trauma Score values range from 1 to 16; the higher the Score, the better the probability of survival. (See Table 2.3.) The Trauma Score has been shown to correlate with survival,[10] to have a high degree of reliability when applied by different personnel during the prehospital phase of care,[11] to aid in identifying an injury severity threshold which merits tertiary care,[12,13] and to be useful in mass casualty triage.[6,7]

Vital sign information from the primary and secondary surveys can be used to compute the Trauma Score which, in turn, can be used as the mechanism for the triage of disaster victims for immediate and definitive care along the following lines.

Table 2.2. The trauma score

		Rate	Codes	Score
A.	*Respiratory Rate*	10–24	4	
	Number of respirations in 15 seconds;	25–35	3	
	multiply by four	≥36	2	
		1–9	1	
		0	0	A. _____
B.	*Respiratory Effort*	Normal	1	
	Retractive—Use of accessory muscles or intercostal	Retractive/		
	retraction	None	0	B. _____
C.	*Systolic Blood Pressure*	≥90	4	
	Systolic cuff pressure—either arm,	70–89	3	
	auscultate or palpate	50–69	2	
		0–49	1	
	No carotid pulse	0	0	C. _____
D.	*Capillary Refill*			
	Normal—Forehead or lip mucosa colour	Normal	2	
	refill in 2 seconds	Delayed	1	
	Delayed—More than 2 seconds capillary refill	None	0	D. _____
	None—No capillary refill			

E. *Glasgow Coma Scale*

				Total GCS Points	*Score*	
1. *Eye Opening*						
Spontaneous	_____4			14–15	5	
To voice	_____3			11–13	4	
To pain	_____2			8–10	3	
None	_____1			5–7	2	
				3–4	1	E. _____

2. *Verbal Response*
    Orientated _____5
    Confused _____4
    Inappropriate words _____3
    Incomprehensible sounds _____2
    None _____1

3. *Motor Response*
    Obeys commands _____6
    Localizes pain _____5
    Withdraw (pain) _____4
    Flexion (pain) _____3
    Extension (pain) _____2
    None _____1

Total GCS Point (1 + 2 + 3)_____   TRAUMA SCORE_____
(Total Points A + B + C + D + E)

Table 2.3. Probability of Survival (P_S) associated with the Trauma Score as determined from 2 844 blunt and penetrating injured trauma patients from the Washington Hospital Center.

Trauma score	P_S
16	99%
15	98%
14	96%
13	94%
12	89%
11	82%
10	72%
9	59%
8	45%
7	31%
6	21%
5	13%
4	7·5%
3	4·3%
2	2·5%
1	1·4%

Immediate Treatment

Generally, patients with a Trauma Score of between 4 and 12 are those who should receive immediate treatment and transport. These individuals will have suffered life-threatening injuries and be in a critical, yet potentially salvageable, condition. Frequently, they will have suffered shock and severe blood loss, been unconscious, or have unresolved respiratory problems, severe open or closed chest and/or abdominal injuries, or major fractures. Also, three levels of burn severity are considered life-threatening and, therefore, warrant expeditious care and transport: (1) burns associated with respiratory compromise; (2) third degree burns of more than 10 per cent of the total body surface; or (3) second degree burns of more than 30 per cent of the total body surface. A triage algorithm for these patients is shown in *Table* 2.4.

Second Priority Treatment

Those individuals, with Trauma Scores of 13, 14 or 15, are considered to be 'urgent', but generally are able to be stabilized at the staging area with appropriate advanced life support interventions. They include those who have suffered back injuries with or without spinal cord damage, moderate blood loss of 500–1000ml, or conscious head-injured patients with a Glasgow Coma Scale greater than 12. Candidates for secondary treatment include burned victims without respiratory compromise, whose third degree burns cover less than 10 per cent total body surface, or whose second degree burns cover less than 30 per cent total body surface. A triage algorithm for these patients is shown in *Table* 2.5.

Table 2.4. Triage: the immediate treatment group.

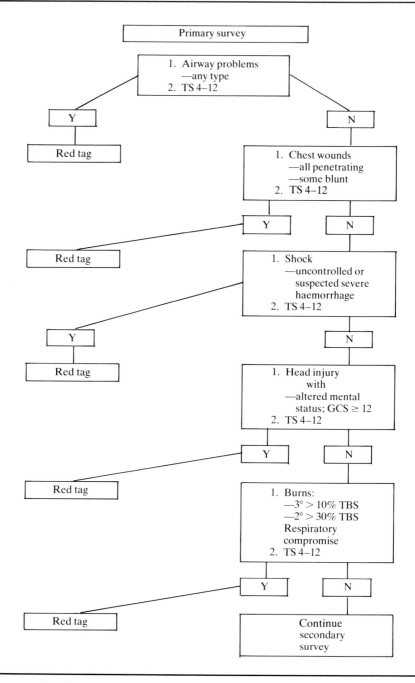

Y = Yes   N = No   TS = Trauma Score

Table 2.5. Triage: the second priority treatment group.

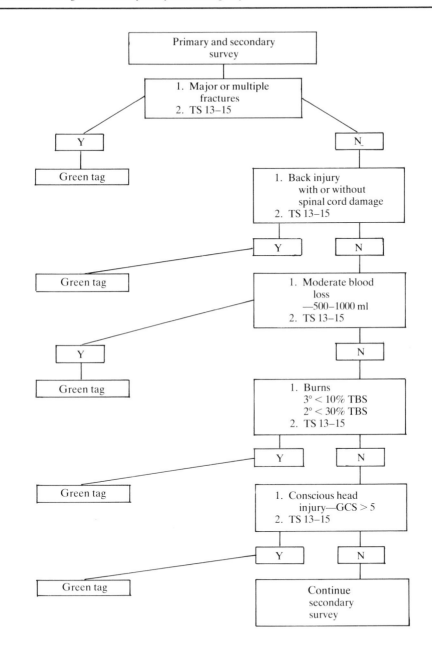

Y = Yes   N = No   TS = Trauma Score

Table 2.6. Triage: the delayed treatment group.

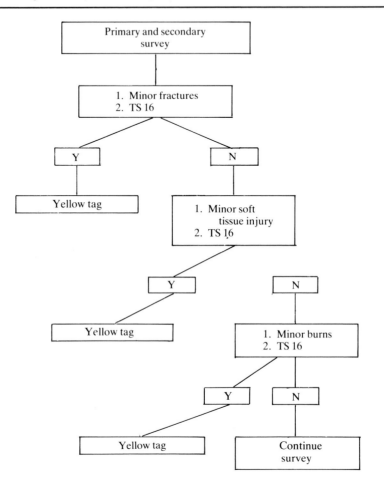

Y = Yes   N = No

Table 2.7. Deceased/will die.

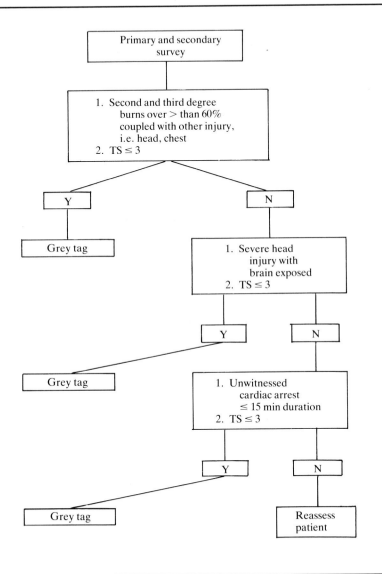

Y = Yes   N = No

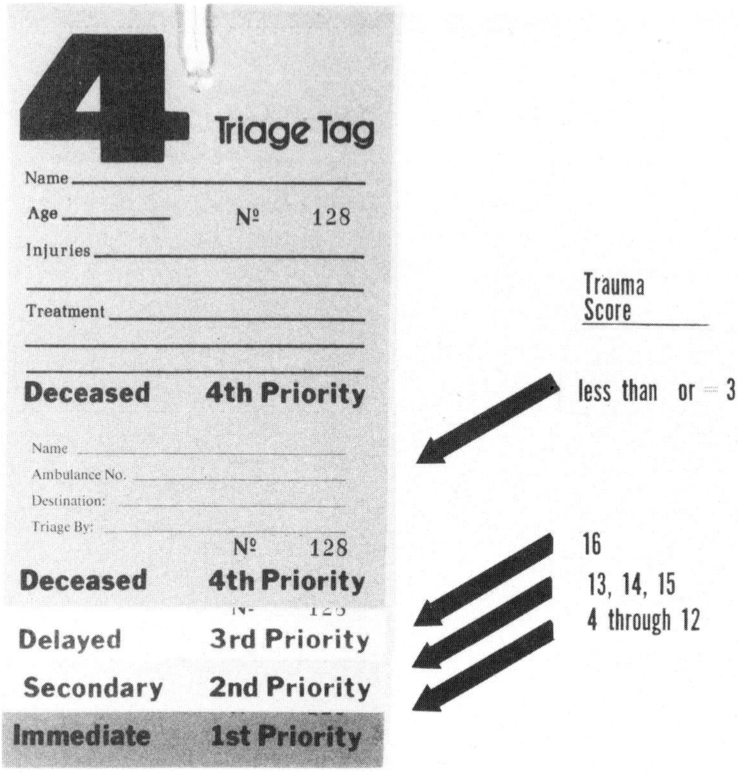

Fig. 2.1. Disaster triage tag.

Table 2.8. Additional factors to be considered in triage.

Mechanism of Injury

Existence of any one of the following mandates rapid transport to tertiary care:

1. Penetrating injury to chest, abdomen, head, neck and groin.
2. Two or more proximal long bone fractures.
3. Combination with burns of ≥ 15 per cent, face or airway.
4. Flail chest.
5. Evidence of high force transfer to the body:
   a. falls 20 feet or more;
   b. crash speed 20 mph or more;
   c. ejection of victim;
   d. pedestrian hit at 20 mph or more;
   e. passenger compartment intrusion ≥ 15 inches;
   f. death of passengers in same vehicle.

Age of Victim

Rapid transport to tertiary care should be considered for any victim who is younger than 5 years of age or older than 55 years of age, especially in the presence of known cardiorespiratory disease.

Delayed Treatment

Those individuals with a Trauma Score of 16 have suffered the least severe injuries, or at least have normal physiology following injury. Their treatment and transport is less urgent. These injuries would include minor fractures, burns and soft tissue injuries, such as abrasions or contusions. A triage algorithm for these patients is shown in *Table* 2.6.

Deceased

This category is reserved for victims who have suffered mortal wounds in which death appears reasonably certain or whose Trauma Score is less than or equal to 3. Examples of these injuries include second and third degree burns of greater than 60 per cent total body surface that are coupled with other major injuries, severe head or chest injuries, or severe head injuries where the brain is exposed. This category also includes those who have had no spontaneous respiratory or cardiac effort for more than 15 minutes and in whom cardiopulmonary resuscitation would be impossible due to the type of injury sustained. A triage algorithm for these patients is shown in *Table* 2.7.

The familiar multicoloured disaster triage tag (the Mettag system) conforms to this hierarchical ordering. The colouring scheme of the tag is as follows: red = immediate; green = secondary; yellow = delayed; and grey = deceased. Use of this tagging system provides a visual indication of both patient condition and which patients should be transported first. An example of a disaster triage tag, with corresponding Trauma Scores, is shown in *Fig.* 2.1. Other triage tag examples are described in Chapters 9 and 25.

Additionally, certain factors, such as mechanism of injury and patient age, need to be considered in the triage decision. By their very nature, certain injuries carry a high risk of death that can be reduced by rapid access to tertiary care. Furthermore, the age of the victim can have a significant impact on outcome, even if the injuries suffered are of a less than severe nature. The American College of Surgeons has identified mechanism of injury and age factors that should be considered in making triage decisions, regardless of the victim's physiological severity.[14] Those factors which are relevant to disaster triage are shown in *Table* 2.8.

DEVELOPING COUNTRIES

Disasters that occur in developing countries present special problems. These countries may have significant primary health care problems even before the disaster occurs (such as limitations in clean water supplies, sanitation facilities or adequate nutrition), which will be further exacerbated by the disaster. Effective treatment for mass casualty victims may be compromised because of a lack of adequately trained and equipped medical personnel at the disaster site and non-availability of sufficient tertiary care centres to provide definitive care. The incidence and transmission of communicable diseases may increase after a disaster.[15] Relocation of disaster victims to refugee camps provides temporary shelter, but may compound existing health care problems.[16]

Such developing countries may have to rely on disaster assistance from neighbouring and developed countries. It is difficult, however, to superimpose an emergency response system from a developed country onto a developing country. There will often be a huge gap in the rescue and medical capabilities of the two countries, support systems (such as blood banks, communication systems, etc.) that are common in more advanced nations will be rare in developing countries, and language and cultural barriers may act to impede further co-operative rescue efforts.

The most effective outside disaster aid may occur in the latter stages of a disaster (i.e. from one day post-disaster onwards) when entities, such as the Office of the United Nations Disaster Relief Co-ordinator, the World Health Organization or the League of Red Cross Societies, provide health relief. Assistance by these entities includes the following:[17]

1. Medical services for those exposed to risk, for evacuees, and for relief workers.
2. Vaccination against transmissible disease (see Chapter 18).
3. Action to relieve subsequent malnutrition.

CONCLUSION

A precise formula that will ensure effective disaster management under all circumstances has yet to be developed. Disaster plans which attempt to delineate a specific emergency response that will be set in motion when a disaster occurs often fail because they lack both flexibility and a realistic method of approaching the tragedies that accompany a disaster. Effective patient assessment and triage techniques are the key factors in reducing the mortality and morbidity that can accompany a disaster. Yet identification of salvageable patients who merit tertiary care is difficult under the most optimal conditions, let alone under the chaotic circumstances created by a disaster. The medical community at large must work with civilian disaster agencies and civil and military defence entities to address the challenge of providing effective care to mass casualty victims. The need for increased attention to patient assessment and triage techniques transcends state, national and ideological boundaries. Only through such collaboration will we reduce the devastating mortality and morbidity that result from a disaster.

REFERENCES

1. Safar P. (1980) Stages of resuscitation and life support in disasters. In: Frey R. and Safar P. (eds.) *Disaster Medicine: Resuscitation and Life Support Relief of Pain and Suffering.* Heidelberg and New York, Springer-Verlag.
2. Emergency care in natural disasters: view of an international seminar. (1980) *WHO Chronicle* **34**, 96–100.
3. Champion H. R. and Sacco W. J. (1986) Triage of trauma victims. In: Trunkey D. D. and Lewis F. R. (eds.) *Current Therapy of Trauma – 2.* Philadelphia, B. C. Decker.
4. Winslow G. R. (1982) *Triage and Justice.* Los Angeles, University of California Press.
5. Moore W. S. (1967) A new classification system for disaster casualties. *Hospitals* **41**, 66–72.

6. Sacco W. J., Champion H. R. and Henderson J. V. (1984) Implementation of severity scores in Navy casualty care. *Proceedings of the 17th Hawaii International Conference on System Sciences, Honolulu, Hawaii.*
7. Sacco W. J. (1983) Application of severity indices to Navy combat casualty care. *Naval Medical Research and Development Command Research Task N00014-82-C-0577.*
8. Champion H. R., Sacco W. J., Carnazzo A. J. et al. (1981) The Trauma Score. *Critical Care Medicine* 9, 672–6.
9. Teasdale G. and Jennet B. (1974) Assessment of coma and impaired consciousness: a practical scale. *Lancet* ii, 81–4.
10. Sacco W. J., Champion H. R., Gainer P. S. et al. (1984) The Trauma Score as applied to penetrating trauma. *Ann. Emerg. Med.* 13, 415–18.
11. Moreau M., Gainer P. S., Champion H. R. et al. (1985) Application of the Trauma Score in the prehospital setting. *Ann. Emerg. Med.* 14, 1049–54.
12. Morris J. A., Marshall G., Bluth R. F. et al. (1984) The Trauma Score: a triage tool in the prehospital setting. (Abstract.) *J. Trauma* 24, 671.
13. Morris J. A., Auerbach P. S., Marshall G. A. et al. (1986) The Trauma Score as a triage tool in the prehospital setting. *JAMA* 256(10), 1319–25.
14. American College of Surgeon's Committee on Trauma. (October 1986) Field categorization of trauma patients (field triage). *American College of Surgeons Bulletin* 71(10).
15. de Ville de Goyet C. (1985) Communicable diseases and epidemiological surveillance in natural disasters, with special emphasis on developing countries. In: Manni C. and Magalini S. I. (eds.) *Emergency and Disaster Medicine.* Heidelberg and New York, Springer-Verlag.
16. Tresalti E., Abdulle F. and Isman H. (1985) Nutritional problems of refugees: three years' experience in the Somali camps. In: Manni C. and Magalini S. I. (eds.) *Emergency and Disaster Medicine.* Heidelberg and New York, Springer-Verlag.
17. Thomas R. G. (1980) WHO's role in emergency relief operations. In: Frey R. and Safar P. (eds.) *Disaster Medicine: Resuscitation and Life Support Relief of Pain and Suffering.* Heidelberg and New York, Springer-Verlag.

Resuscitation Medicine including the Management of Severe Trauma

INTRODUCTION

Resuscitation Medicine

Resuscitation medicine may be defined as 'the science, technology and practice of efforts to reverse acute terminal states and clinical death'. Resuscitation consists of emergency resuscitation and long-term resuscitation (i.e. intensive care, intensive therapy). Resuscitology (or reanimatology) is the science of resuscitation. Emergency medicine (EM) and critical care (intensive care) medicine (CCM) are needed for the delivery of resuscitation.

The steps of cardiopulmonary-cerebral resuscitation (CPCR) (*Table* 3.1) are grouped into basic, advanced and prolonged life support.[1] A strict separation of these life-supporting steps into 'cardiac'[2] vs. 'trauma' life support[3] is not advisable, since the pathophysiological derangements to be treated and the techniques to be used are similar.[4] Nevertheless, one may find in literature and teaching texts the abbreviations for basic cardiac and trauma life support (BCLS, BTLS), followed by advanced cardiac and trauma life support (ACLS, ATLS), which often must be extended to prolonged life support (PLS) (intensive care), which should include cerebral resuscitation.[5,6] Physicians involved in disaster medicine should remain informed about the current results of resuscitation research.

In disasters, of course, trauma life support for victims with a pulse is more often needed than cardiac life support for victims without a pulse. The principle resuscitative measures for disaster victims are grouped into life-supporting first aid (LSFA) (*Fig.* 3.1), i.e BTLS; and ATLS.[1] LSFA by lay bystanders within minutes offers a greater life-saving cost-effectiveness than ATLS by experts after hours or days, particularly in mass disasters. ATLS includes fluid resuscitation, endotracheal intubation(*Fig.* 3.2), cricothyrotomy (*Fig.* 3.3), advanced artificial ventilation patterns, pleural drainage (*Fig.* 3.4), resuscitative thoracotomy (*Fig.* 3.5) and a variety of other invasive measures. ATLS should be subdivided into measures that require physicians and those which do not. With external haemorrhage controllable by LSFA, ATLS should ideally include resuscitative surgical interventions which are essential to prevent death and disability from controllable intracranial, intrathoracic and intra-abdominal haemorrhage.

LSFA-ATLS measures should be accompanied by a primary survey of the key pathophysiological derangements, to be followed by a secondary survey of regions injured (*Table* 3.2). (*See* Chapter 2.) After stabilization of airway,

Table 3.1 Phases, steps and measures of cardiopulmonary-cerebral resuscitation

Phases	Steps	Measures performed	
		Establish unresponsiveness—Activate EMS system	
		WITHOUT equipment	**WITH equipment**

I
BASIC LIFE
SUPPORT—BLS
(Emergency
 oxygenation)
	Airway control	1. Backward tilt of head*
		  Supine aligned position*
		  Stable side position*
		2. Lung inflation attempts*
		3. Triple airway manoeuvre
		  (jaw thrust, open
		  mouth)*
		4. Manual clearing of
		  mouth and throat*
		  Back blows—
		  manual thrusts
			5. Pharyngeal suction
			6. Pharyngeal intubation
			7. Endotracheal intubation
			  Tracheobronchial
			  suction
			8. Cricothyrotomy
			  Translaryngeal
			  O₂ jet insufflation
			9. Tracheotomy
			  Bronchoscopy
			  Bronchodilation
			  Pleural drainage

	Breathing support	Mouth-to-mouth (nose) ventilation*	Mouth-to-adjunct with or without O₂ Manual bag-mask (tube) ventilation with or without O₂ Hand-triggered O₂ ventilation Mechanical ventilation
	Circulation support	Control of external haemorrhage* Position for shock* Pulse checking Manual chest compressions	Mechanical chest compressions Open chest direct cardiac compressions Pressure pants (MAST) for shock
II ADVANCED LIFE SUPPORT—ALS (Restoration of spontaneous circulation)	**Drugs and fluids**		i.v. line
	Electrocardiography		ECG monitoring
	Fibrillation treatment		Defibrillation
III PROLONGED LIFE SUPPORT—PLS (Cerebral resuscitation and post-resuscitation intensive therapy)	**Gauging**		Determine and treat cause of demise Determine salvageability
	Human mentation		Cerebral resuscitation
	Intensive care		Multiple organ support

* Life supporting first aid

(Reproduced with slight modification from: Safar P. and Bircher N. (1987) *Cardiopulmonary-Cerebral Resuscitation*, 3rd ed. Stavanger, Laerdal; Philadelphia, Saunders.)

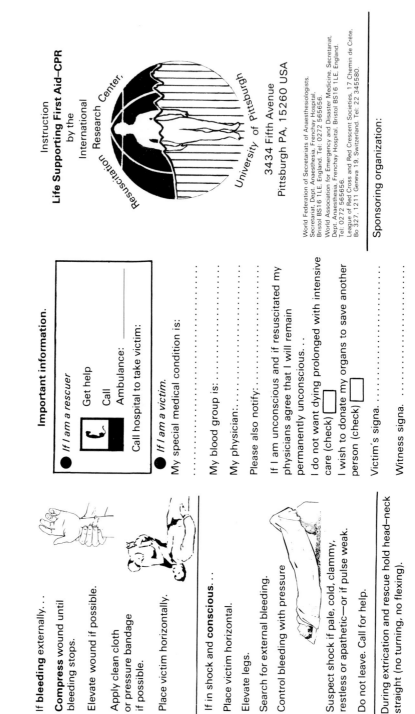

Instruction

Life Supporting First Aid–CPR

by the
International
Resuscitation Research Center,
University of Pittsburgh
3434 Fifth Avenue
Pittsburgh PA, 15260 USA

Important information.

● *If I am a rescuer*

Get help
Call
Ambulance:
Call hospital to take victim:

● *If I am a victim.*

My special medical condition is:

....

My blood group is: ....

My physician: ....

Please also notify: ....

If I am unconscious and if resuscitated my physicians agree that I will remain permanently unconscious. . .

I do not want dying prolonged with intensive care (check)

I wish to donate my organs to save another person (check)

Victim's signa. ....

Witness signa. ....

If **bleeding** externally. . .

Compress wound until bleeding stops.

Elevate wound if possible.

Apply clean cloth or pressure bandage if possible.

Place victim horizontally.

If in shock and **conscious**. . .

Place victim horizontal.

Elevate legs.

Search for external bleeding.

Control bleeding with pressure

Suspect shock if pale, cold, clammy, restless or apathetic—or if pulse weak.

Do not leave. Call for help.

During extrication and rescue hold head–neck straight (no turning, no flexing).

World Federation of Secretariats of Anaesthesiologists. Secretariat, Dept. Anaesthesia, Frenchay Hospital, Bristol BS16 1LE. England. Tel: 0272 565656.
World Association for Emergency and Disaster Medicine. Secretariat, Dept. Anaesthesia, Frenchay Hospital, Bristol BS16 1LE. England. Tel: 0272 565656.
League of Red Cross and Red Crescent Societies, 17 Chemin de Crête, Bo 327, 1211 Geneva 19, Switzerland. Tel: 22 345580.

Sponsoring organization:

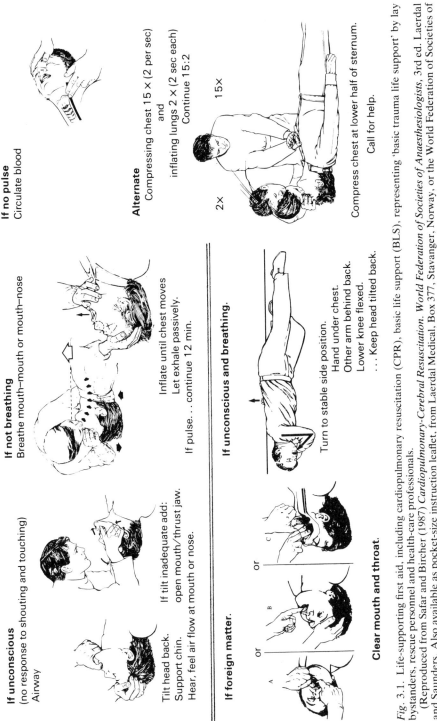

If unconscious
(no response to shouting and touching)
Airway

Tilt head back.
Support chin.
Hear, feel air flow at mouth or nose.

If tilt inadequate add:
open mouth/thrust jaw.

If not breathing
Breathe mouth–mouth or mouth–nose

Inflate until chest moves
Let exhale passively.

If pulse. . . continue 12 min.

If no pulse
Circulate blood

Alternate
Compressing chest 15 × (2 per sec)
and
inflating lungs 2 × (2 sec each)
Continue 15:2

2×   15×

Compress chest at lower half of sternum.
Call for help.

If unconscious and breathing.

Turn to stable side position.
Hand under chest.
Other arm behind back.
Lower knee flexed.
. . . Keep head tilted back.

If foreign matter.

or   or

A   B   C

Clear mouth and throat.

Fig. 3.1. Life-supporting first aid, including cardiopulmonary resuscitation (CPR), basic life support (BLS), representing 'basic trauma life support' by lay bystanders, rescue personnel and health-care professionals.
(Reproduced from Safar and Bircher (1987) *Cardiopulmonary-Cerebral Resuscitation. World Federation of Societies of Anaesthesiologists,* 3rd ed. Laerdal and Saunders. Also available as pocket-size instruction leaflet, from Laerdal Medical, Box 377, Stavanger, Norway, or the World Federation of Societies of Anaesthesiologists CPR Committee, c/o Dr P. Baskett, Frenchay Hospital, Bristol, UK—for distribution by organizations and agencies.)

breathing and blood pressure, the severity of the victim's condition may be evaluated and scored. Evaluation, accompanied by support of vital functions, should be performed at the scene, and at various steps in the life support chain to the hospital ICU. The available, always finite resources, should be allocated according to maximum need and life-saving potential. The BTLS, ATLS and PLS measures carried out at the scene, during transportation and in the hospital emergency department, operating room and ICU, should be brain-orientated,[5,6] since achieving survival with an intact brain is the overriding goal. Finally, results will depend not only on the weakest step of CPCR, but also on the weakest link in the life support chain. The latter reaches from the scene (including extrication and rescue), via transportation and staging areas, to the hospital—the emergency and critical care medicine (ECCM) continuum.[7]

LSFA capability at the scene depends on large scale public education.[1,8] ATLS must be delivered by the regional ECCM system.[7] Many industrialized countries have advanced trauma hospitals. Resuscitative surgery requires medical teams with special knowledge, skills, experience and judgement in advanced resuscitation, anaesthesiology and trauma surgery. In disasters with delayed evacuation, resuscitative surgery at the scene could be life-saving. This might be facilitated with the use of mobile ICU-type operating rooms transportable by helicopter.

Table 3.2. Primary and secondary surveys of trauma victims

Primary Survey
Airway
Breathing
Circulation (pulse? skin? haemorrhage?)
Disability (consciousness)
Exposure (undress)

Secondary Survey (External, internal, penetrating injuries?)
Head (scalp, skull)
Face (eyes, pupils, fundi, lens, mouth, nose)
Cervical spine. Neck
Chest (external, internal)
Abdomen (external, internal). Rectum (sphincter, blood)
Extremities (wounds, fractures)
Neurological (consciousness, eyes, motor, sensory, coma score)
X-rays. Lab tests. Special studies. Surgery.

Disaster Medicine

Disaster medicine may be defined as 'health care efforts in which the number or severity of acutely ill or injured persons exceeds the capacity of the local emergency medical services (EMS) system'.[7,9]

Disasters can be classified into three categories:[9]

1. Multi-casualty incidents, such as transportation accidents or fires, for which the local EMS system is overtaxed, but responds by implementing its disaster plan, sometimes with help from neighbouring EMS systems.
2. Mass disasters, which include major earthquakes, floods and conventional wars, in which the local EMS system is destroyed and in which LSFA must be provided by uninjured bystanders and ATLS delivered from the outside.

3. Endemic–epidemic disasters, usually in poor developing countries which have no modern EMS systems.

The latter can be the result of drought with starvation and dehydration, infections and revolution. They require ongoing socio-politico-economic rather than merely medical solutions.

Multi-casualty incidents and mass disasters may be subclassified into natural and man-made disasters. Natural mass disasters include major earthquakes, floods, hurricanes and fires. Man-made mass disasters include major fires, industrial accidents, wars and nuclear accidents. The potential magnitude of the problem encountered by disaster resuscitology is illustrated by the commonly used scenario for planning national disaster medical systems: a major earthquake. One such major earthquake killed about 80000 people in Peru in 1970, and 100000 in China in 1976. Earthquakes injure about 2–3 times as many people as they kill.[10]

Disaster medicine concerns itself with resuscitation, public health and rehabilitation of people and regions. Until recently, many poor developing countries have had no EMS systems. No effective, realistic disaster plans exist even in many countries and communities with EMS systems, not even to meet the resuscitative challenges of multi-casualty incidents. Mass disasters have, until recently, been the domain of public health, sociology and Red Cross organizations, which focus on helping uninjured survivors. In earthquakes, response times for medical relief has been 2 days or more, too slow for resuscitation to have a life-saving impact. Since the founding of the Club of Mainz in 1976, interest has been aroused in exploring the addition of modern resuscitation to the planning for medical response to mass disasters such as major earthquakes.

Disaster Resuscitology

In 1981, disaster resuscitology was initiated as a new field of inquiry and service.[11] Interview studies of physician-survivors of earthquakes have suggested a significant, realistic life-saving potential of modern resuscitation medicine.[1] About one-third of those counted ultimately as dead in major earthquakes die slowly and are potentially accessible for LSFA and ATLS. Among these about 40 per cent would not have died if uninjured, lay co-victims had had LSFA capability and ATLS medical teams had reached the victims within 6 hours. This estimated resuscitation potential in 10–15 per cent of those killed in earthquakes exists only with very rapid (but feasible) response times. This should not be a deterrent, but rather a challenge to overcome logistic obstacles. The life-saving potential of resuscitation medicine's BLS and ALS for victims of conventional wars has been proven.[12] Major conventional wars can kill and maim even more people than earthquakes, but usually allow time for preparations and are spread out over long periods. Military medicine and airlift capabilities are essential for response to national mass disasters.[13] In a full-scale nuclear war, medicine in general and resuscitation medicine in particular would have no chances to offer help.

In everyday EMS, about 50 per cent of trauma deaths occur before the patient reaches the hospital.[3] The majority of these deaths are the result of external or internal exsanguination or complete airway obstruction within the first few minutes to one hour post-trauma. The majority of the ultimately unresuscitable deaths are due to massive brain injury. Certain patterns of dying are also characteristic of disaster victims and can be studied to determine the patho-physiological bases for resuscitation.[1,4]

In major earthquakes,[12,14] death can be instantaneous, as from crushing of the head or chest, exsanguination from external or internal haemorrhage, or drowning; rapid (within minutes or hours), as from asphyxia, hypovolaemic shock or exposure hypothermia; or delayed for days, as from crush syndrome (crushing of muscle tissue) or sepsis. The release of crushed extremities, abdomen or pelvis has sometimes been followed by cardiac arrest. Coma secondary to head injury or shock can cause asphyxia due to upper airway soft tissue obstruction, aspiration or hypoventilation. Head injury, even of non-crippling severity (concussion or minor contusion), can cause one or more minutes of impact apnoea,[1] followed by coma with airway obstruction when breathing movements return. This results in asphyxia, which worsens the brain damage caused by the initial trauma, unless airway control and exhaled air ventilation are initiated immediately. Asphyxia can also occur secondary to aspiration or pulmonary oedema, and as a result of dust inhalation, electric shock from broken electric lines, and smoke inhalation and burns from fires. Early survivors of traumatic shock have died from dehydration, hypothermia, hyperthermia, starvation, diarrhoea and sepsis. Combinations of dying mechanisms seem to be common, but have been inadequately studied (see Chapter 20).

In major floods, people have died from combinations of trauma, drowning and hypothermia with or without submersion. Cold water submersion of up to about 40 minutes has occasionally been reversed to complete recovery.[15] Death from cold exposure without drowning has an even better chance of being reversed by resuscitation. These conditions of clinical death require extraordinary advanced resuscitative measures, which may not be available for days following a mass disaster (see Chapters 17, 21 and 26).

In disasters caused by intoxicating gases, dying processes include combinations of upper airway burns, pulmonary oedema, bronchospasm, and bronchial secretions and oedema.

In disasters involving burns, there can be a mixture of carbon monoxide poisoning, traumatic shock, asphyxia from inhalation injury and late sepsis. They lead to dying processes which are very complex, some of which are beyond the scope of this chapter. The logistics of giving modern burn care to a large number of casualties are enormous. The scarcity of burn ICU facilities and specialized teams is a major limiting factor in the preparedness for mass disasters involving burns, such as major fires and industrial accidents.

Resuscitation of radiation victims must be included in the preparedness for mass disasters. Radiation injuries might happen as a result of technological failure, human error or terrorism. One should consider the whole range of possibilities, from the subtle leak of radioactive material from a nuclear reactor or power plant into air, water and ground, to the explosion of a small nuclear device (see Chapter 30).

This chapter reviews the fundamentals of resuscitation methods which have been shown to save lives in everyday EMS and which might thus save lives in disasters of various kinds too. After some fundamental considerations on LSFA (BLS), general ALS steps and ATLS, specific considerations for selected pathological conditions associated with disasters are reviewed.

LIFE-SUPPORTING FIRST AID (LSFA) (Basic Life Support)

Introduction

Basic life support (BLS) for both cardiac and trauma cases is also called 'life-supporting first aid' (LSFA). We believe that LSFA should include cardio-pulmonary resuscitation (CPR), steps A, B and C, without equipment (*Fig.* 3.1) and (*Table* 3.1). LSFA must be provided at the scene, during transport and throughout the hospital. LSFA should and can be mastered by all lay persons above 10–12 years of age, and all health care professionals.[1,8]

LSFA includes the following steps (*Fig.* 3.1):

1. Control of external haemorrhage by compression and elevation, without surgical measures.
2. Positioning of the shocked conscious victim horizontally with legs elevated.
3. Airway control, by backward tilt of the head (moderate backward tilt in the unconscious victim with suspected cervical spine injury), if necessary with additional forward displacement of the mandible and holding the mouth slightly open.
4. Manual clearance of foreign matter from mouth and pharnyx as needed.
5. Mouth-to-mouth or mouth-to-nose ventilation.
6. Positioning of the unconscious, spontaneously, adequately breathing victim on his side with the head tilted backward.
7. Palpation of the pulse and, when absent, performing external chest (heart, sternal) compressions, realizing that in the traumatized victim with severe blood loss external CPR will not circulate blood.
8. 'Rescue pull', i.e. extrication of the victim to safety while holding head, neck and chest aligned.

Evaluation and resuscitation must go hand-in-hand and be continued in the emergency department and other areas of the hospital. While an adequate airway is being established, as soon as personnel capable of delivering advanced trauma life support (ATLS) arrive, an intravenous (i.v.) route should be established for fluid resuscitation; in selected cases medical anti-shock trousers (MAST) should be applied; and a search for signs of internal haemorrhage in cranium, chest, abdomen, pelvis and crushed extremities should be carried out (*Table* 3.2). A history should be obtained from the patient, if conscious, and from bystanders, ambulance personnel and relatives. Undue patient movements should be avoided before transfer to the most appropriate hospital. Within the hospital transfer to radiology and other areas away from the critical care facilities should be minimized. Patients in need of immediate surgery should be taken directly to the operating room.

External Haemorrhage (*Fig.* 3.1)

Control of external haemorrhage must be immediate, since the loss of 1 l of blood or more in an adult (much less in children) can be life-threatening. External bleeding from veins and capillaries, as well as most pulsating bleeding from arteries, can be controlled by sealing, with pressure, the torn vessels against solid tissues underneath and, if possible, by elevating the bleeding site. Compressing arterial pressure points proximal to the extremity wounds is less reliable and more difficult to learn.

Tourniquets should be used only as a last resort and only in cases of extreme trauma to the extremities in which major vessels have been injured. Even in traumatic amputations, severed vessels may retract and stop bleeding. When the tourniquet is in place for extended periods, nerves, blood vessels and the entire extremity may be permanently damaged. When applied too loosely, the tourniquet can increase bleeding by impeding venous drainage. If a tourniquet is used, a cravat or folded handkerchief is better than a rope or wire. Apply a pad over the artery to be compressed (pressure point), wrap the tourniquet twice around the extremity and tie a half knot. Place a stick, pencil or similar object on top of the half knot and tie the ends of the tourniquet in a square knot above the stick. Twist the stick to tighten the tourniquet until the bleeding stops, securing it in that position. Write on the patient's forehead 'T' and the time the tourniquet was applied.

Airway Control (Fig. 3.1)

Airway obstruction must be immediately recognized (no air flow, silent or noisy breathing, suprasternal or intercostal retractions) and be corrected. After trauma, obstruction due to coma or airway injury must be considered. In coma from any cause, soft tissue obstruction at the hypopharyngeal level by the tongue and epiglottis, or due to malpositioning of head, neck and jaw, is most common.[16] Obstruction may also be due to aspiration of vomitus, mucus or blood; laryngospasm; or airway injury with subsequent bleeding and swelling of tissues.

The emergency airway control steps (Table 3.1) should be pursued swiftly and vigorously until the airway is open. Mid-position or flexion of the head causes airway obstruction. Maximum backward tilt of the head relieves hypopharyngeal obstruction in about 80 per cent of cases.[16] In coma associated with trauma, head and neck injury cannot be ruled out at the scene. Exaggerated backward tilt of the head, as well as flexion and turning of the head and neck, may aggravate a cervical spinal cord injury. Therefore, maximum head tilt should be modified to moderate head tilt. This often requires additional opening of the mouth and jaw thrust (triple airway manoeuvre). An open mouth is needed because of commonly occurring nasal obstruction. Jaw thrust may be necessary to regain the necessary stretch of anterior neck structures lost by opening the mouth. The triple airway manoeuvre, which entails holding head-neck-chest in the aligned position, is the most important life-saving step for traumatized victims. It can be learned even by lay personnel.

When trained health professionals arrive, they can replace jaw thrust with an oro- or nasopharyngeal tube. A nasopharyngeal tube is better tolerated and is preferred when there is trismus, but is not recommended when a basal skull fracture is suspected.

The oesophageal obturator airway[17] is of value in cases of cardiac arrest outside the hospital treated by personnel not trained in tracheal intubation. However, it is a poor substitute for endotracheal intubation. Its use is contraindicated in the spontaneously breathing unconscious patient, and certainly in the conscious patient, because its insertion can provoke vomiting, regurgitation, aspiration and laryngospasm. Moreover, it does not permit satisfactory endotracheal suctioning. Airway control with the use of devices is part of advanced life-support.

When head tilt plus mouth open plus jaw thrust and mouth-to-mouth (or mouth-to-nose) positive pressure inflation attempts meet obstruction, or when vomit or other foreign matter appears in the mouth, the upper airway must be cleared of foreign matter. Force open the mouth and clear foreign material from the mouth and pharynx by a finger sweep (*Fig.* 3.1), until pharyngeal suction is possible. The definitive ALS measures include pharyngolaryngoscopy, suctioning and removal of foreign material under vision, endotracheal intubation, tracheobronchial suction, and bronchoscopic removal of foreign material.

If the patient is conscious, and is suspected of having aspirated foreign material, and is only partially obstructed, i.e. can talk, he should be encouraged to take deep breaths, cough and spit foreign matter out. Digital probing, thrusts and back blows should be avoided, as such manoeuvres may aggravate the obstruction.

If the patient is conscious or unconscious, and with suspected foreign body aspiration but is completely obstructed, i.e. with cyanosis, ineffective cough or unable to talk or cough, any possibly effective measure should be used rapidly as an act of desperation. No single method should be taught to the exclusion of others. Sudden complete obstruction can cause unconsciousness from hypoxia within 1–2 minutes. Thrusts and back blows have been recommended, in attempts to loosen the object impacted in the upper airway.[2] Data about these indirect manoeuvres are controversial and mainly anecdotal.

The rationale for use of subdiaphragmatic abdominal thrusts (Heimlich manoeuvre)[18] is that it pushes the diaphragm upward and thereby creates an artificial cough to expel an obstructing foreign body. Physiological evidence indicates that abdominal thrusts produce very weak increases in airway pressure when the airway is closed and very low airflow rates when the airway is open, like a weak natural cough. Back blows produce higher airway pressures than thrusts when the airway is closed, and might either loosen the object, or impact it further into the standing or sitting victim. Abdominal thrusts are being promoted by the originator[18] and are taught by the American Heart Association[2] and the American Red Cross. These organizations recently removed back blows from the list of measures to be taught. In contrast, the International League of Red Cross Societies[8] and the World Federation of Societies of Anesthesiologists' guidelines do not recommend the teaching of abdominal thrusts, because of their dubious efficacy and the risk of aggravating injuries.

The most effective and definitive methods for relieving airway obstruction due to aspiration of foreign material require extra advanced life support equipment and special training:

1. Use of a laryngoscope or tongue blade plus flashlight, for looking at the mouth, pharynx and larynx.
2. Extraction of the foreign material under direct vision by Kelly clamp, Magill forceps, or suction.
3. If complete obstruction persists, endotracheal intubation (*Fig.* 3.2), cricothyrotomy (*Fig.* 3.3), or translaryngeal jet insufflation. Such equipment should be employed only by trained health care professionals. Blind extraction attempts with instruments are hazardous.

Ventilation and Oxygenation (*Fig.* 3.1)[1]

Cessation of breathing can be the result of coma, asphyxia, drug overdose, as well as other causes. Accidental injury, particularly head trauma, can cause transient sudden coma, breath-holding and hypoventilation. At the scene, treatment of the comatose trauma victim includes moderate backward tilt of the head plus mouth open and jaw thrust, and exhaled air ventilation,[1] starting with mouth-to-mouth ventilation. In cases of trismus, mouth-to-nose ventilation may be required. Each inflation attempt should be over 1–2 seconds, until the chest expands, removing the mouth to allow passive exhalation. Continue with about one inflation every 5 seconds. Mouth-to-mouth ventilation has replaced the back-pressure arm-lift methods of the 1950s.

Ambulance and hospital personnel, and even 'first responders' (e.g. police, lifeguards), should switch as soon as possible to ventilation with 50–100 per cent oxygen using advanced life-support techniques. Spontaneous, assisted and controlled ventilation with oxygen are possible with use of a pocket mask with oxygen nipple (*Fig.* 3.1). This device leaves both hands free for support of mask and airway.

Positioning

Shock is defined as a 'reduction in overall tissue perfusion, resulting in vital organ systems malfunction'. Trauma can result in rapid exsanguination. If either nature or a rescuer stops moderate or severe bleeding before the pulse disappears, the usual result is hypovolaemic shock. The clinical picture of hypoperfusion associated with hypovolaemia includes a faint peripheral pulse, tachycardia (which may be absent in infancy, old age, or during general anaesthesia), cold, moist skin, oliguria, tachypnoea and CNS excitation, possibly progressing to hypoventilation and CNS depression. The arterial blood pressure may be normal in fit persons until 20–30 per cent of the blood volume has been lost because of compensatory vasoconstriction. Rapid loss of about 50 per cent of blood volume can be followed by cardiac arrest.

A seriously injured person should not be moved by personnel who are not trained in field rescue, unless it is essential for LSFA, to avoid aggravating his injuries, or to protect both victim and first aiders from further accidents. If the shocked patient is conscious, he should be placed in the horizontal and supine (face up) position with legs elevated (*Fig.* 3.1). This may have a slight autotransfusion effect and counteracts postural hypotension. Normal body temperature should be maintained, avoiding overheating as well as hypothermia. Light-weight thermal blankets are useful. The head-down position is not recommended. If the shocked patient is unconscious and breathing adequately, he should be placed in the supported supine position or moved with head/neck/chest aligned into the stable side position (*Fig.* 3.1). Do not give anything to drink, as an anaesthetic may be needed later. Even when conscious, vomiting and aspiration may occur.

If the victim needs to be moved to safety, the 'rescue pull', i.e. extrication without equipment, should be applied. Move the injured limbs as little as possible; and immobilize the head, neck and chest in the aligned position preferably with helpers simultaneously providing head-tilt, open mouth and jaw thrusts in unconscious patients. Ambulance personnel, whenever possible, should extricate with the help of a short backboard applied before moving the patient gently onto a long backboard, using established methods of pre-hospital trauma care.

External Cardiac Resuscitation (Fig. 3.1)[1,19]

Cardiac arrest is defined as 'the clinical picture of sudden cessation of circulation in a patient who was not expected to die at that time'. Cessation of circulation is verified when all the following conditions are present: unconsciousness, apnoea or gasps, death-like appearance, and no pulse in the carotid or femoral artery. Absence of heart sounds and the presence of dilated pupils are unreliable signs.

Irrespective of the ECG pattern of cardiac arrest, the absence of a pulse calls for an immediate start of standard external (closed-chest) CPR. The recommended method[1,2] calls for 15 chest (cardiac) compressions (at a rate of 80–100/min) alternated with 2 successive lung inflations (allowing for about 1–2 s for each inflation). If there are 2 CPR-trained health care professionals present, they may use one interposed lung inflation after every 5 chest compressions (again at a rate of 80–100/min), with a pause after every 5th compression to allow for the lung inflation. A combination of IPPV plus chest compressions should be continued until a spontaneous pulse returns. IPPV should start with exhaled air and switch to 100 per cent oxygen when it becomes available. IPPV via an endotracheal tube does not have to be synchronized with sternal compressions, which should be without interruption.

Standard closed-chest CPR produces variable borderline blood flow for cerebral viability, even in pulseless victims without blood loss but is the only emergency measure available for use by laymen in case of lack of pulse. When no pulse is present, blood volume must be restored and even expanded. This requires ALS by paramedics, nurses or physicians.

Attempts to improve, in terms of outcome, the efficacy of external CPR-BLS by various 'pneumatic' modifications without the need for equipment have so far failed.[2] Chest compressions, by raising central venous pressure peaks as high as aortic pressure peaks, produce very low perfusion pressures, particularly through the myocardium. Lung inflations simultaneous with chest compressions and abdominal binding ('new CPR') may result in improved carotid blood flow, but can increase intracranial pressure and reduce brain oxygenation. As this method requires both a tracheal tube and a mechanical ventilator, it is not a BLS method.

Patients who develop witnessed sudden ventricular fibrillation, who immediately begin (spontaneously or coached) vigorous repetitive coughing, can thereby circulate enough blood to remain conscious until defibrillation 1–2 min later. Cough CPR is based on spontaneous pneumatic 'thoracic diastole' (deep gasp) followed by forceful 'thoracic systole' (Valsalva manoeuvre cough).

External CPR alone, in the exsanguinated victim, is futile.[1,3] The patient with no pulse and hypovolaemia (trauma-haemorrhage) needs rapid i.v. fluid replacement and epinephrine simultaneously with CPR to reverse clinical death (see below: special considerations, exsanguination cardiac arrest).

GENERAL ADVANCED LIFE SUPPORT

Advanced life support (ALS) (*Table* 3.1) begins with BLS steps A, B and C. In absence of pulse, this must be followed by rapid attempts at restarting spontaneous circulation, using the ALS steps D (drugs and fluids), E (electrocardiography) and F (fibrillation treatment, defibrillation). Closed-chest (external) CPR is more often indicated for ACLS; open-chest CPR for ATLS (see below).

In the absence of a pulse due to asphyxia or exsanguination, CPR steps A, B and C plus correction of the cause of arrest can sometimes restart heart action; but in most cases of cardiac arrest, ALS by a combination of defibrillation, epinephrine (adrenaline), and i.v. fluids is required.

Endotracheal Intubation (*Fig.* 3.2)

For both ACLS and ATLS, in the comatose patient, endotracheal intubation is the definitive step of emergency airway control. It is indicated when the patient has lost consciousness, unless his upper airway protective reflexes are intact, coma is expected to be brief, and he is attended continuously by experienced personnel. Endotracheal intubation is also indicated in the conscious patient who has inadequate spontaneous clearing of the tracheobronchial tree, suspected aspiration, upper airway areflexia, or a need for prolonged mechanical ventilation. Improved endotracheal tubes and cuffs have minimized laryngotracheal damage.

In cases of suspected *head injury*, endotracheal intubation is the ultimate step in emergency airway control. However, it does *not* have first priority prior to arrival in the hospital. Reflex hypertension and unskilled intubation attempts accompanied by straining, asphyxia and aspiration, can cause intracranial pressure to rise and lead to intracranial disaster. To intubate the trachea successfully without causing intracranial complications following head trauma, requires special techniques and an experienced operator. If head injury is suspected and an experienced operator is not available, oxygenation and assisted ventilation by mouth-to-mask with O_2 enrichment or by bag-mask-O_2 are safer than attempts at endotracheal intubation. In suspected head injury with coma, neck injury is also possible. If assisted IPPV without an endotracheal tube fails, intubation becomes an essential act of desperation. The goal is to intubate orally, without causing coughing or straining, after hyperventilation by mask with 100 per cent O_2, with relaxation by succinylcholine and cricoid pressure to prevent regurgitation. However, failed intubation attempts by the novice with the use of a muscle relaxant can be lethal.

For emergency airway control, orotracheal intubation is preferred over nasotracheal intubation, which is less predictable, more time-consuming, and potentially more traumatic. Nasal tubes are contraindicated in suspected basilar skull fracture. Nasotracheal intubation, however, may be the only possible method in the spontaneously breathing patient, without asphyxia, who has trismus or in whom tilting the head backward maximally is contraindicated, as in suspected cervical fracture. For difficult intubations, tactile orotracheal intubation with use of the lighted stylet should be practised.[20]

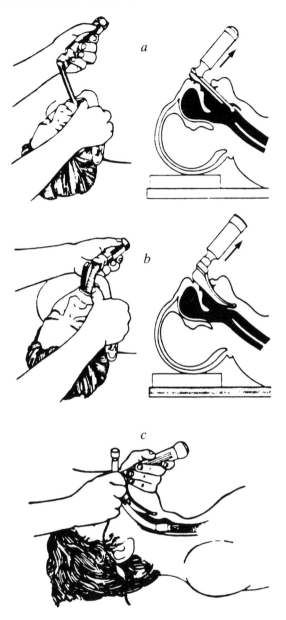

Fig. 3.2. Technique of orotracheal intubation: *a*, Laryngoscopy for endotracheal intubation with straight laryngoscope blade. *Left*, insertion of blade. *Right*, larynx exposed. Note elevated occiput with head tilted backward (sniffing position). Note direct elevation of epiglottis with tip of blade. Do not use teeth as fulcrum. Keep pressure off upper teeth and lip; *b*, Laryngoscopy for endotracheal intubation with curved laryngoscope blade. *Left*, insertion of blade. *Right*, larynx exposed. Note indirect elevation of epiglottis by tip of blade elevating base of tongue. Note also direction of lift, which is anteriorly and inferiorly at 45° to vertical (coronal) plane. *c*, Exposure of the larynx with curved blade and insertion of cuffed tube through right corner of mouth, while looking along laryngoscope blade. For detailed instructions, *see* Safar and Bircher, op. cit.

(Reproduced with permission of authors and publishers.)

Cricothyroid membrane puncture (*Fig.* 3.3) or translaryngeal oxygen jet insufflation can be used as an alternative to tracheal intubation, but is rarely essential. Tracheotomy (below the cricoid cartilage) is not for emergency airway control; it should be considered for long-term airway care, after a translaryngeal tube has been in place for several days, or earlier when coma is expected to last longer than about one week. Conscious patients are more comfortable with a tracheostomy tube, which permits them to talk.

Fibreoptic bronchoscopy can be lifesaving. Bronchoscopy is indicated in cases of aspiration, for clearing solid foreign matter or thick mucus or blood from the tracheal broncheal tree. However, for clearing such materials, the rigid bronchoscope, with a ventilation-oxygenation attachment, is more effective than the fibreoptic bronchoscope.

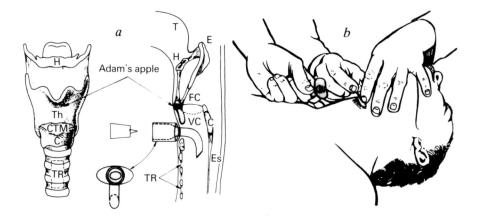

Fig. 3.3. Cricothyrotomy: *a*, Anatomy with cannula in place. H, hyoid cartilage; Th, thyroid cartilage; C, cricoid cartilage; TR, trachea; CTM, cricothyroid membrane; E, epiglottis; T, tongue; FC, false cords; VC, vocal cords; Es, oesophagus. Bevelled curved cannula with knife blade (with handle rubber stopper, to be carried safely within 15 mm slip joint of cannula). The cannula shown can be self-made from curved endotracheal tube slip joints (6 mm outside diameter for adults; 3 mm outside diameter for large children), with 15 mm male adaptor to connect ventilation equipment. Special cannula not essential. Regular small bore cuffed endotracheal or tracheostomy tube with 6 mm outside diameter is satisfactory in adults. For small children and infants use smallest size uncuffed endotracheal or tracheostomy tube catheter-outside-needle of i.v. supplies, 12–14 gauge. *b*, Technique of cricothyroid membrane puncture via small horizontal skin incision.

(Reproduced from Safar and Bircher, op. cit. with permission of authors and publishers.)

Pleural Drainage (*Fig.* 3.4)

Emergency pleural drainage is discussed in this section relating to airway control (*Table* 3.1) because tension pneumothorax kills by collapsing the lung, bronchial compression and asphyxia.[4] Tension pneumothorax should be suspected when chest injury or IPPV is followed by tracheal shift, progressive inability of the chest to deflate, progressive abdominal distension (inversion of diaphragm and

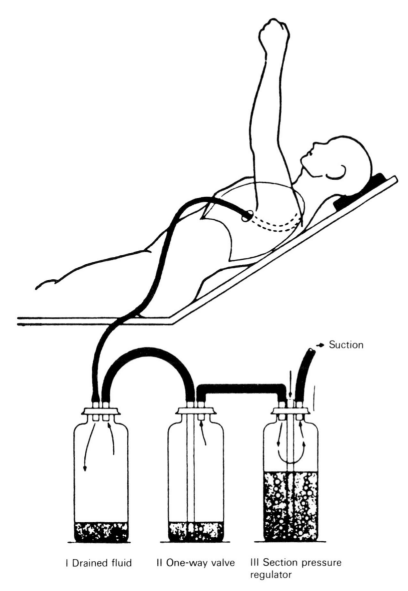

→ Suction

| I Drained fluid | II One-way valve | III Section pressure regulator |

Fig. 3.4. Technique of pleural drainage. The appropriate size chest tube is inserted through a stab incision in the skin and into the pleural cavity, with the open technique (blunt Kelly clamp pierced through the intercostal space and prised open for tube insertion) or the closed technique (using a trocar). The latter technique requires greater skill to avoid complications. One lateral-to-posterior chest tube, with multiple holes, is usually sufficient. The tube is connected via a Y-tube to a bottle system consisting of bottle 1 for collection of fluids; bottle 2, a one-way valve; and bottle 3 to keep a constant controllable negative pressure. For transportation a one-way valve instead of the three-bottle system is used. In hospitals the three-bottle system may be replaced by a chest suction device, provided it permits control of negative pressure and a high flow rate. If negative pressure is not required a thoracic drainage bag (Portex) may be used which is more convenient for transport.

(Reproduced from Safar and Bircher, op. cit. with permission of authors and publishers.)

pneumoperitoneum), progressive hypotension, and mediastinal shift to percussion. Proof is by needle puncture via the second intercostal space anteriorly. Treatment is by drainage via a large-bore tube.

Ventilation and Oxygenation [21]

In the hands of pre-hospital personnel not trained in anaesthesia, use of the pocket mask is more effective than use of the bag-valve-mask unit, since the former leaves both hands available to provide mask fit and jaw thrust. When the bag-valve-oxygen unit is used with a tracheal tube, a positive end-expiratory pressure (PEEP) valve may be attached. Use of a simple portable mechanical ventilator acceptable in cases with normal lungs. However, if the patient has abnormal lungs, use of a more sophisticated volume-set time-cycled ventilator, with PEEP and IMV attachments, is preferred for controlled ventilation, at least after hospital admission.

By the time the injured patient in shock arrives in the emergency room, he may be hyperventilating spontaneously. Nevertheless, he should continue to receive 50–100 per cent oxygen. In cases of severe polytrauma, irrespective of the state of consciousness, controlled mechanical hyperventilation with an inhaled oxygen concentration (FIO_2) of 50–100 per cent stabilizes ventilation and oxygenation during control of haemorrhage, fluid resuscitation and emergency surgery. A muscle relaxant may be necessary, and 'softening' doses do not hamper recognition of an intracranial lesion and assessment of the state of consciousness. Weaning from controlled ventilation can be accomplished with intermittent mandatory ventilation (IMV) or assisted ventilation with pressure support, gradually progressing to spontaneous breathing.

Assessment of the pulmonary status requires measurement of arterial PO_2 in relation to FIO_2. Normal PaO_2 values are 75–100 mmHg with FIO_2 21 per cent; over 250 mmHg with FIO_2 50 per cent; and over 500 mmHg with FIO_2 100 per cent. Arterial PO_2 should be kept at a minimum of 60 mmHg (the knee of the haemoglobin oxygen dissociation curve) in the conscious patient, or at a minimum of 100 mmHg in the unconscious patient. Pulmonary oxygen toxicity can be prevented by limiting the use of FIO_2 100 per cent to less than 6–12 hours. FIO_2 50 per cent appears safe for unlimited periods. Shunting per se increases the tolerance by the lungs of an FIO_2 of 100 per cent.[22]

The adequacy of alveolar ventilation is determined by arterial PCO_2. Normal $PaCO_2$ values are 35–45 mmHg. Most spontaneously breathing patients in shock hyperventilate. Since shock can decrease, and trauma as well as resuscitation can increase oxygen consumption and CO_2 production, ventilation requirements in terms of tidal volumes and rates are unpredictable. They should ideally be adjusted to obtain the desired $PaCO_2$. During controlled ventilation, moderate hyperventilation to $PaCO_2$ of about 30 mmHg is desirable. This can usually, in the patient with normal cardiac output and oxygen consumption, be accomplished by tidal volumes of 15 ml/kg at a rate of 12/min.

In shock, mean airway pressure should be kept as low as possible, since increased mean intrathoracic pressure tends to reduce further return of blood to the heart. If spontaneous breathing is inadequate, IPPV is recommended.

High frequency oxygen jet ventilation[23] is a new technique. One hundred per cent oxygen is intermittently insufflated via a thin catheter inserted into the endotracheal tube or percutaneously through the cricothyroid membrane.

Cycling rates of 100–1000/min, delivering 100 per cent oxygen with a tidal volume smaller than the estimated dead space, can restore and maintain the normal arterial P_{O_2} and P_{CO_2} values of non-breathing subjects with normal lungs. This technique allows simultaneous spontaneous breathing to occur, lowers mean airway pressure with less risk of causing barotrauma or reduction in cardiac output, enables ventilation in the presence of large pulmonary leaks, and if used via a cricothyroid or transtracheal cannula, lessens chances of injury to the tracheal mucosa. The ability of this technique to recruit alveoli and increase arterial P_{O_2} in the presence of reversible shunt (e.g. aspiration, pulmonary oedema) depends on additional PEEP and intermittent deep lung inflations.

Drugs and Defibrillation [1,2]

Electrical asystole and electromechanical dissociation call for epinephrine (adrenaline); ventricular fibrillation and ventricular tachycardia call for electric countershocks; and recurrent ventricular fibrillation or tachycardia calls for lidocaine or bretylium in addition to countershocks. For external electric defibrillation, recommended energy levels start with about 3 watt second/kg body weight, which should be increased for repeated shocks. New automatic external defibrillators which 'read' the ECG and give computer-programmed countershocks, are in use by ambulance technicians and are now available for laymen.

Precordial thumping cannot reliably defibrillate; it can actually cause ventricular fibrillation. During asystole or severe bradycardia due to heart block, however, repetitive precordial thumping in the conscious patient or external cardiac compressions in the unconscious patient (the latter being too painful for the conscious patient) can be used effectively to pace the oxygenated heart into contractions, while waiting for atropine, isoproterenol (isoprenaline), and a pacemaker.

In sudden primary ventricular fibrillation, the ideal treatment is immediate electric defibrillation; during the first 30 s after disappearance of the pulse neither basic life support, nor drugs, are needed before an initial trial of electric defibrillation. After circulatory arrest of 30 s, BLS is recommended in the first instance. After 1 min, epinephrine is indicated. Intravenous drugs should be given into a central vein and circulated by chest compressions for about 1 min before a countershock is applied.

Epinephrine (adrenaline) (0·5–1 mg in adults) should be given as the first drug, either i.v. or in 10 ml of water via the endotracheal tube, without waiting for an ECG diagnosis. Although epinephrine can produce ventricular fibrillation in a non-fibrillating heart, it facilitates defibrillation. Epinephrine stimulates sympathetic alpha- and beta-receptors. The alpha-receptor stimulation increases peripheral vascular resistance without constricting the coronary and cerebral vessels. The resulting increase in diastolic pressure improves myocardial and cerebral perfusion during CPR and makes the heart more resuscitatable. The beta-receptor stimulation is not important during CPR, but may be advantageous when spontaneous circulation returns, at which time it enhances cardiac contractility and cardiac output. In asystole and electromechanical dissociation, epinephrine helps restart spontaneous cardiac action by elevating perfusion pressure and increasing myocardial contractility.

Vasoconstrictors, i.e. predominantly alpha-receptor agonists, may be considered helpful in restoring a spontaneous circulation. They have not been studied and used as extensively as epinephrine. They include norepinephrine (noradrenaline), metaraminol, phenylephrine, methoxamine, and dopamine in high doses, and all have been used effectively after the restoration of spontaneous circulation.

Cardiac stimulants, which are predominantly beta-receptor agonists, do not enhance restoration of a spontaneous circulation during cardiac compressions but may be useful in intractable electromechanical dissociation. After restoration of a spontaneous circulation, they may overcome intractable hypotension due to a low cardiac output. These drugs include isoproterenol (isoprenaline), dopamine in low doses, dobutamine and calcium chloride.

Lidocaine (lignocaine) is the second drug to be considered in sudden cardiac death. Lidocaine raises the ventricular fibrillation threshold. It is the drug of choice for the prevention and treatment of ventricular extrasystoles and ventricular tachycardia. It is usually given in bolus doses of 1 mg/kg i.v., when ventricular fibrillation or ventricular tachycardia continue after the first 3 countershocks. It may also be administered via the tracheal tube. Lidocaine may be repeated as necessary in 1 mg/kg i.v. doses and as an i.v. infusion of $1–4 \text{ mg} \cdot 70 \text{ kg}^{-1} \cdot \text{min}^{-1}$. In ventricular fibrillation lidocaine, or other antiarrhythmic agents are not substitutes for CPR and electric countershocks. In recurrent ventricular fibrillation, lidocaine is indicated in addition to repeated countershocks. Bretylium is a new, promising antiarrhythmic agent that should be considered when lidocaine fails; recommended doses are 5 mg/kg i.v. repeated to a maximum of 30 mg/kg.

Sodium bicarbonate ($NaHCO_3$) is the third drug to be considered during CPR-ABC for i.v. administration (not intratracheally!). The recommended initial dose is 1 mmol/kg of body weight i.v. given 15–20 min after a sudden arrest. Without arterial pH monitoring, not more than $0 \cdot 5$ mmol/kg should be given, to avoid severe alkalaemia, hyperosmolality and CO_2 release from $NaHCO_3$. Transient hyperventilation is needed to eliminate the CO_2 that has accumulated in tissues and that being released from the bicarbonate. Excessive $NaHCO_3$ makes the heart non-resuscitatable. As soon as possible, $NaHCO_3$ administration should be guided by arterial pH values, which should be maintained between $7 \cdot 3$ and $7 \cdot 6$. With near-normal arterial pH, there is no evidence that base deficit itself must be corrected. Moderate acidaemia may be beneficial. Bicarbonate alone does not enhance restoration of spontaneous circulation, but it enhances the effect of epinephrine, which is inactivated by tissue acidosis occurring after prolonged arrest.

Cerebral Resuscitation

Cerebral resuscitation attempts[6,24] are indicated in comatose cardiac arrest survivors. They should start immediately after restoration of spontaneous normotension, or perhaps even before restoration of spontaneous heart beat.

Until recently, the concept prevailed that normothermic cardiac arrest of longer than 4–5 min is invariably followed by permanent brain damage. This concept was based on laboratory, intra-hospital, and pre-hospital observations.[25] The discovery of post-ischaemic secondary derangements of cerebral and extra-cerebral function[26] raised the possibility of special regimes which might improve the chance of a good cerebral outcome, by prevention or amelioration of these secondary changes. With post-arrest control of normotension and normal blood gas values, and with general brain-orientated intensive care, renal and pulmonary derangements can be prevented, but secondary cardiovascular and cerebral changes are still present.[27]

Special cerebral resuscitation regimes that could be added to standard brain-orientated life-support (*Table* 3.3) have been studied in animals[1] and patients. The first such treatment found effective in a long-term animal model was a combination of immediate post-arrest induced arterial hypertension, haemo-dilution and heparinization, particularly when delivered by cardiopulmonary bypass.[6] The efficacy of barbiturate therapy after cardiac arrest was suggested by good results with barbiturates after incomplete ischaemia and focal ischaemia. In patients with cardiac arrest, thiopental loading proved feasible and safe, even after cardiac arrest, but overall cerebral outcome was not significantly enhanced. Therapy with a calcium entry blocker immediately after cardiac arrest or global head ischaemia appears promising. Calcium entry blockers ameliorate cerebral vasospasm. Combinations of 'blocking drugs' have been tried before, but not under controlled conditions. The most effective protective agent against anoxia, if induced before the insult, is hypothermia. Post-cardiac arrest hypothermia, however, may be beneficial or detrimental and is in need of investigation.

General brain-orientated life support has the potential to extend the reversible period of normothermic cardiac arrest from 5 min to a potential 15 min or more.[6] This calls for increasingly accurate prognosis of permanent brain damage. Neurological dysfunction at 6–12 hours post-arrest is not fully reliable. A chemical brain biopsy, consisting of CSF analysis for leaking brain enzymes, seems a reliable indicator of severity of insult and permanent brain damage after cardiac arrest, but not after focal brain lesions. Patients found in persistent vegetative state should be permitted to die.

ADVANCED TRAUMA LIFE SUPPORT

Introduction

In disasters, advanced trauma life support (ATLS) is more important than advanced cardiac life support (ACLS). Both include the same steps of resusci-tation (*Table* 3.1), but have different emphases.[1] Disaster resuscitology is based on everyday LSFA and ATLS. In major earthquakes, an estimated 10–15 per cent of those killed could have been saved with LSFA plus ATLS.

Trauma is the leading cause of death in those under 40 years of age in many industrialized countries; malnutrition, infectious diseases and trauma are the leading causes of death before old age in the Third World. Trauma is the predominant cause of death and disability from multi-casualty incidents and mass disasters. In the USA there are about 10 million disabling injuries per year, and accidents cause 150000 deaths per year. Although trauma was recognized as a major public health problem in the 1950s,[28] serious medical efforts to combat the problem on a large scale did not start until the 1960s in Europe[29] and 1970s in the USA.[3,7,30-32]

Not every trauma victim 'dead on admission to hospital' is a hopeless case.

Table 3.3. Standard brain-oriented life support guidelines for coma

A. Extracranial homeostasis

For cardiovascular-pulmonary support.

1. Control MAP and normalize blood volume with i.v. vasopressor/vasodilator and fluids. Post-anoxia plasma volume expansion (e.g. Ringer's solution, Haemaccel or Dextran 40, 10 ml/kg) optional.
   a. Induce brief mild hypertension (MAP 120–140 mmHg) for 1–5 min, desirable with restoration of spontaneous circulation (often automatic owing to epinephrine during CPR). Hypertension contraindicated after cerebral trauma.
   b. Maintain normotension (MAP 90 mmHg; systolic AP 120–130 mmHg, or normal for patient) throughout coma; accept spontaneous slight hypotension (MAP 60–90 mmHg) after cerebral trauma. If ICP monitored, keep CPP (MAP–ICP) over 50 mmHg.
   c. Insert bladder-CVP-arterial catheters; pulmonary arterial balloon catheter optional.
   d. Position head up 10–30 degrees, turn entire patient side/side every 2 hours without causing straining.
2. Immobilize with softening (not fully paralysing) doses of relaxant (e.g. pancuronium) if necessary during controlled ventilation. Maintain controlled ventilation for at least 2 hours post-arrest, longer if necessary.
3. Control (essential) or prevent (optional) restlessness, straining, seizures:
   a. Thiopental or pentobarbital 5 mg/kg/hr (aim for plasma level 2–4 mg/dl), total 30 mg/kg (more for recurrent seizures).
      or
   b. Diphenylhydantoin (Dilantin, phenytoin) 7 mg/kg i.v. bolus + 7 mg/kg/24 hr maintenance.
      or
   c. Diazepam (Valium) 5 mg/70 kg i.v. titrated as needed. For pain (when awake) narcotic by i.v. titration.
4. Maintain arterial Pco_2 at 25–35 mmHg during controlled ventilation, 20–40 mmHg during spontaneous breathing.
5. Maintain arterial pH at 7·3–7·6 (with ventilation and $NaHCO_3$ i.v. as needed).
6. Maintain arterial Po_2 over 100 mmHg, with FIO_2 90–100%; after 1–6 hours FIO_2 50%.

7. Give corticosteroid (optional):
   a. Methylprednisolone 1 mg/kg i.v. followed by 0·5 mg/kg/6 hr i.v.
      or
   b. Dexamethasone 0·2 mg/kg i.v. followed by 0·1 mg/kg/6 hr i.v.
   c. *Stop* or taper corticosteroid at 48–72 hours.
8. Blood variables—control:
   a. Haematocrit 30–35%; electrolytes normal.
   b. Plasma COP over 15 mmHg, serum albumin over 3 gm/dl.
   c. Serum osmolality 280–330 mOsm/litre.
   d. Glucose 100–300 mg/dl.
9. Maintain normothermia; avoid hyperthermia.
10. Give fluids i.v.—no dextrose in water alone.
    a. Use dextrose 5–10% in 0·25–0·5% NaCl i.v., 30–50 ml/kg/24 hr (100 ml/kg/24 hr, in infants); add potassium as needed.
    b. Give alimentation: dextrose 20%, amino acids, electrolytes, vitamins. (Start at 24–48 hours, i.v.—g.i.)

B. Intracranial Homeostasis

1. Rule out mass lesion: history, clinical picture; x-ray film; CT or NMR scan or cerebral angiogram in selected cases. Prevent straining during examination with use of partial paralysis (pancuronium).
2. Monitor ICP (only if safe technique established); optional after CPR; recommended after cerebral trauma and in encephalitis:
   a. Hollow skull screw preferred in non-traumatic coma.
   b. Ventricular catheter preferred in traumatic coma.
   c. Control ICP at or below 15 mmHg. by:
   a. Further controlled hyperventilation ($Paco_2$ to 20 mmHg) with relaxation and sedation (no coughing!).
   b. Ventricular CSF drainage.
   c. Mannitol 0·5 gm/kg i.v. plus 0·3 gm/kg/hr, i.v., short-term; or mannitol 1 gm/kg once i.v., empirical, without ICP monitoring, immediately following restoration of spontaneous circulation after cardiac arrest, and at neurological deterioration (optional).

Table 3.3. Standard brain-oriented life support guidelines for coma (*continued*)

  d. Loop diuretic i.v. (e.g. furosemide, 0·5–1·0 mg/kg i.v.)
  e. Thiopental or pentobarbital 2–5 mg/kg i.v.; repeat as needed.
  f. Corticosteroid (above).
  g. Hypothermia, 30–32°C, short-term (with controlled ventilation, relaxant, anaesthetic, vasodilator); short-term hypothermia optional; long-term hypothermia not recommended.
3. Monitor (optional).
  a. Regular EEG.
  b. Computerized EEG (cerebral function monitor).
  c. Evoked potentials (experimental).
  d. Treat EEG seizures (A-2, A-3 above).
4. Monitor neurological recovery and prognosis.
  a. Determine CSF CPK-BB at 48–72 hr.
  b. Monitor depth of coma by Glasgow Coma Score or Pittsburgh-Glasgow Coma Score.
  c. Monitor cerebral blood flow and metabolism (experimental).
5. Determine and manage outcome.
  a. Determine periodically cerebral and overall performance categories No. 1 to 5.
  b. Determine accurately and certify brain death (CPC 5), starting 6 hours after cardiac arrest. If brain death is certified, consider removing donor organs with permission and discontinue IPPV.
  c. Determine persistent vegetative state (CPC 4). If unresponsive 1–2 weeks after cardiac arrest (1 year postcerebral trauma) consider 'letting die'.

* For unconscious, critically ill, or injured patients; for use after global ischaemic-anoxic insult, modify guidelines for other causes of coma.

Instantaneous death is often the result of exsanguination from a large vessel or irreparable destruction of the brain causing apnoea. Cases of rapid exsanguination are occasionally salvageable, at least in cities within a few minutes of a trauma centre. Deaths early after injury are often due to airway obstruction, severe blood loss, or head injury. Many of these deaths are preventable by LSFA (plus ATLS) within the first 'golden hour' after injury, at the scene, during transport and in the hospital. Late deaths (days to weeks) are usually the result of sepsis or multiple organ failure following the inadequately controlled initial sequence of trauma-hypovolaemia-infection-sepsis.

Immediately following an incident, uninjured laymen or 'first responders' (e.g. police, fire-fighters, lifeguards) should apply LSFA. Making an injured person accessible for resuscitation may require a simple pull or elaborate procedures carried out by skilled rescue personnel. Immediately health professionals arrive, more advanced resuscitation and stabilization should begin, accompanied by primary and secondary surveys, the latter preferably done by a physician. The decision as to which invasive measures of ATLS the trained non-physician is permitted to apply outside or inside hospitals, varies between countries and communities.

After stabilization at the scene, the decision as to when to transport and to which hospital is a matter of judgement based on experience. There is evidence that patients with severe life-threatening trauma, particularly of head, chest, abdomen, pelvis or femur, or with polytrauma, should have the airway and ventilation controlled at the scene and then be rushed to the closest major trauma centre, with on-going life support. Prolonged efforts at stabilization in the field, as recommended for cardiac emergencies, are *not* recommended for cases of trauma, as uncontrollable internal haemorrhage may continue to exsanguination and absence of pulse before the facilities and teams necessary for resuscitative surgery are reached. The decision on whether a trauma victim should be transferred to a special trauma centre can be aided by rapid assessment in the field, using a primary survey, a secondary survey, assessment of consciousness with a coma scale[33] and determination of a trauma scale.[34] (*See* *Table* 3.4 on p. 76 and Chapter 2.)

After initial assessment, the paramedic or physician at the scene should speak directly to the physician in the trauma centre which is to receive the patient. A record of relevant individual data, injury mechanism, general history if available, vital signs and emergency management and stabilization, should accompany the patient if possible. Transfer from scene to trauma centre or from primary hospital to trauma centre should be with full life support, controlled by a physician experienced in traumatology, or by paramedics or nurses guided by a physician via radio or standing orders.

The *primary survey* (*Table* 3.2) is the initial assessment accompanied by LSFA of the airway, breathing and circulation. (*See also* Chapter 2.) The patient should be undressed, and disabilities which may indicate neurological or bony injury noted. Assume cervical spine injury in any patient with injury above the clavicle. Airway control in maxillofacial trauma may be difficult and must be improvised. Patients with maxillofacial trauma and head trauma are also cervical spinal cord injury suspects. The absence of neurological deficit does not rule out cervical spine injury. It should be presumed until ruled out by X-ray examination.

Hypovolaemic shock is recognized by palpation of the pulse, and noting skin colour, capillary refill and blood pressure. If the radial pulse is faint or absent and the femoral or carotid pulse palpable, the systolic blood pressure will probably be 60–70 mmHg. External bleeding should be controlled by pressure, pneumatic splints (or leg portion of a MAST suit), or (rarely) a tourniquet. Internal bleeding in the chest or abdomen or around major fractures or penetrating injuries, requires surgical control in an operating room; transportation to such a facility should not be delayed. For major external or internal bleeding below the diaphragm, with signs of shock, many emergency physicians favour early application of the MAST[35] in the field or during transportation. During transportation, large bore i.v. infusions should be started with salt or colloid solution. Most traumatic shock is due to hypovolaemia. Blood should be drawn for cross-matching later. Salt solution i.v. in the field may be followed by a colloid solution and then by blood or red blood cells to keep the haematocrit above 20 per cent. Traumatic hypovolaemic shock is not to be treated with drugs. A vasopressor is only justified transiently to sustain a pulse when cardiac arrest is threatened due to exsanguination, while the lost blood volume is replaced.

A nasogastric tube should be inserted in the severely traumatized, stuporous or comatose patient, unless a basal skull fracture is suspected. A urinary catheter should be inserted unless urethral transection is suspected. ECG monitoring should be used if available.

The *secondary survey* (*Table* 3.2) should be conducted by a physician, if one is available. (*See also* Chapter 2.) It starts with detailed examination of the head (eyes, pupils, fundi, lens, penetrating injuries, face, skull), and continues with examination of face, cervical spine and neck, with continuous support of head, neck and chest. A sports helmet should be removed with great care if cervical injury is suspected and, in the absence of other vital factors, may be left in place until an X-ray is taken. Then follow examination of chest, abdomen, rectum (sphincter tone, blood), extremities (wounds, fractures) and the neurological picture. Neurological examination during the secondary survey includes repeated assessment of the level of consciousness, pupils, and, in the conscious victim, motor and sensory function; in unresponsive patients, coma scoring is performed. Until ruled out, any severe injury calls for immobilization on a long spine board, with cervical collar, sand bags and tape to prevent head-neck motion. In suspected intracranial haemorrhage, rapid transfer to an appropriate facility is essential. Suspicion of intracranial haemorrhage and drainage of epidural or subdural haematoma by the closest competent surgeon, within 1 hour of injury, are crucial. The secondary survey ends with appropriate X-rays, laboratory tests, special studies and surgery.

Primary and secondary surveys must be accompanied by control of external haemorrhage and steps A, B and C of resuscitation, and follow general principles of wound care. These include prevention of contamination by the application of sterile dressings in the field; thorough cleaning, removal of devitalized tissue and foreign bodies in the ATLS facility or hospital; and tetanus prophylaxis.[3] Most patients will have had 2 or more prior injections of tetanus toxoid. They should be given 0·5 ml of 'absorbed toxoid' for both tetanus-prone and non-tetanus-prone wounds. No passive immunization is needed. Patients without previous toxoid and non-tetanus-prone wounds should receive 0·5 ml of toxoid, but in the case of tetanus-prone wounds 0·5 ml of toxoid, plus human tetanus immunoglobulin (250 units) and antibiotics. Tetanus antitoxin prepared from horse serum should not be used. It is assumed that increasingly more people will have had 4 injections of diphtheria-pertussis-tetanus immunization in early childhood, a 5th dose at 4–6 years of age and a booster every 10 years; a previously non-immunized adult will have had 3 injections of toxoid and a booster every 10 years.

Open-Chest CPR[1]

Before the 1960s, open-chest cardiac compression was widely used in hospitals, with good results. It is now a forgotten art, but it should be revived to be taught in training programmes for physicians and for wider use in hospitals. It produces significantly better perfusion pressures and blood flows than closed-chest compression, since direct heart massage (in contrast to chest compressions) does not increase venous pressures and, if prolonged, provides a better chance to restart the heart and for the brain to recover. Other advantages are the ability to feel and visualize the heart, to inject cardiac drugs directly into the heart, and to recognize and treat intrathoracic pathology, such as haemorrhage. It also gives access to a pulmonary embolus.

Physicians treating trauma victims should consider an early switch from the closed-chest to the open-chest CPR technique in circumstances for which it may be the only effective method of restoring life. These include suspected intrathoracic pathology, such as tension pneumothorax or haemorrhage, and and inability to produce a palpable femoral or carotid pulse with chest

a

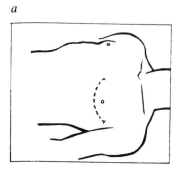

b

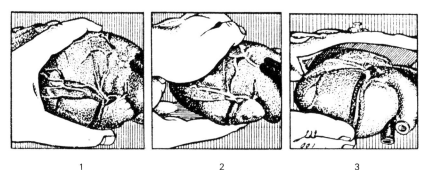

1   2   3

c

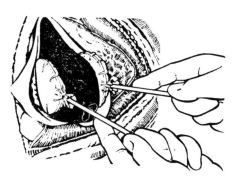

Fig. 3.5. Open-chest cardiopulmonary resuscitation. *a*, Open the chest through the 4th or 5th left intercostal space. Grasp and rhythmically compress the heart. *b*, Hand positions for open-chest CPR. Operator stands on patient's left side facing cephalad. After thoracotomy, insert left hand and pump heart (first without opening pericardium) either with thumb posteriorly over left ventricle and fingers anteriorly over right ventricle (1); or with two hands, using palm of left hand over right ventricle and fingers 2–5 of right hand over left ventricle posteriorly (2); or using fingers 2–5 of right hand posteriorly over left ventricle compressing the heart against the sternum upward (3). Methods shown in (2) and (3) give better blood flow and are less fatiguing and less traumatic than methods shown in (1). *c*, Internal direct electric defibrillation. When fibrillation is felt, apply the electrodes and counter-shock, first with the pericardium closed. (If possible, have electrodes prepared with tied-on, saline-soaked gauze). Apply the internal electrodes as illustrated, wearing rubber gloves, and release the shock. Use shocks of about 0·2–0·5 J/kg body weight.

(Reproduced from Safar and Bircher, op. cit. with permission of authors and publishers.)

compressions, as is occasionally the case with chest injury, chest or spine deformities. In addition, it is indicated in intractable ventricular fibrillation or mechanical asystole, as may occur in hypothermia.

The technique of open-chest cardiac compression is as follows (*Fig.* 3.5): cut through skin and muscles under the left breast over approximately the fourth intercostal space; pierce the intercostal space open with a blunt instrument or your fingers; insert a rib spreader when available; compress the heart immediately before opening the pericardium by placing the fingers of one hand behind the heart and the thenar eminence and thumb in front of the heart; use a wringing action with 80–100 compressions per minute; take care not to pierce the atrium with the thumb; compress large hearts with one hand behind and one hand in front of the heart; if the heart feels empty, speed up intravenous fluids and compress the descending aorta during massage.

When ventricular fibrillation is felt or seen on the ECG, defibrillate using two paddle electrodes placed directly on the heart (with saline-soaked pads if immediately available)—one behind the left ventricle, the other over the anterior surface of the heart. Start with 0·5 J/kg body weight. High energy shocks applied directly to the heart can cause thermal damage. In intractable ventricular fibrillation or when intra-cardiac drugs are needed, open the pericardium. Inject epinephrine into the cavity of the left ventricle. Do not give norepinephrine or sodium bicarbonate via the intra-cardiac route.

In suspected cardiac tamponade, if time permits and the patient still has a pulse, rapid drainage of the pericardial sac by needle puncture may obviate the need for thoracotomy.

Circulatory Shock[4,38,49]

Shock is a low flow state with a 'clinical picture of overall tissue perfusion inadequate to meet tissue needs'. Shock, if not reversed in time, may lead to lethal multiple organ failure due to hypoperfusion. Vital organs may become irreversibly damaged before circulation ceases entirely.

Shock states may be classified as follows:
1. Hypovolaemia (oligaemia).
2. Cardiac pump failure (cardiogenic shock).
3. Total blood flow obstruction (pulmonary embolism, cardiac tamponade).
4. Altered blood flow distribution (septicaemia, intoxication, sympathetic paralysis).

Traumatic shock may consist of a sequence of 3 insults: (*a*) tissue injury; (*b*) hypovolaemic shock; and (*c*) sepsis. With prompt treatment of (*a*) and (*b*), (*c*) can often be prevented.

In shock states, there is usually time for compensatory mechanisms to come into play. These may give short-term protection through cerebral and coronary vasodilation and vasoconstriction in other vascular beds, producing ischaemia of skin, muscles, kidneys and the hepato-gastrointestinal system. In spite of these mechanisms, however, the brain may suffer permanent damage if the mean arterial pressure drops below about 30–40 mmHg for prolonged periods, particularly if accompanied by low arterial Po_2. Shock states predispose the sick heart to ventricular fibrillation or asystole, which can be triggered by minor interventions, such as transportation or airway suction.

In the treatment of shock from crushing injuries, which includes myoglobinuria, deliberate fluid overloading has been effective in increasing urine flow and restoring oxygen transport.[12]

While hyperglycaemia at the time of cardiac arrest worsens cerebral acidosis and seems to worsen outcome, optimal post-cardiac arrest blood glucose levels have not been determined. In the treatment of the incomplete ischaemia of shock, however, induced hyperglycaemia might be beneficial.

Haemodilution[36,37]

Adequate concurrent treatment of acute haemorrhage with plasma substitutes (Ringer's solution, dextran, hydroxyethyl starch, polygelatin, albumin) is essential in the absence of blood and leads to acute normovolaemic haemodilution. Four sequential phases of response during haemodilution without hypovolaemic shock have been demonstrated.[37]

1. Complete compensation of arterial oxygen transport through an increase in cardiac output down to a haemoglobin of approximately 5·5 g/dl (about 20 per cent haematocrit).
2. Partial compensation with a haemoglobin of 4–5·5 g/dl (about 15 per cent haematocrit).
3. Reversible decompensation with a haemoglobin of 3–4 g/dl (about 10–15 per cent haematocrit); at this point, cardiac output declines from its peak, heart failure occurs, and blood lactate increases. Animals can survive without requiring blood transfusion if haemodilution is with colloid, but not if it is with Ringer's solution.
4. Irreversible decompensation with a haemoglobin below approximately 3 g/dl (10 per cent haematocrit) breathing air or below about 2 g/dl (6 per cent haematocrit) breathing 100 per cent oxygen. A dramatic decrease in cardiac output, oxygen consumption and venous oxygen values is followed by cardiac arrest in asystole.

Patients with oligaemia or cardiopulmonary disease may decompensate earlier. Monitoring may include central *or* mixed venous Po_2 and base deficit. When the mixed venous Po_2 reaches 30–35 mmHg, metabolism in vital organs can be assumed to become anaerobic, and there is consequently a need to increase the arterial oxygen-carrying capacity by infusion of blood or red blood cells. In most patients treated for blood loss with normovolaemic (or hypervolaemic) haemodilution, it is wise not to let the haematocrit fall below 30 per cent. The widely accepted sequence of action is: Ringer's solution or isotonic NaCl (up to about 10 ml/kg × 4) followed by a colloid plasma substitute (1:1 blood volume lost) accompanied or followed by red cells or whole blood to prevent a drop of haematocrit to below 25–30 per cent.

Fluid Resuscitation[36–38]

For fluid resuscitation the largest possible cannula should be inserted, in order of preference, in: arm vein—external jugular—subclavian—right internal jugular—femoral vein. In some cases, a venous cutdown is required. Each trauma hospital should have available rapid infusion devices with blood warmers. Those with roller or pressure pumps are particularly effective, permitting infusion of 1–10 l/min.[39]

During CPR and during treatment of shock, fluid loading is required. Even a cardiac arrest without blood loss is followed by vasodilation and capillary leakage. An initial intravenous load of 10 ml/kg of a plasma substitute such as Ringer's solution is indicated.

The choice of i.v. fluid for resuscitation from hypovolaemia remains controversial.[1,3] Nonetheless, it is clear that replacing all blood loss with blood is neither sound nor necessary. Bank blood can transmit hepatitis and acquired immune deficiency syndrome (AIDS), and can cause haemolytic reactions as a result of incompatability, although modern blood banking techniques minimize these risks. Moreover, typing and cross-matching delays availability of blood. Fresh, type-specific cross-matched whole blood would be ideal, but usually is not immediately available and would be expensive. Stored, bank blood is also expensive, and entails additional risks, particularly in massive transfusions.[40] These risks include hypothermia,[40] deficiency of clotting factors, high potassium ion concentration, low pH, and microemboli. In general, safe blood and blood product services are expensive and may not be available in all regions of the world. Thus, the first line of therapy in blood loss and for blood volume expansion is a plasma substitute without red blood cells.

In moderate haemorrhage (not exceeding about 20 per cent of blood volume loss) electrolyte solutions alone, such as isotonic sodium chloride (0·9 per cent) or Ringer's solution, are adequate to maintain blood volume and homeostasis temporarily. If an electrolyte solution alone is used, it should be given in a volume 3–4 times the blood volume lost, as it equilibrates throughout the extracellular space. More must be added to compensate for urine output. Thus, the plasma volume supporting effect of salt solutions in severe blood loss is either brief or depends on the creation of interstitial oedema, before intravascular volume can be maintained. Although pulmonary oedema is rapidly cleared from healthy lungs, particularly during IPPV, some studies suggest that the use of salt solutions instead of colloid contributes to pulmonary oedema and consolidation after traumatic shock. Lactated Ringer's solution with its many physiological ions, and balanced salt solutions with normal pH, are theoretically more physiological than 'physiological' (0·9 per cent) sodium chloride solution. The latter, however, is cheaper and equally effective in treating acute moderate extracellular fluid loss.

Hypertonic sodium chloride solution (4–6 per cent) attracts interstitial fluid into the intravascular space. It is being investigated for emergency treatment of hypovolaemia under military field conditions. Small volumes (e.g. 250 ml) have been effective in animal experiments in preventing cardiac arrest from an otherwise lethal haemorrhage. The volume effect is brief, unless 4–6 per cent saline is combined with a colloid, such as dextran or polygelatin. This may help in keeping the injured alive until they can receive full fluid resuscitation and be transported to a surgical facility. The possible risks of hypertonic saline (e.g. effects on blood cells and endothelium) remain to be investigated.

In severe haemorrhage (over 30 per cent of blood volume loss) the use of electrolyte solutions alone is unphysiological, as it produces tissue oedema if enough is given to maintain plasma volume. Indeed, salt solutions alone under such circumstances may be incapable of maintaining blood volume, cardiac output, arterial pressure, and tissue oxygenation, even in 3–4 times replacement volumes; while colloid plasma substitutes in a one to one ratio of replacement to volume lost, are effective. The choice of a specific colloid solution is controversial. The normal colloid osmotic pressure of 25 mmHg is maintained primarily by a serum albumin concentration of 5 gm/dl. A reduction of serum albumin concentration to half of normal reduces colloid osmotic pressure by two-thirds, at which level tissue oedema tends to develop.

The controversy about electrolyte vs. colloid plasma substitutes is unresolved because both seem to be needed. In normovolaemic haemodilution (blood volume replaced while being lost) without a shock state, colloid in the same volume as that lost is superior to Ringer's solution at three times that lost.[37,38] In shock with capillary leakage, there may be no difference, or colloid may even be worse. In the treatment of established hypovolaemic shock, electrolyte solution in addition to blood is needed because of 'sequestration' of body fluids in extravascular interstitial and intracellular compartments.

The ideal colloid plasma substitutes are human serum albumin, 5 per cent, in isotonic saline, or commercial plasma protein fractions which contain mainly albumin plus a small amount of globulins. They are very expensive and often unnecessary, since serum albumin and globulin levels are fairly rapidly restored from body pools. Therefore, dextrans, gelatin, starch solutions, or other adequately tested synthetic colloids are also recommended. These products are inexpensive and suitable for long-term storage, and they support survival as well as albumin, and better than salt solutions. Dextran 70, 6 per cent in isotonic saline, has a 30 per cent intravascular retention after 24 hours; Dextran 40, 10 per cent in isotonic saline, has a shorter retention time, but reduces sedimentation rate and may have a more potent antisludging effect.[41] Dextran 40 should, however, be given only after urine flow has been restarted with electrolyte solution, since it tends to plug renal tubules. Hydroxyethyl starch, 6 per cent in isotonic saline, has characteristics similar to Dextran 70. All plasma substitutes and electrolyte and colloid solutions produce hypo-coagulability by diluting the clotting factors. Dextrans and starches (particularly Dextran 40), in addition, coat platelets, thus adding further to the anticoagulant effect. This is good for the microcirculation and bad in cases of trauma with incomplete haemostasis. Although synthetic colloids have caused anaphylactic reactions, such reactions are rare and unimportant for emergency resuscitation. For dextrans, haptenes are available for optional prevention of allergic reactions. The dextrans may interfere with typing and cross-matching of blood (therefore, draw blood first), unless a cell washing laboratory technique is used. Hypertonic glucose was found beneficial in shock states. It needs re-evaluation, since hyperglycaemia at the onset of experimental ischaemia worsens brain damage.

Polygelatins have proved eminently satisfactory in clinical practice, particularly in the UK and Europe. They have no direct effect on clotting factors, satisfactory intravascular retention (6–8 h half-life) and a low index of allergic reactions. They do not interfere with blood-typing and cross-matching.

Plasma pooled from multiple donors may transmit hepatitis. Pasteurized plasma preparations (e.g. 5 per cent plasma protein fraction) are safe, except when occasionally found to contain vasodilator substances. Fresh frozen plasma or cryoprecipitate is indicated in certain haemorrhagic diatheses.

For severe ongoing haemorrhage, warmed fresh whole blood, type specific and cross-matched, would be the ideal resuscitation fluid, but is not immediately available. Banked whole blood or banked packed red blood cells should be used to sustain the haematocrit at or above 30 per cent. In the absence of haematocrit determinations, whole blood or red cells should be added to plasma substitutes, when estimated blood loss reaches and exceeds 30 per cent of blood volume, or if the patient was anaemic prior to haemorrhage. The preservative-anticoagulant citric-acid-phosphate-dextrose (CPD) and saline adenine glucose-mannitol (SAG-M) have replaced citric-acid-citrate-dextrose (ACD).

During massive infusions of banked blood or red cells, calcium administration is usually not needed, but blood should be warmed to near body temperature during transfusion. Sodium bicarbonate may be given to correct a large measured base deficit. To prevent coagulation problems, it has been suggested that fresh frozen plasma (250 ml/70 kg) be added to every 1500 ml/70 kg of stored blood infused.

Packed red blood cell solutions, because of their high haematocrit, need dilution with isotonic saline solution added to the bag or infused simultaneously, to enhance flow rate in the infusion for haemorrhage. Undiluted packed red cells are recommended in anaemia associated with heart failure or hypertension.

Artificial red cells with haemoglobin encapsulated in liposomes are currently being assessed in animals, and may prove suitable for human use.[42]

The physician charged with responsibility for resuscitation should be familiar with coagulation problems caused by protracted shock states and massive blood transfusion. He should be conversant with simple clotting tests available for bedside use (e.g. clotting time at 37°C in glass tube, clot retraction and clot lysis), and with the indications for certain blood components and heparin. Such techniques are beyond the scope of this chapter.

Oxygen carrying blood substitutes, such as stroma-free haemoglobin,[43] and fluorocarbons, have been under laboratory and clinical investigation in recent years. In 1988, neither stroma-free haemoglobin nor Fluosol appears ready for widespread clinical use, as available preparations have not yet been perfected. Improvements may influence the treatment of massive blood loss in the future. Stroma-free haemoglobin is rapidly lost from the circulation and causes pulmonary hypertension and other complications attributed to the impurity of the haemoglobin preparation. A polymerized version (Biotest) showed good retention, blood pressure support and oxygen carrying capability in a haemorrhagic shock monkey model. Stroma-free haemoglobin is more promising than fluorocarbons, which have no advantage over plasma substitutes in subjects breathing air. The fluorocarbon solution (Fluosol DA 20 per cent) that has been under clinical trials, requires inhalation of 100 per cent oxygen and carries less oxygen at Po_2 600 mmHg (8 ml O_2/dl Fluosol), than haemoglobin at Po_2 100 mmHg with 15 g haemoglobin (20 ml O_2/dl blood). Fluosol, however, carries more oxygen than other plasma substitutes (0·3 ml O_2/dl per 100 mmHg). The latter, however, promote blood flow better as they have a lower viscosity. Fluorocarbons may have carcinogenic effects on tissues in which they accumulate.

Emergency resuscitation for hypovolaemic shock is required not only in cases of trauma, haemorrhage, and burns, but also in cases of severe diarrhoea (e.g. cholera). In the out-of-hospital treatment of mass outbreaks of diarrhoeal disease or of traumatic shock in conscious victims of mass disasters, when i.v. fluid administration is not possible, oral fluids have a place in the treatment of mild to moderate hypovolaemic shock. Commercially available oral replacement powders, when diluted as recommended, yield isotonic or one-half isotonic Ringer's solution plus carbohydrates (e.g. 5 per cent dextrose), vitamins, amino acids, and flavouring to give them an acceptable taste. The Red Cross recommends adding 1 teaspoon of sodium bicarbonate to each litre of water to be taken by mouth. Fluids should not be given by mouth when the patient is stuporous or comatose, because of risk of aspiration, or when an operation may be needed.

The most appropriate treatment strategy for blood volume or plasma volume loss is to start with (lactated) Ringer's solution up to about 4000 ml/70 kg body weight (4 × replacement of 20 per cent blood loss). This is followed by a colloid plasma substitute (1 × additional blood volume lost). Packed red blood cells or whole blood are used to restore and maintain haematocrit at about 30 per cent. Haemorrhagic diatheses are best treated with fresh frozen plasma and fresh whole blood.

SPECIAL CONSIDERATIONS

Alveolar Anoxia[4]

Alveolar *anoxia* is relatively rare. Examples occur in patients who have inhaled anoxic gas (e.g. laboratory, industrial, mining or anaesthetic accidents), or who have suffered rapid decompression (in high altitude flying). A sudden switch from breathing air or oxygen to breathing oxygen-free inert gas results in spontaneous hyperventilation, and within 1 minute, in coma (perhaps with convulsions), hypotension, bradycardia, and pupillary dilatation. Within 3–7 minutes, cardiac arrest develops in asystole. Clinical death, after up to about 5 minutes, is completely reversible with CPR.

Alveolar *hypoxia* is common, as in exposure to high altitude or inhalation of gas mixtures of reduced oxygen concentration. Alveolar hypoxia kills by the same mechanism as hypoxia from pulmonary disease. At an arterial Po_2 of 30 mmHg, the cerebral vessels are maximally dilated and a further decrease in Pao_2 leads to cerebral anaerobiosis. Cardiac arrest may occur at a Pao_2 of 15–25 mmHg, in fit persons, and at a higher level in sick people.

Carbon Monoxide Poisoning[44]

Carbon monoxide (CO), an inert odourless gas, is probably not a cellular poison per se; by virtue of its affinity for haemoglobin, however, it produces acute normovolaemic 'anaemic' hypoxia. Haemoglobin binds CO about 200 to 300 times more readily than it binds oxygen; the carboxyhaemoglobin produced is subsequently not available for oxygen transport. In CO poisoning there is a normal arterial Po_2 with a low available O_2 content. CO poisoning may occur with exposure to products of combustion in closed spaces (e.g. fires, explosions, automobile exhaust, industry).

As little as $0 \cdot 2$ per cent CO inhaled will form CO haemoglobin at a rate of 1 per cent/min. If the patient is doing heavy work, this rate will increase to $2 \cdot 4$ per cent/min, and within about 45 minutes CO will saturate 76 per cent of the haemoglobin, a lethal concentration. Conscious dogs inhaling 1 per cent CO reach 80 per cent CO haemoglobin saturation almost instantaneously, and death is sudden. There is no hyperventilation, since the chemoreceptors are sensitive to a decrease in arterial P_{O_2}, not O_2 content, and no compensatory increase in cardiac output, since viscosity (haematocrit) is unchanged. CO shifts the oxyhaemoglobin dissociation curve to the left. Respiratory enzymes have a greater affinity for CO than for oxygen.

Irreversible cerebral damage apparently occurs before cardiac arrest. Hypotension seems to be a more crucial parameter in determining the outcome for the brain than the percentage of CO haemoglobin and duration of exposure. The organism tolerates normovolaemic haemodilution better than CO poisoning.

Humans breathing low concentrations of CO develop a sequence of headache, vertigo, yawning, dimmed vision, tachycardia and vomiting. Higher concentrations or longer exposure result in coma, twitching, collapse, pupillary dilatation, Cheyne-Stokes respirations, apnoea and cardiac arrest (asystole). The skin is warm; a cherry-red colour of the skin, while pathognomonic of CO poisoning, is seen only rarely. The treatment includes IPPV with 100 per cent oxygen and CPR when indicated. Inhalation of CO_2 has not proved valuable; hyperbaric oxygenation has, but is rarely available early enough to influence the outcome. After exposure to CO, coma extending more than 30–60 min during 100 per cent O_2 breathing is indicative of hypoxic encephalopathy. Cerebral resuscitation measures may be worth trying (e.g. early calcium entry blocker, hypertension, hypothermia).

Asphyxia[4]

Asphyxia is a combination of a reduced arterial P_{O_2} and an increased arterial P_{CO_2} due to a reduction in alveolar ventilation (minute volume minus deadspace minute ventilation). The extremes of hypoventilation are complete airway obstruction and apnoea, and these comprise the two principal causes of asphyxia.

Causes of upper airway obstruction include trauma with soft-tissue obstruction or inhalation of blood, inflammatory swelling of tissues and food bolus obstruction. Laryngospasm may result in hypoxia-induced apnoea, but usually the larynx relaxes just before cardiac arrest occurs. Foreign matter may trigger reflex laryngospasm. If started prior to cardiac arrest, skilfully applied positive pressure artificial ventilation can usually revive the patient, even if the foreign matter was not removed.

Partial airway obstruction, as in bronchospasm, first stimulates increased respiratory efforts. When the patient becomes exhausted or the obstruction worsens, asphyxia develops, with rapidly progressive hypoxaemia and hypercarbia leading to secondary apnoea and cardiac arrest.

Complete airway obstruction results in increased breathing efforts (exaggerated intrathoracic pressure fluctuations causing intercostal and suprasternal retractions) and sympathetic discharge (arterial hypertension and tachycardia). This leads to unconsciousness within about 2 min, when the P_{aO_2} reaches about 30 mmHg (arterial oxygen saturation 50 per cent). Apnoea occurs after

2–6 min, and absence of pulse (asystole) at 5–10 min. Hypoxia and acidosis combine to cause circulatory failure.

Sudden apnoea without airway obstruction, in an air-breathing patient, results in a similar course toward asphyxial cardiac arrest, but events proceed at a somewhat slower pace than in complete airway obstruction, because in apnoea the absence of struggling means a lower oxygen consumption during the dying process. Sudden apnoea may occur as a result of a high-energy electric shock; the intravenous injection of a paralysing dose of a muscle relaxant; sudden severe increase in intracranial pressure with brain herniation; and large doses of anaesthetics, narcotics or hypnotics.

Hypercarbia without hypoxaemia can be produced by inhalation of an oxygen-enriched atmosphere prior to hypoventilation or apnoea (apnoeic diffusion oxygenation). The rate of $Paco_2$ rise in apnoea is about 5 mmHg/min. Preventilation and complete denitrogenation with 100 per cent oxygen can initially produce a $Paco_2$ of over 600 mmHg while sustaining the Pao_2 above 75 mmHg for 20–30 min during apnoea, provided the oxygen-filled alveoli and airways remain connected to an oxygen reservoir without other gases. Apnoeic diffusion oxygenation is a principle applied in prophylactic oxygen inhalation for patients whose respiratory movements or airway patency are at risk (e.g. convulsive states).

Exsanguination Cardiac Arrest [3,4]

Exsanguination usually leads to an agonal state (no pulse, gasping) and, after loss of more than 50 per cent of blood volume, to clinical death in asystole. Resuscitative efforts may subsequently produce ventricular fibrillation (VF).

Resuscitation from exsanguination consists of the *simultaneous* application of the following:

1. Ventilation with oxygen if available.
2. External cardiac compressions.
3. Control of haemorrhage—by external compression of the bleeding sites, tourniquet, shock trousers (MAST), laparotomy, or thoracotomy.
4. Massive i.v. infusions, through large-bore cannulae of the most immediately available plasma substitute, from a rapid infusion system[39] ready in emergency room or operating room.
5. Epinephrine (1 mg) and sodium bicarbonate (1 mmol/kg) i.v., added to the plasma substitute (4, above).
6. ECG monitoring; if ventricular fibrillation or ventricular tachycardia occurs, apply external defibrillation.
7. Open-chest CPR with haemeostasis if 1–5 above not immediately effective or if intrathoracic haemorrhage is suspected.

Rapid exsanguination leaves 40–50 per cent of total red cell mass in the body. Continued blood loss, accompanied by further wash-out of haemoglobin with plasma substitutes, however, may reduce haematocrit below 20 per cent. If this is the case, typed and cross-matched blood, immediately available, should be used in conjunction with plasma substitutes. After restoration of spontaneous circulation and control of haemorrhage, a haematocrit of about 30 per cent should be restored eventually and clotting factors replaced as needed.

Intra-abdominal haemorrhage should be treated, to prevent cardiac arrest, with application of a MAST suit. The suit should stay inflated at 100 mmHg until the team is ready for laparotomy and massive infusion. In case of cardiac arrest, left thoracotomy and clamping of the lower thoracic aorta can stop the haemorrhage before deflation of the pressure suit.

Hypothermia[14,15,45,46]

Man is homeothermic through a delicate mechanism that maintains core body temperature near 37°C.[4] The hypothalamic temperature-regulating centre controls the required balance of heat production (primarily from muscular work and hepatic metabolism) and heat retention or elimination (primarily through cutaneous vasoconstriction and vasodilatation, sweating and pulmonary ventilation).

By reducing the consumption of oxygen, hypothermia protects vital organs during apnoea and circulatory arrest. However, hypothermia can itself cause cardiac arrest in man when the heart temperature reaches about 22–28°C. Healthy, unmedicated humans, exposed to low environmental temperatures without protection, fight the cold with cutaneous vasoconstriction, shivering and catecholamine release, which result in a transient increase in oxygen consumption, heart rate, arterial pressure and cardiac irritability. The latter can cause cardiac arrest in patients with heart disease even before core temperature decreases. With persisting exposure, the defence mechanism finally becomes depressed and the body core temperature decreases. When core temperature falls to 30–33°C, a further decrease in temperature will usually be unopposed by shivering and vasoconstriction. CNS depressant and vasodilating drugs (including alcohol) and muscle relaxants foster a more rapid downward drift in core temperature in a cold environment. The decline in body temperature is accompanied by a decline in total and cerebral oxygen consumption, cardiac output, cerebral blood flow, microcirculation (hence, increased blood sludging and viscosity), arterial pressure, heart rate, respiratory minute volume, and electrical activity of the brain. While hypothermia endangers the myocardium, it protects the brain, through reduction in brain metabolism and acidosis and preservation of cerebral enzyme and membrane functions.

Oxygen consumption falls to about 50 per cent of normal at a core temperature of 30°C and to 15 per cent of normal at 20°C, at which point the EEG is isoelectric. Core temperatures below about 22–28°C stop the human heart in asystole or ventricular fibrillation. Restoration of a spontaneous circulation, including defibrillation, may be difficult unless the heart temperature is rapidly increased during cardiac compressions; this may require thoracotomy and direct rewarming of the heart, or extracorporeal circulation with a heat exchanger. During rewarming, VF may occur, triggered by shivering with increased oxygen consumption, uncontrolled acidaemia, mechanical stimulation of the heart by CPR, or other factors. To prevent this, rewarming under spontaneous circulation should be slow, with control of shivering by drugs, blood gas and pH. Rewarming methods during resuscitation include, in order of increasing effectiveness, surface warming, warming of inhaled gas, warm i.v. fluids, warm gastric or peritoneal lavage, and venoarterial pumping via an oxygenator and heat exchanger (emergency cardiopulmonary bypass).

The basic pathophysiological differences in hypothermic states encountered in clinical medicine are:

1. Induced hypothermia during *surgery* for elective cardiac arrest or temporary vessel occlusion for surgical operations, preceded by normal circulation and oxygenation. This permits complete cerebral recovery after circulatory arrest of up to about 30 min at 30°C, 60 min at 20°C or 90 min at 15°C, but requires extracorporeal cooling and warming by cardiopulmonary bypass.

2. Accidental hypothermia from *exposure*, without submersion, without asphyxia. This results in cardiac arrest at 25–28°C, and in further cooling; there are anecdotal reports of complete recovery when bodies with a 10–15°C core temperature were rewarmed and ventilated after apparent clinical death of several hours. In the presence of a spontaneous (possibly very slow) pulse, slow rewarming should be accompanied by gentle artificial ventilation, but *no* chest (heart) compressions, as the latter can induce ventricular fibrillation. If there is no pulse, the patient should be transported, with on-going external CPR and slow rewarming (which is controversial), to a facility where controlled external and pulmonary warming, thoracotomy for intrathoracic warming, and extracorporeal circulation are available to raise the core temperature to the 28–30°C required for defibrillation and restoration of spontaneous normotension. Warming from 30°C to 36°C should be slow. Undocumented reports from Russia and Germany suggest benefit from rapid immersion warming to 37°C.

3. Cold water *drowning* results in cooling during asphyxiation.[15] Cardiac arrest can occur without water in the lungs (associated with laryngospasm or air lock), with fresh water in the lungs (which may be absorbed), or with seawater in the lungs (which causes severe lung damage) (*see* Chapter 26). Cardiac arrest in cold water drowning is less easily reversible than exposure hypothermia, because of tissue acidosis and anoxia at the time of hypothermic cardiac arrest, but recovery of humans after up to 40 min of ice water submersion has been reported.[15]

In maritime disasters in icy waters, many victims with lifejackets may be immersed without submersion of the face, without drowning. In ordinary clothes, they can cool within 2–5 min to apnoea and cardiac arrest!

Hyperthermia[47]

Emergencies arising from increased body temperature vary from benign electrolyte imbalance to rapidly lethal derangements of several organ systems (*see* Chapter 18). These reflect both normal (but exaggerated) and defective responses to increased temperature. Each year in the United States, 4000 to 9000 persons die from hyperthermia-related crises, such as heat stroke and febrile convulsions.

Usually most marked in the muscles of the legs and abdomen, *heat cramps* are relatively benign sequelae of electrolyte loss through sweating.

Heat exhaustion is a form of hypovolaemic shock caused by the body's exaggerated response to high environmental temperatures; massive fluid loss through sweating leads to peripheral vasomotor collapse. The patient has a pale, cold, clammy skin, wide pupils, arterial hypotension, tachycardia and an increased core temperature. Nausea and vomiting frequently accompany this syndrome and further exacerbate hypovolaemia. Emergency treatment is aimed at restoring vascular volume, providing a cool environment, positioning the patient supine with legs raised, and infusing isotonic saline or Ringer's solution.

Heat stroke (heat pyrexia)[47] represents a failure of heat regulation through sweating. The pathogenesis of heat stroke is usually a combination of external heat, severe exercise, dehydration and (viral) infection. The patient has a flushed, hot, dry skin. Cardiac output, arterial pressure, heart rate, minute volume of breathing and core temperature are all increased. Blood glucose levels may be very low. The cerebral cortex can suffer irreversible heat damage, especially at temperatures of about 40°C or above. The insult to the brain depends on the duration and degree of hyperthermia above 40°C, as well as on the adequacy of Pao_2, cardiac output and blood glucose. Treatment consists of rapid cooling; ventilation with oxygen; intensive therapy for shock, respiratory failure, and brain failure; and CPR when appropriate, which can restore spontaneous circulation. Cooling should be cautiously carried to the point of normothermia—using external means, cold i.v. and rectal fluids, and perhaps extracorporeal circulation with a heat exchanger. A core temperature of about 42°C or higher results in an irreversible shock state resembling the clinical picture of a combination of hypovolaemic, cardiogenic and septic shock, in spite of correction of blood glucose, temperature and other monitored variables.

Electric Shock[2,4,48]

In electric shock several special considerations apply. Household alternating current (110 V in the USA, 220 V in Europe) may cause ventricular fibrillation. High voltage current passing through the heart causes a contraction only as long as the current flows, and passing through the brain can cause apnoea. Apnoea leads to secondary asphyxial cardiac arrest which may be reversed by CPR without the need for defibrillation. In addition, electric shock can cause tissue burns.

The likelihood of electric current producing ventricular fibrillation depends on the intensity of the current, its frequency of oscillations, its path (whether or not the heart is included), and the duration of contact. Direct current is more injurious than alternating current of the same voltage, as d.c. produces electrolytic tissue damage and burns. Chances of recovery are best when neither brain nor heart lies directly in the path of the current.

Household voltage of 110 or 200 V a.c. (50–60 Hz), when it traverses the human heart from hand to foot, usually results in ventricular fibrillation. In hospitalized patients, even very low currents have killed due to improperly earthed apparatus connected to patients with catheter or wire leads going into the heart. In patients with heart disease, low-voltage currents may cause arrhythmias without cardiac arrest, which in turn can subsequently trigger ventricular fibrillation.

Household voltage seems to produce little long-term deleterious effect on the myocardium if exposure is only momentary. Noxious effects depend on resistances which determine the amperage going through the heart. The resistance of an adult person's thorax is about 70–100 ohm and varies with the type of skin contact. Dry skin offers resistance of several thousand ohm. Inside the body, bone tissue and air-filled lungs offer high resistance, but the extracellular fluid is an excellent conductor.

At 110 V, a 60-cycle alternating current in humans of less than 0.01 A, applied from hand to foot, will cause merely a 'funny' sensation; with 0.01 A, the person will experience tetanic muscle contraction. Between 0.1 and 1 A, the likelihood of inducing ventricular fibrillation and sudden death is greatest. With more than 1 A, the myocardium contracts fiercely and if the episode results in ventricular fibrillation, may be defibrillated. High-voltage line accidents result in either ventricular fibrillation, or the pattern described below for lightning, depending on the amount of current traversing heart and brain.

The treatment of victims of electric shock includes the following:

1. The rescuer should make sure the victim is no longer in contact with the current source to avoid receiving a shock himself. If possible, shut off the source, or dislodge the victim from contact using a stick, rope or other non-conductive implement.
2. Administer CPR steps A, B and C and steps D, E and F as needed.
3. Remember that tetanic muscle spasms may cause fractures and that the magnitude and severity of internal tissue damage cannot be gauged from external burns. Thus, even patients who wake up quickly after electrocution must be admitted to hospital.

Lightning may produce millions of volts.[4,48] Many persons struck by lightning are merely stunned and may have transient difficulty in moving, hearing or feeling. Some suffer burns, primarily at the entry and exit points of the erratic paths travelled by lightning current. If the current passes through brain and heart, the victim suddenly loses consciousness (electronarcosis) and becomes apnoeic, probably because of instantaneous cessation of metabolism. At the same time, the heart is thrown into a sustained contraction. Soon after termination of the lightning shock, the contracted heart relaxes and resumes spontaneous contractions with sinus rhythm, while the respiratory centre remains paralysed. Then, owing to the apnoea, the heart is asphyxiated, leading to secondary asystole unless artificial ventilation is started before the onset of cardiac arrest. Usually, the brain arrest is reversible. Very high voltage, however, can burn and destroy brain tissue. On the other hand, some victims of lightning stroke have survived more than 10 min of clinical death when treated by CPR and prolonged critical care, with complete CNS recovery.[48]

Drowning[15,49,50]

Submersion accidents kill more than 100000 people per year worldwide (*see* Chapter 26). Near-drowning implies that the victim was removed from the water with a pulse present, and drowning that the victim was removed with an absent pulse in clinical death. In either case, the victim may or may not survive, depending on resuscitation and numerous other factors. Victims removed from the water with a pulse, and before anoxic relaxation of the larynx and agonal gasps occur, are easily resuscitated with artificial ventilation since the lungs are usually normal. If water or vomitus is inhaled, the picture becomes more complicated.

Inhaled *fresh water* rapidly passes into the circulation, so that a subject removed prior to circulatory arrest may have dry lungs. The results of fresh water aspiration are not only hypoxaemia, hypercarbia, and acidaemia, but also hypervolaemia, haemodilution, with reduced serum electrolyte concentrations, haemolysis, and hyperkalaemia from acidaemia and haemolysis. Dogs with fresh water flooding of the lungs developed ventricular fibrillation within less than 3 min. At the moment of ventricular fibrillation, the dogs had inhaled and absorbed about 40 ml/kg of water (50 per cent of blood volume). With CPR, IPPV/100 per cent oxygen, epinephrine and electric countershock, most dogs could be fully resuscitated. It appears that ventricular fibrillation is primarily the result of anoxia and hypervolaemia, not of the moderate hyperkalaemia and haemolysis to which it was attributed in the past. Chlorinated water, in the customary swimming pool concentration, has the same effect as fresh water.

Inhaled *sea water*, which is hypertonic (3–5 per cent salt), leads in dogs to transudation of fluid from the circulation into the alveoli, resulting in hypovolaemia, about 30 per cent decrease in blood volume, haemoconcentration and increases in the serum of sodium, magnesium, potassium and chloride. Sea water damages the capillary-alveolar membrane, resulting in plasma protein loss into the alveoli and fulminating pulmonary oedema with hypoxaemia, which is proportional to the quantity of sea water inhaled. Hypoxaemia, bradycardia and oligaemic hypotension lead to systole. If resuscitation is started before the pulse fails, prolonged IPPV with 100 per cent oxygen and plasma volume restoration should result in survival. About twice as much inhaled sea water as fresh water is needed to cause cardiac arrest. Sea water is worse for the lungs; fresh water is worse for the heart; both damage the brain through asphyxiation.

In human victims of near-drowning with evidence of fresh or sea water inhalation, who are rescued *before* cardiac arrest, electrolyte disturbances are minimal or absent ½ to 1 h after removal from the water. Apparently, the organism can rapidly correct the electrolyte changes and clear the free plasma haemoglobin. The main limiting factor in human near-drowning is severe and prolonged hypoxaemia from the damage any type of water causes in the lungs. The pulmonary lesion, however, is usually reversible with modern respiratory care. The brain can survive often very low Pa_{O_2} values, provided there is good cardiac output and arterial pressure. As little as 2 ml/kg of any type of water inhaled can produce hypoxaemia, bronchospasm and pulmonary vasospasm. Larger amounts of fresh or brackish water cause alveolar atelectasis from loss of surfactant, whereas sea water produces pumonary oedema in addition. Additional regurgitation and aspiration of gastric contents, which is not uncommon, complicates the pulmonary pathological changes.

The main limiting factor during resuscitation attempts in human drowning cases rescued after the onset of cardiac arrest, is brain damage. Prevention of brain damage calls for immediate special post-resuscitative therapy. Absence of early awakening is no reason to give up, particularly if drowning occurred in *cold water,* which protects the brain. This is illustrated by the documented survival with normal CNS of a 5-year-old boy after 40 minutes of submersion in ice-cold fresh water; his heart was restarted by external CPR and rewarming, his pulmonary oedema was controlled by respiratory care, and he regained consciousness within about 2 days.[15] At least 25 case reports have been published about victims of cold water drowning, with submersion times of 7–30 minutes, who survived with good brain function. This is most likely due to protective brain temperatures (30°C or less) reached before heart action ceases due to asphyxia.

In victims of near-drowning, with a pulse,[49] or drowning, without a pulse,[50] reoxygenation should not be delayed by attempts to drain fluid from the lungs.

A good swimmer can start mouth-to-mouth or mouth-to-nose resuscitation while treading water. Otherwise mouth-to-mouth ventilation can be started when the rescuer is standing in shallow water, placing the victim's head and chest over his knee. Chest compressions are not possible until the victim is removed from the water. If the abdomen is distended after the victim has been removed from the water, he may be turned briefly on his side and the upper abdomen compressed to expel water and gas. Some recommend turning quickly into the prone position and lifting the abdomen to force water out ('breaking' the victim). Abdominal thrusts[18] should not be routine, as they may delay reoxygenation and do not seem to enhance recovery of the lungs. Ventilation should be switched from exhaled air to 100 per cent oxygen as soon as possible because pulmonary changes occur with even small amounts of inhaled water. Hospital admission is mandatory, even if the victim recovers consciousness at the scene or during transport. Late pulmonary oedema is not unusual. Victims of sea water submersion should have early intratracheal IPPV with 100 per cent O_2 and plasma substitute infusion. After submersion to absence of pulse, resuscitation started early and continued throughout coma has occasionally resulted in recovery.

If neck injury is suspected following diving into shallow water, the victim should be floated onto a backboard before removal from the water. If mouth-to-mouth ventilation is needed, jaw thrust with moderate backward tilt of the head is used, asking a helper to hold head-neck-chest aligned, to avoid aggravating a possible spinal cord injury. The neck should not be flexed.

Rescue from water should be attempted only by stronger swimmers. Others should quickly find a floating device. Teaching rapid rescue from water is as important as teaching resuscitation. 'Reach' with a pole. 'Row' a boat or surfboard. 'Throw' a life-preserver, and 'Go' (swim) toward a drowning person only as a last resort.

Scuba divers may drown as a result of dysbaric complications which may cause coma and loss of reflexes. These hyperbaric injuries can be due to the following:

Nitrogen narcosis may occur below 68 m (200 ft) depth when breathing air.

Decompression sickness (the 'bends') causes nitrogen bubbles to be released into all tissues, including the brain, during rapid ascent after nitrogen loading at a depth of over 10 m (30 ft). Decompression sickness can be avoided by slow ascent according to decompression tables.

Cerebral air embolism is fortunately rare, but is the most threatening potentially lethal complication, because it cannot always be avoided, even with sound diving practices. This accident can be caused by rapid ascent for just a few metres, resulting in the expansion of trapped gas in the lungs and alveolar rupture. This may lead to entry of air into the pulmonary veins, causing cerebral and/or coronary air embolism and sudden death.

Severe Polytrauma[51,52]

The fate of the victim of severe multiple injuries is usually determined by the location and extent of brain tissue destruction, the degree and rate of initial haemorrhage, and whether or not there is a cardiac arrest due to exsanguination before help arrives. Ameliorating factors include early haemostasis and fluid resuscitation, initial airway and breathing control, ATLS within the first hour, and rapid resuscitative surgery for intracranial, intrathoracic or intra-abdominal trauma. Early fluid resuscitation, immobilization and wound care can prevent late deaths after polytrauma due to fat embolism, thromboembolism, sepsis and multiple organ failure. The latter include acute tubular necrosis of the kidney (ATN) and adult respiratory distress syndrome (ARDS) in the absence of chest injury. It is not hypovolaemia alone but probably its combination with tissue trauma and sepsis which cause so-called 'irreversible shock'.

All the subsequent sub-headings represent conditions which contribute to the mortality of polytrauma. The interaction of multiple organ derangements includes brain trauma, where increased intracranial pressure (ICP) can cause neurogenic pulmonary oedema, and cardiovascular failure reduces perfusion pressure both of which minimize the chance of recovery. Airway problems or hypoxaemia after chest injury can add to brain failure, and abdominal trauma with peritoneal spillage of intestinal contents can be associated with sepsis and mediator effects contributing to hypovolaemic shock. Gastrointestinal-hepatic tissue injury can cause overall microcirculatory disturbances, including ATN and ARDS; tissue injury and hypovolaemic hypotension cause gastro-intestinal ischaemia, which can progress to stress ulcers, gastric haemorrhage and gut necrosis often as the final cause of death. Neutralizing gastric acidity is important, in addition to preventing and promptly correcting hypovolaemic shock.

For effective treatment of polytrauma, a general trauma surgeon should remain the co-ordinator of multidisciplinary surgical intervention; and the most experienced and skilled anaesthesiologist should guide resuscitation.

Cerebral Trauma[33,53,54]

Mortality among head injury patients, who remain unconscious for over 6 hours, has been reduced with intensive care management, including artificial ventilation, monitoring and control of ICP, and rapid evacuation of accessible intracranial haemotomas. The main factors causing mortality and morbidity are early post-insult arterial hypoxaemia and hypotension, and petechial haemorrhages in the midbrain and brainstem after acceleration/deceleration injury. Gastric ulcers and other extracerebral complications can increase mortality.

When the impact of head injury results in a brief period of apnoea, which may be associated with airway obstruction, a bystander should immediately use the triple airway manoeuvre and mouth-to-mouth or mouth-to-nose ventilation. Routine administration of oxygen is recommended as soon as possible. Definitive airway control with endotracheal intubation should be accomplished by the most experienced physician available. Straining, coughing and reflex hypertension as a result of protracted intubation attempts can cause cerebrovascular engorge-ment with ICP rise, leading to further damage to the already injured brain.

Intracranial haemorrhage does not produce oligaemic shock, but results in a rise in ICP, which reduces cerebral perfusion pressure and eventually leads to brain herniation and apnoea.

'Concussion' implies no significant anatomical brain injury. The hallmarks are brief depression of the CNS and retrograde amnesia, headache, dizziness and nausea, without localizing signs. The pupils may be fixed and dilated in the early phase just after injury, even in salvageable patients. 'Contusion' implies more prolonged unconsciousness and often focal signs. All patients with a head injury should be evaluated in the hospital emergency department and considered as possible candidates for admission.

After initial resuscitation, one should determine the level of consciousness, pupillary reaction, vital signs and extracranial injuries. A skull roentgenogram is less helpful to guide management than clinical signs and CT imaging. Life support by experts must be uninterrupted during transport.

Extradural (epidural) haemorrhage must be detected promptly. Immediate surgical intervention is indicated. The prognosis is excellent only if the extradural haematoma is drained within 1–2 hours. Subdural, usually venous, haemorrhage is also life-threatening, but symptoms develop more slowly. Evacuation by emergency burr holes or craniotomy is more effective in extradural than in subdural haematoma. If this is not possible in a trauma centre with neurosurgery, the general trauma surgeon should be trained to perform these life-saving procedures. Subarachnoid haemorrhage results in bloody CSF and may not require immediate surgery. Haemorrhages within the brain substance can be recognized by CT scanning.

If the patient remains in coma after initial resuscitation, life support should be brain-orientated (*Table* 3.4). This should include ICP monitoring, although the indications for this measurement are not fully agreed.

The assessment of head-injured patients requires continuous monitoring and titrated life support, accompanied by on-going reassessment to be compared with the initial clinical picture. Arterial pressure is usually high (or low if accompanied by extracranial injuries), and should be controlled at normotensive or slightly below normotensive levels. A progressive bradycardia, usually accompanied by hypertension, suggests a cerebral lesion in need of surgery.

Table 3.4. Trauma scoring. One of several popular trauma scales (scoring system) is the following:[34]

	Trauma score	Points/score
Respiratory rate	36/min or greater	2
	25–35/min	3
	10–24/min	4
	0–9/min	1
	none	0
Respiratory expansion	normal	1
	shallow	0
Systolic blood pressure	90 or greater	4
	70–89	3
	50–69	2
	0–49	1
	no pulse	0
Capillary refill	normal	2
(fingernail bed)	delayed	1
	none	0

Note: Trauma score of 8 or less calls for transfer to trauma centre.

(Reproduced from: Champion H. R. et al. (1981) The trauma score. *Crit. Care Med.* **9**, 672.)

Head injury tends to cause hyperthermia, which should be reversed to moderate hypothermia. A simple way of following the neurological dysfunction is use of the Glasgow Coma Scale.[33] Lumbar puncture, EEG and radiotracer techniques are not helpful in the initial management of cerebral trauma, but CT and NMR imaging are highly useful diagnostic and prognostic tools.

Head injury as well as ischaemic anoxia and other brain insults can be followed by generalized seizures, which can cause asphyxia from pharyngolaryngospasm and apnoea. Neurons suffer not only from hypoxaemia secondary to impaired oxygenation during convulsions, but also from the hypoxic acidosis induced by the increased metabolic activity. Thus, management of generalized convulsions requires IPPV with O_2, if necessary with the aid of a muscle relaxant. Soon thereafter, administration of a CNS depressant such as diazepam, thiopental or pentobarbital, for rapid action, and phenobarbital or phenytoin, for prolonged effect, can minimize the electric discharges from the brain. Seizure disorders can also stimulate cardiac dysrhythmias.

Spinal Cord Trauma [30,31,55,56]

Any victim of trauma with an injury above the clavicle should be suspected of having a cervical spine injury. This calls for assessment, resuscitation and life support with head-neck-chest aligned in the neutral position and without moving the spine during transport. Moderate backward tilt of the head is acceptable, but maximal backward tilt, flexion or rotation of the head must be avoided. As soon as possible, with head-neck-chest aligned manually, the patient should be placed on a spine board and immobilized with cervical collar, sandbags and tape, for transport, ideally, to a spinal cord injury centre. Management of spinal injury requires specialized knowledge and experience.

Initial assessment should include a search for neck deformity, pain, tenderness, motor and sensory disturbances of the extremities, bladder and rectal control, and spinal shock, that is, hypotension without tachycardia. Lateral cervical spine and chest roentgenogram, and CT scanning should be performed if available. Management includes immobilization and general life support with maintenance of arterial normotension. Experimental attempts to save the integrity of the spinal cord include surgical decompression, local hypothermia, and a variety of pharmacological and physical agents.

Thoracic Trauma [3,31]

Blunt thoracic trauma rarely requires resuscitative surgery. It is the cause of about one quarter of trauma deaths, many of which are preventable. The predominant cause of death is progressive hypoxia from pulmonary contusion, atelectasis, consolidation and shunting, worsened at times by flail chest and/or pneumothorax. Tension pneumothorax and cardiac tamponade are summarized below.

Blunt or penetrating intrathoracic injury can result in exsanguination. Open pneumothorax, or a sucking chest wound, also leads to atelectasis and hypoxia. The defect should be promptly closed with a sterile occlusive dressing taped on three sides, leaving the fourth side open to function as a valve. A chest tube should be placed away from the defect (*Fig.* 3.4). Surgical closure is performed later. Massive haemothorax is usually caused by a penetrating injury, less commonly by blunt trauma. It should be detected by percussion, auscultation, and a shock state. Treatment requires rapid pleural drainage and restoration of blood volume. An autotransfusion device should be used if available. Sometimes emergency thoracotomy may be required.

Flail chest was thought in the past to cause progressive hypoxia and hypercarbia from 'pendel air'. This is now thought to be less important than pulmonary contusion and consolidation, which may require higher negative intrathoracic pressures for lung expansion than the flail chest will permit. Some patients can be managed without endotracheal intubation, with titrated increase in F_{IO_2} by mask, perhaps with CPAP. Pain control and monitoring of blood gas values, particularly the alveolar-arterial P_{O_2} gradient, are important. Intercostal nerve or thoracic epidural blocks should be considered. When there is significant shunting during spontaneous breathing, controlled hyperventilation is capable of re-expanding the lungs by increasing the FRC, counteracting flailing and shunting, stabilizing the chest wall and reducing pain.

Besides flail chest and pulmonary contusion, causes of death are traumatic aortic rupture, tracheobronchial injury, and traumatic diaphragmatic hernia. They all usually require emergency surgery. Myocardial contusion requires ECG and haemodynamic monitoring and management similar to that of myocardial infarction. If the patient with crushed chest develops a cardiac arrest, closed-chest CPR is indicated, switching to open-chest CPR if intrathoracic haemorrhage is suspected.

Tension pneumothorax is an opening into the pleural space, either through the chest wall or through the lung, with pressure in the pleural space rising above atmospheric throughout the respiratory cycle. This collapses the ipsilateral lung. Previously healthy individuals will become hypoxic with a 40–50 per cent shunt, even breathing 100 per cent O_2. If the opening operates as a one-way valve, for instance in a contused lung, rupture of alveolar blebs, or air trapping in asthma or emphysema, positive-pressure ventilation or coughing can force increments of gas into the pleural space, where it cannot escape and a tension pneumothorax develops. Alveoli may also rupture into the pulmonary interstitial spaces, resulting in mediastinal and subcutaneous emphysema, noticed in the form of crepitation about the neck, and subserosal blebs, which can rupture secondarily into the pleural space.

Tension pneumothorax should be suspected when there is progressive difficulty in ventilating the lungs, progressive inability of the lungs to deflate passively, progressive deterioration of the circulation, mediastinal shift, and progressive distension of the abdomen. There is no time or need for roentgenographic diagnosis. Circulatory arrest seems to be due to a combination of severe hypoxia and compression and kinking of bronchi and great veins. The treatment of suspected pneumothorax consists of confirmation by needle puncture and drainage by a large bore tube (*Fig.* 3.4). When, in the absence of a pulse, tube drainage fails to relieve the tension pneumothorax, open-chest cardiac resuscitation is indicated (*Fig.* 3.5).

Cardiac tamponade should be suspected under circumstances that may disrupt the integrity of the myocardium like a stab wound, gunshot wound, intracardiac needle injection, or catheterization after cardiac surgery or myocardial infarction.

There are signs of compromized cardiac output with arterial hypotension, elevated CVP with venous distension and exaggerated pulsations, muffled heart sounds, and pulsus paradoxus, i.e. during deep inhalations the arterial pressure decreases markedly. There may be substernal pain. If time permits a roentgeno- gram, it will show a widened heart shadow. Arterial pressure, particularly pulse pressure, and cardiac output decline, while venous pressure and heart rate increase. Death in asystole or ventricular fibrillation is due to progressive inability of the heart to fill during diastole. Progress depends on the speed with which blood accumulates in the pericardium. Treatment starts with pericardial needle aspiration via the paraxyphoid approach, preferably under ECG monitoring. Aspiration may have to be repeated and perhaps followed by the surgical creation of a pleural-pericardial window. In absence of pulse, suspicion of cardiac tamponade is an indication for open-chest CPR with incision and drainage of the pericardial sac and direct control of the bleeding site.

Abdominal Trauma [3,31,51,52]

About 25 per cent of penetrating injuries involve the abdomen. Blunt abdominal injuries (which represent 6 per cent of all trauma) constitute up to 25 per cent of all trauma deaths.

Because of the dome shape of the diaphragm, injuries to the abdomen may involve the thorax and vice versa. Abdominal trauma should be suspected from the location of bruises and wounds and the type of accident. Emergency laparotomy, which may be life-saving, requires assessment of the shock state, and examination of the abdomen and lower part of the thorax, including rectal and vaginal examination. There may be retroperitoneal vascular injuries or catastrophic haemorrhage into the abdomen from the aorta or vena cava, and less rapid bleeding from the liver, spleen or kidneys. Penetrating injury often causes haemorrhage or perforation of the bowel, and is an indication for laparotomy. Blunt abdominal trauma is an indication for peritoneal lavage. Resuscitation should not be delayed with X-ray examinations when the patient is in shock.

Limb Trauma [3,30,31]

Patients with only fractures and soft tissue injuries of the extremities are rarely in need of major resuscitative efforts, except to prevent or correct immediately hypovolaemia from major external or intra-tissue blood volume loss. This can be life-threatening in bilateral femoral fractures, traumatic amputations, crushing trauma of the pelvis, major open fractures of any kind, and polytrauma with multiple fractures. A closed femur fracture can result in internal blood loss of 1–2 litres. In general, extremity trauma should not receive priority attention during emergency resuscitation and primary survey. Immobilization of fractured extremities before moving the patient, however, is important to prevent further injury, pain, fat embolization, shock and morbidity. One can effectively improvise immobilization, even without splints. Resuscitation has priority over splinting!

Burns[3,31,57]

In the USA, about 12000 persons burn to death every year. Most burn injuries are due to flame; some are due to scalds, electric current, chemicals or radiation. Life support must have priority over treatment of the skin lesions, which do not need treatment prior to definitive care in hospital. Most dangerous are upper and lower airway burns due to heat, ash, gases and other combustion products. While providing life support, a brief history of the circumstances of the injury should be obtained and assessment of the extent and degree of the burn injury and associated injuries made. Suspected airway burns call for continuous respiratory observation, diagnostic-prognostic fibreoptic bronchoscopy, and perhaps intubation and mechanical ventilation. In the hospital, the burnt patient, particularly if unconscious, must be examined for carbon monoxide poisoning, and for associated head-neck injury and pneumothorax. The patient should be weighed for subsequent fluid therapy. Pulmonary care should be guided by frequent arterial P_{O_2} measurements on a constant F_{IO_2}, to detect early shunting. Non-invasive monitoring using a pulse oximeter can often be substituted for arterial catheterization.

The extent of surface burns should be assessed by the rule of 9s. Each arm counts as 9 per cent, each leg as 18 per cent; the front of the trunk as 18 per cent; the back of the trunk as 18 per cent; and the head as 9 per cent, though in a child as 18 per cent.

Eventually the depth of the burn wounds should be determined, assessing first degree (erythema), second degree (red or mottled skin with swelling and blisters), and third degree (full thickness burn with leathery appearance, dry or moist, coagulation necrosis, no bleeding) injury. Water loss through skin areas with third degree burns may be over 10 times the normal water loss through skin (about 1000 ml 70 kg^{-1} day^{-1}). Besides fluid loss, major burns result in heat loss, paralleled by greatly increased O_2 consumption. Gastric tube feeding is preferred to i.v. alimentation, provided there is gastrointestinal motility. Gastric feeding, H_2 blocker therapy and an antacid help prevent haemorrhage from gastric stress ulcers.

The criteria for admission to a burn centre include the following:
1. Any burn involving over 25 per cent of the body surface area.
2. Third degree burns of more than 10 per cent of body surface area.
3. All burns of the face, eyes, ears, hands, feet or perineum.
4. Suspected pulmonary burns of any extent.
5. Associated major injuries
6. Lesser burns in patients with pre-existing major disease.
7. Burns of over 20 per cent of the body surface area in the young or the old.
8. High voltage electric burns.

Some patients have survived 70–80 per cent surface area burns after aggressive resuscitation and advanced intensive care, and multiple plastic operations. With improved early treatment of shock, the principal cause of early mortality from burns has been due to smoke inhalation, airway burns and hypoxic brain damage from CO poisoning. The latter requires early aggressive cerebral resuscitation efforts.[1,6]

Hypovolaemic shock must be promptly corrected. If the treatment of shock is delayed, acute tubular necrosis of kidneys and multiple organ failure may follow. Increased capillary permeability occurs first in the burn area, but in extensive surface burns, can become systemic. In contrast to mechanical trauma, whole blood is not lost in large quantities. Thus, a combination of balanced salt solution (e.g. lactated Ringer's) and colloid solution (e.g. polygelatin, plasma protein fraction or albumin) is needed. A negative nitrogen balance calls for early oral or parenteral hyperalimentation. Pulmonary oedema may develop as the result of pulmonary burns, overinfusion and overall increased capillary permeability.

Early i.v. fluid resuscitation is recommended for any degree burn greater than 20 per cent of body surface area, titrated according to hourly urinary output and measurements of body weight. Urine flow should be maintained at about 1 ml kg^{-1} h^{-1} for children and 0·5 ml kg^{-1} h^{-1} for adults. Usually, electrolyte solution 2–4 ml kg^{-1} per cent^{-1} body surface burn is required over 24 h (Baxter formula).

The Brooke US Army Hospital guidelines call for more electrolytes than colloid solution during the initial 24 h, and an emphasis on colloid during the second 24 h. Over the first 24 h, lactated Ringer's solution 1·5 ml kg^{-1} per cent^{-1} body surface area burn (up to a maximum of 50 per cent), plus a colloid (albumin, plasmanate, fresh frozen plasma, dextran 10, polygelatin, or hydroxyethyl starch) in a dose of 0·5 ml kg^{-1} per cent^{-1} body surface burn, including 2000 ml of water should be given. More should be administered in the first 8 h and the rest in the subsequent 16 h. During the second 24 h electrolyte solution 0·75 ml kg^{-1} per cent^{-1} body surface burn is given, plus the same amount of colloid and water as in the first 24 h. Several other fluid resuscitation formulae are also acceptable. Hypertonic salt solutions for initial burn shock therapy are controversial. If they are used, the serum sodium should be maintained below 158 mmol/l. Most burn centres follow isotonic salt solutions with a colloid solution. Maintaining urine flow may require aggressive fluid replacement. Serum albumin should be maintained above 2·5 g/dl.

Other considerations for the acute management of burn victims include:
1. Early life support to follow the principles of this chapter (above).
2. Cold water application for minor burns, but not for extensive burns. Sterile moist dressings may be applied in the field. Second degree burn blisters should be preserved intact. Narcotic analgesics should be given i.v. in titrated doses.
3. Cleaning of all burn wounds with mild antiseptic solution. Early conservative debridement should be undertaken. For severely burnt patients, topical antimicrobial agents, e.g. silver sulfadiazine, or (for better eschar penetration) mafenide acetate should be applied.
4. Definitive burn wound care, prevention and treatment of sepsis (the major cause of late deaths), and reconstructive plastic surgery are beyond the scope of this chapter. Neomycin dressings are used by some after grafting.
5. Laboratory blood tests include haematology, clotting data and arterial blood gas values. Chest roentgenograms should be taken at regular intervals.
6. Circulation in burned swollen extremities should be preserved by escharotomy and fasciotomy. Topical enzymes (e.g. Travase) may be substituted for escharotomy in milder cases.

SUMMARY

Resuscitation potentials have been documented for everyday emergency medical services, multicasualty incident type disasters, and conventional wars. Resuscitation potentials in mass disasters, like major earthquakes, are highly suspect; for nuclear power plant accidents are unknown but must be prepared for; and for nuclear war are zero. Prevention is the only effective treatment for nuclear war. Modelling studies are needed to evaluate the cost-effectiveness of resuscitative preparedness for major industrial disasters, earthquakes, volcanic explosions, floods, storms, major fires and other mass disasters.

Effective planning for resuscitation response in disasters is made so difficult because not only does each disaster have a different set of demands and opportunities, but also mass disasters are rare, and time factors are crucial. For example, planning in the USA is for the scenario of a major earthquake, which could generate within minutes up to 100 000 severely injured people in need of emergency medical care and hospitalization.

To save victims who develop cardiac arrest at the scene, a rapid advanced trauma life support (ATLS) team response would be required. This may be difficult to mobilize without help from the military. Triage concepts may distract ATLS teams away from victims who have no pulse to those more likely salvageable. Exsanguinated disaster victims with polytrauma arriving at an advanced facility without a pulse, might be saved by haemostasis via thoracotomy and open-chest CPR, or even in the future with use of emergency cardiopulmonary bypass. ATLS teaching for general or specialized surgeons should include resuscitative interventions for lethal haemorrhage into the cranium, the chest and the abdomen.

Life-supporting first aid (LSFA) is ready for innovative research. Unanswered questions go beyond control of external haemorrhage, airway control, and appropriate positioning. For example, could the pulse be sustained longer in the hypovolaemic victim, while waiting for an ambulance or helicopter with a medical team to arrive, by keeping the victim warm or cold, quiet or stimulated, with or without oral or rectal fluid administration, and with or without oxygen inhalation? What is the optimal positioning?

ATLS and resuscitative surgery could also benefit from innovative research. Investigation of the pathophysiology of dying processes could lead to new therapeutic concepts.

Most important for disaster resuscitology is the need for novel, immediately available, rapidly transportable tools for finding victims in collapsed buildings; and for extricating victims who need life support without adding injury.

Improving life-saving potentials in disasters through use of modern resuscitation medicine must consider the limiting time factors:

1. For control of external haemorrhage and airway control by LSFA to be effective, these measures have to be applied usually within seconds to minutes of injury: this calls for LSFA-trained, uninjured, lay co-victims, provided through widespread public education.
2. For traumatic-hypovolaemic shock to be reversed in time to avoid delayed multiple organ failure, early haemostasis may require resuscitative surgery, and fluid resuscitation would have to be started immediately. However there are doubts whether, for example in earthquakes, ATLS delivered beyond 6–12 h could save lives.

The limiting time factors call for military-civilian collaboration, particularly for the transport of ATLS teams and for rescue and evacuation. The basis for resuscitation in disasters, however, is the capability of regional everyday emergency medical services (EMS) systems. Everyday EMS have gone through three decades of development, at least in industrialized countries. If most of what is known about methods, personnel, education, organization, communication and evaluation were applied throughout regions and states, the basis for resuscitation delivery in disasters would exist. The combined local-regional systems would then make up the National Disaster Medical Systems (NDMS) capability.

Unanswered questions in need of research, concerning the delivery in disasters of LSFA, ATLS and resuscitative surgery, include:

—What is the role of hospitals other than trauma centres in NDMS plans?
—Do field hospitals and staging areas, proven effective in wars, which require 24–72 hours to be set up, have any life-saving potential in NDMSs designed for major earthquakes?
—What is the advisability of sending medico-surgical resuscitation teams to the scene?
—Could such teams perform resuscitative surgery in the field, using ICU-type operating rooms which could be airlifted?
—Which lessons learned from everyday EMS and from wars are relevant to major earthquakes, fires, or industrial accidents?

In attempts to answer these and many other questions, NDMS plans should not be made from the armchair, but rely heavily on the advice of resuscitation experienced health professionals who have had experience in disasters.

Resuscitation medicine, if applied with reason and compassion, by trying to achieve useful survival for as many victims as possible, should be considered not only on the basis of numerical results, but also for its philosophical impact. Medicine in general and resuscitation medicine in particular represent an imposition of human values on the species-orientated random processes of nature on earth. Resuscitation implies a commitment by individuals, a devotion to the restoration of lives cut short before fulfilment. Even where the therapeutic impact of resuscitation affects only a few, its moral impact may have a significant influence in a world where human life is often regarded as expendable.

To conclude with the words of Rudolph Frey: 'As the globe is becoming smaller, we must convince politicians to mobilize medical, military and governmental resources toward a common goal. The opportunities are real. Therefore, physicians and non-physician leaders should commit themselves to the improvement of global emergency and critical care medicine.'

ACKNOWLEDGEMENTS

Asmund and Tore Laerdal helped initiate the book from which this chapter is based.[1] The authors' research has been supported by the US Army's Surgeon General, the National Institutes of Health, the Pennsylvania Department of Health, and the Asmund S. Laerdal Foundation. Sections of this chapter have been adapted from the authors' previous publications[1,6] and the American College of Surgeons Advanced Trauma Life Support material.[3] W. B. Saunders

Company have permitted the use of previously published material.[1,4] Ms Lisa Cohn helped with editing. Ms Fran Mistrick and Ms Tancy Crawford helped with the preparation of the manuscript.

REFERENCES

1. Safar P. and Bircher N. (1987) *Cardiopulmonary-Cerebral Resuscitation. World Federation of Societies of Anaesthesiologists.* 3rd edition. Stavanger, Laerdal; Philadelphia, Saunders.
2. American Heart Association (AHA) 1985 National Conference (Montgomery W. H., Chairman, Donegan J., McIntyre K. M. et al.) (1986) Standards and guidelines for cardiopulmonary resuscitation (CPR) and emergency cardiac care (ECC). *JAMA* **255** (suppl.), 2841.
3. American College of Surgeons Committee on Trauma (Collicott P. E. et al.): (1984) *Advanced Trauma Life Support Course for Physicians.* American College of Surgeons (55 East Erie Street, Chicago, IL 60611, USA).
4. Safar P. (1986) The mechanisms of dying and their reversal. In: Schwartz G., Safar P., Stone J. et al. (eds). *Principles and Practice of Emergency Medicine.* Philadelphia, Saunders.
5. Grenvik A. and Safar P. (eds.) (1981) Brain failure and resuscitation. *Clin. Crit. Care Med.* New York, Churchill Livingstone.
6. Safar P. (1986) Cerebral resuscitation after cardiac arrest. A Review. *Circulation* **74** (suppl. IV), 138.
7. American Society of Anesthesiologists, Committee on Acute Medicine (Safar P., Chairman) (1968) Community-wide emergency medical services. *JAMA* **204**, 595.
8. Caroline N. L. (1984) *Life Supporting Resuscitation and First Aid: A Manual for Instructors of the Lay Public. Guidelines of the League of Red Cross and Red Crescent Societies (LRCS) and the World Federation of Societies of Anaesthesiologists (WFSA).* Geneva, LRCS Publications, 17 Chemin des Crets, 1211 Geneva 19, Switzerland.
9. Safar P. (1976, 1980, 1985) Resuscitation potentials in mass disasters. (*a*) In: Frey R., Nagel E. and Safar P. (eds.) *Mobile ICUs (1973). Anesthesiology and Resuscitation,* Vol. 95. Heidelberg, Springer-Verlag; (*b*) In: Frey R. and Safar P. (eds.) *Resuscitation and Life Support in Disasters (1977). Disaster Medicine,* Vol. 2. Heidelberg, Springer-Verlag; (*c*) In: Manni C. and Magalini S. I. (eds.) *Emergency and Disaster Medicine* (1st R. Frey Memorial Lecture, 1983). New York, Springer-Verlag, p. 28.
10. Manni C. and Magalini S. I. (eds.) (1985) *Emergency and Disaster Medicine. Proceedings of the Third World Congress, Rome, May 24–27, 1983.* Berlin, Springer-Verlag.
11. Safar P. (ed.) (1985) Disaster resuscitology. Proceedings of the Second World Congress on Emergency and Disaster Medicine (Club of Mainz), Pittsburgh, USA, 1981. *J. Wld. Assoc. Emerg. Disaster Med.* **1** (Suppl. 1).
12. Adler J. (ed.) (1984) *Proceedings International Symposium on Disaster Medicine, Jerusalem, Israel.* (J.A., Share-Zedek Hospital, Jerusalem, Israel.)
13. Bisgard J. C. (1985) The role of the military in international military-civilian collaboration for disaster medicine in the USA. *J. Wld. Assoc. Emerg. Disaster Med.* **1**(1), 21.
14. Villazon A. (1986) The Mexico City earthquake of 1985, an international disaster. *J. Wld. Assoc. Emerg. Disaster Med.* **2**, 1–4.
15. Siebke H., Rod T. and Breivik H. (1975) Survival after 40 minutes submersion without cerebral sequelae. *Lancet* **i**, 1275–7.
16. Safar P., Aguto-Escarraga L. and Chang F. (1959) A study of upper airway obstruction in the unconscious patient. *J. Appl. Physiol.* **14**, 760.
17. Don Michael T. A. (1986) The role of the esophageal obturator airway in cardiopulmonary resuscitation. *Circulation* **74** (Suppl. IV), 134.
18. Heimlich H. J. (1975) A life-saving maneuver to prevent food choking. *JAMA* **234**, 398.
19. Kouwenhoven W. B., Jude J. R. and Knickerbocker G. G. (1960) Closed-chest cardiac massage. *JAMA* **173**, 1064.
20. Stewart R. D. (1984) Tactile orotracheal intubation. *Ann. Emerg. Med.* **13**, 175.
21. Safar P. and Caroline N. (1986) Respiratory care techniques and strategies. In: Schwartz G., Safar P., Stone J. et al. (eds.) *Principles and Practice of Emergency Medicine.* Philadelphia, Saunders, Chapter 11.

22. Winter P. M. and Miller N. J. (1984) Oxygen toxicity. In: Shoemaker W. C., Thompson W. L., Holbrook P. R. (eds.) *Textbook of Critical Care*. Philadelphia, Saunders.
23. Klain M. (1984) High-frequency ventilation. In: Shoemaker, W. C., Thompson W. L., Holbrook P. R. (eds.) *Textbook of Critical Care*. Philadelphia, Saunders, p. 323.
24. Safar P. (ed.) (1978) Brain resuscitation. (Special Symposium Issue.) *Crit. Care Med.* **6**, 199.
25. Eisenberg M. S., Hallstrom A. and Bergner L. (1982) Long-term survival after out-of-hospital cardiac arrest. *N. Engl. J. Med.* **306**, 1340.
26. Negovsky V. A., Gurvitch A. M. and Zolotokrylina E. S. (1983) *Postresuscitation Disease*. Amsterdam, Elsevier.
27. Safar P. (1985) Effects of postresuscitation syndrome on cerebral recovery from cardiac arrest. Review and hypotheses. *Crit. Care Med.* **13**, 932.
28. Seeley S. (1966) *Accidental Death and Disability: the Neglected Disease of Modern Society*. Committee on Trauma and Committee on Shock, Division of Medical Sciences. National Academy of Sciences (National Research Council, 2101 Constitution Avenue, Washington, DC 20418, USA.)
29. Frey R., Nagel E. and Safar P. (eds.) (1976) Mobile intensive care units. Advanced emergency care delivery systems. Symposium, Mainz 1973. *Anesthesiology and Resuscitation*, Vol. 95. Heidelberg, Springer-Verlag.
30. American Academy of Orthopaedic Surgeons, Committee on Injuries (1971) *Emergency Care and Transportation of the Sick and Injured*. American Academy of Orthopaedic Surgeons, 430 North Michigan Avenue, Chicago, Il. 60611, USA.
31. American College of Surgeons (1980) *Early Care of the Injured Patient*. Philadelphia, Saunders.
32. Caroline N. L. (1986) *Emergency Care in the Streets*. Boston, Little Brown.
33. Teasdale G. and Jennett B. (1974) Assessment of coma and impaired consciousness. A practical scale. *Lancet* **ii**, 81.
34. Champion H. R., Sacco W., Carnazzo A. J. et al. (1981) The trauma score. *Crit. Care Med.* **9**, 672.
35. Kaplan B. C., Civetta J. M., Nagel E. L., et al. (1973) The Military Anti-Shock Trouser in civilian pre-hospital emergency care. *J. Trauma* **13**, 843.
36. Messmer K. (ed.) (1976) Hemodilution: a symposium. *Der Anästhesist* **25**, 123.
37. Takaori M. and Safar P. (1967) Treatment of massive hemorrhage with colloid and crystalloid solution. *JAMA* **199**, 297.
38. Shoemaker W. C. (1984) Pathophysiology and therapy of shock syndromes. In: Shoemaker W. C., Thompson W. L. and Holbrook P. R. (eds.) *Textbook of Critical Care*. Philadelphia, Saunders, p. 52.
39. Sassano J. (1986) The rapid infusion system. In: Winter P. M., Kang Y. G. (eds.) *Hepatic Transplantation: Anesthetic and Perioperative Management*. Philadelphia, Praeger.
40. Boyan C. T. (1964) Cold or warmed blood for massive transfusions. *Ann. Surg.* **160**, 282.
41. Gelin L. W., Solvell L. and Zederfeldt A. (1969) The plasma volume expanding effect of low viscous dextran and macrodex. *Acta Chir. Scand.* **122**, 309.
42. Hunt C., Burnette R. R., MacGregor R. D. et al. (1985) Synthesis and evaluation of a prototypal artificial red cell. *Science* **230**, 1165–8.
43. DeVenuto F. (ed.) (1982) (Symposium Issue) Acellular oxygen-delivering resuscitation fluids. *Crit. Care Med.* **10**, 237.
44. Forbes W. H. (1962) Carbon monoxide. In: Whittenberger J. L. (ed.) *Artificial Respiration*. New York, Hoeber (Harper and Row), p. 194.
45. Ledingham I. McA., Douglas I. H. S., Routh G. S. et al. (1980) Central rewarming systems for treatment of hypothermia. *Lancet* **i**, 1168.
46. Reuler J. B. (1978) Hypothermia: pathophysiology, clinical settings, and management. *Ann. Intern. Med.* **89**, 519.
47. Shibolet S., Lancaster M. C. and Dannon Y. (1976) Heat stroke: a review. *Aviation Space Envir. Med.* **47**, 280.
48. Ravitch M., Lane R., Safar P. et al. (1961) Lightning stroke. Recovery following cardiac massage and prolonged artificial respiration. *N. Engl. J. Med.* **264**, 36.
49. Modell J. H. (1986) Near drowning. *Circulation* **74** (Suppl. IV), 27.
50. Redding J., Cozine R. A., Voigt G. C. et al. (1961) Resuscitation from drowning. *JAMA* **178**, 1136.
51. Cowley R. A. and Trump B. F. (eds.) (1981) *Pathophysiology of Shock, Anoxia, and Ischemia*. Baltimore, Williams and Wilkins.

52. Cowley R. A. and Dunham C. M. (1982) *Shock Trauma/Critical Care Manual. Initial Assessment and Management.* Baltimore, University Park Press.
53. Jennett B. and Bond M. (1975) Assessment of outcome after severe brain damage: a practical scale. *Lancet* **i**, 480.
54. Jennett B., Teasdale G., Galbraith S. et al. (1977) Severe head injuries in three countries. *J. Neurol. Neurosurg. Psychiatry* **40**, 291.
55. Albin M. S. (1984) Acute spinal cord trauma. In: Shoemaker, W. C., Thompson W. L., Holbrook P. R. (eds.) *Textbook of Critical Care.* Philadelphia, Saunders, p. 928.
56. Wagner F. C. (1977) Management of acute spinal cord injury. *Surg. Neurol.* **7**, 346.
57. Artz C. P., Moncrief J. A. and Pruitt B. A. (1979) *Burns: A Team Approach.* Philadelphia, Saunders.

J. Restall and R. J. Knight

4

Analgesia and Anaesthesia in the Field

INTRODUCTION

This chapter presents a distillate of experience gained since 1945 in providing aid to victims of one of the world's more enduring man-made disasters—armed conflict between nations. In the 1980s there have been invasions of Afghanistan, Grenada and the Falkland Islands, and continuing wars in Central America, Lebanon and Iran/Iraq. In the latter conflict alone it has been reliably estimated that 1·5 million casualties have occurred. The requirement for a nation's anaesthetists to be able to work in the field would therefore seem to be universal and the military experience in war has many applications in the civil major disaster in the provision of pain relief and anaesthesia in the field.

THE PROBLEM

Modern weapons systems are considerably more sophisticated in the rate of fire (rounds/min) and in lethality compared with those used in the last major European war of 1939–45. The projectile fired from the present generation of small arms, the 5·56 weapon, weighs less than the old ·303 round, 9·4 g as against 11·2 g, but has a much greater velocity, 970 m/s as against 300 m/s. Consequently, the present generation of weapons create considerably more kinetic energy (KE = ½ Mass × Velocity^2), than those used previously: this kinetic energy (KE) is dissipated throughout the casualty's body when the projectile strikes its target. High speed cine radiography has demonstrated the various phenomena which occur when a high velocity round (HVR) strikes its target. On impact, the HVR moves rapidly through tissues, generating a vacuum cavity into which external debris is sucked, causing contamination of the wound. The KE of the impacting projectile is transmitted equally in all directions within the fluid filled systems of the body. The pressure wave so generated produces capillary rupture throughout the tissues.

The probability of a casualty surviving a wound from a HVR is related to, firstly, the KE of the projectile at the moment of impact and, secondly, to the point of entry into the body. A casualty with a peripheral limb wound, even with a shattered long bone, is much more likely to survive than one with a thoraco-abdominal wound. Head wounds sustained with a HVR or even a HVR fragment have a very poor survival rate. The fluid nature of the brain is an ideal trans-mission medium for the HVR's KE.

The immediate psychology of the battle casualty and the implications of his wounds require special understanding. The authors have seen wounds, which would be deemed as horrendous in civilian practice, utterly disregarded by the men sustaining them. Often the situation appears to change postoperatively when frequent and large doses of analgesia are demanded by the same man. This marked change in pain threshold, or attitude, occurs as the significance of being an amputee at the age of 20 for example, takes root in the patient's mind. The euphoria of survival and the repression of pain gives way to the intense anxiety of trying to project a return to civilian life, to marriage and family. How best to manage this sequence of events is considered in the chapter 'Psychological Response to Disasters' (Chapter 16).

The problems inherent in providing analgesia and anaesthesia will depend on the following factors:

1. The nature and kinetic energy of the missile striking the casualty.
2. The point of impact of the missile and the subsequent trauma produced.
3. The extent and availability of immediate care.
4. The delay likely before evacuation for surgical treatment.

ANALGESIA IN THE FIELD

Alcohol and alkaloids of *Papaver somniferum* traditionally have provided relief to the battle field casualty; rum to the navy and laudanum to the infantry. In more recent times, the emphasis has moved towards refined components of the latter, and morphine sulphate or papaveretum in small self-administered syrettes have been the drugs of first choice for most armies.

The Route of Administration

The accepted guidelines for using opium alkaloid syrettes are for either the wounded man or his 'buddy' to inject the contents of the syrette (morphine 15 mg or papaveretum 30 mg) into a muscle mass, the vastus lateralis or the deltoid being the normal choices. No attempt is to be made at cleaning the skin and injection through clothing is not actively discouraged.

Much criticism has been levelled at these syrettes for many years. Foremost amongst these were the complaints that the needle was too short for adequate intramuscular penetration and the dose of the drug squeezed from the malleable toothpaste tube-like syrette was highly variable. There was little criticism directed at the choice of the drug; opium alkaloids are inexpensive and, if used correctly, provide both analgesia and a degree of euphoria to their recipients. Recent technological advances in the design and construction of a spring-loaded single-use syringe with a longer needle have removed the former points of criticism. Currently at issue is the choice of the most appropriate analgesic and whether intramuscular injection is the best route for the administration of an analgesic.

The average infantry soldier, and often his officer, has an excessive respect for, and an overvalued opinion of, morphine, frequently viewing the drug as potentially life-saving in its own right. Nonetheless, the intramuscular injection of an opiate into a wounded comrade is something that a soldier can be readily trained to do, and does so willingly because the act of injecting the drug is perceived as a duty. In his reviews of the analgesia requirements of American soldiers, Beecher[1,2] questioned whether analgesia needed to be offered to all wounded combatants. The question can be reconsidered today in the light of the increased lethality of the HVR, as to whether a casualty who may have lost 50 per cent of his intravascular volume will be able to perfuse peripheral muscle sufficiently to absorb an intramuscular injection of an opiate. The question might be extended to ask whether the central nervous system in a hypovolaemic patient is significantly further depressed by the absorption of papaveretum 20–30 mg. It has been the authors' experience that the absorption of opiates given in the front line is often delayed until adequate resuscitation is provided. As peripheral perfusion improves, so the one or several doses of opiate are absorbed and may precipitate complete respiratory failure which becomes apparent only at the end of operation or in the immediate postoperative period.

Unless the anaesthetist is aware of this sequence of events, a 'clouding of the consciousness' in the resuscitated casualty may occur. It is not unknown for papaveretum 90–120 mg to have been given en route to a Field Surgical Team (FST) and the reduction in level of consciousness be misinterpreted as resulting from closed intracranial trauma. This error can cause the casualty's priority grading for surgery to be changed and result in a delay or postponement of operation. The judicious use of naloxone under these circumstances can frequently help to clarify the casualty's clinical status.

Considerable interest has been shown in the potential role of sublingual analgesics, not least because of their simplicity in administration. The ability of buprenorphine to provide satisfactory postoperative analgesia has been demonstrated in a series of studies.[3] The authors cannot envisage this technique as being of immediate value in the severely wounded casualty, but its role in both the less severely traumatized preoperative and the postoperative casualty possibly warrants further consideration.

Subcutaneous injection of morphine is an alternative approach; the teaching of this technique to soldiers could be a stumbling block, as would the uncertain rate of absorption in the shocked casualty. Transcutaneous absorption and absorption via the nasal mucosa are further potential routes for the administration of analgesics which have not yet been fully exploited, perhaps because of the potential for addiction in civilian life. In civilian practice, the inhalational route has been used very satisfactorily in the form of 50 per cent nitrous oxide/oxygen premixed in a single cylinder (Entonox) which is self-administered by the patient using a mask or mouthpiece attached to a demand apparatus.[4,5] All emergency ambulances in the UK and many in other countries are equipped with the Entonox apparatus which has proved safe and effective in the hands of ambulancemen over more than 17 years of clinical experience.

However, the relatively bulky and heavy apparatus required makes Entonox unsuitable for field military use but it should be possible to devise an aerosol spray which would permit absorption of a measured dose of analgesic from the lungs. Such a device would have several theoretical advantages, especially in ease of administration in the conscious casualty and in certainty of absorption. Absorption from the bronchi could well approximate to the intravenous absorption profile. Logically, however, the most effective route for the administration of analgesics is directly intravenously. This offers the advantages of speed of onset and accurate control over the dose of drug given. However, it is currently the most difficult practical technique and certainly the most dangerous because of the potential for overdosage prior to the casualty coming under medical supervision. It is suggested that a continuous infusion of low dose opiates has a definitive role in the postoperative management of the casualty but not in the preoperative evacuation phase. Similarly, although a sustained release preparation of morphine could find a place in either situation, careful patient selection is required.[6]

Given that the reliability and performance of the spring-loaded self-administered syringe is now seemingly of a high order, it is considered that, despite its many disadvantages, the intramuscular route of injection, complete with the injection placebo effect on the recipient and sense of duty done for the injector, will remain for the time being the technique of choice for the provision of analgesia in the field.

The Choice of Analgesic

Whether morphine or its derivatives continue to be the correct choice of analgesic drug warrants brief consideration. Morphine and its cogenors are the traditional choice; their many actions are well known and understood, and their reliability proven. The principal disadvantage is depression of depth and rate of respiration, with nausea and vomiting as troublesome side-effects. Morphine is a pure agonist and thought to act upon the Mu and Kappa opioid receptors, to produce analgesia.[7] Two benzomorphan derivatives, pentazocine and nalbuphine, are agonist–antagonist in their central actions; both can precipitate

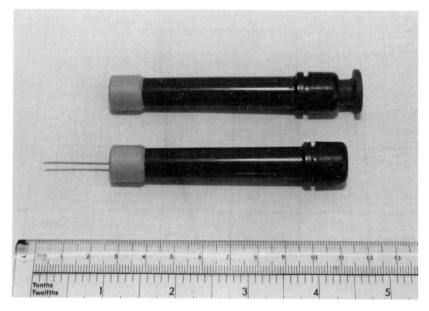

Fig. 4.1. A spring-loaded, self-administered syringe before and after use. (Manufactured by Medimech Ltd, London.)

psychomotor phenomena (pentazocine more than nalbuphine), yet neither possess the analgesic potency of morphine. It should not, however, be possible to depress the respiratory centre to the same extent as with morphine, despite a second or even third dose being injected and absorbed while en route to surgical treatment. It is the authors' contention that, because of the increased safety margin over pure agonist agents, an analgesic such as nalbuphine with agonist–antagonist properties,[8] currently represents the safest approach to the difficult problem of providing analgesia for the battle wounded casualty before he comes under medical supervision.

The British Army has decided to replace the morphine and papaveretum syrettes previously used in battle situations with spring-loaded automatic syrettes filled with nalbuphine (*Fig.* 4.1). Nalbuphine has a low abuse potential and therefore is not subject to the same stringent regulations as morphine. It is important that the contents of an emergency treatment kit are freely available and not locked away in a protected cupboard. Nalbuphine has analgesic properties equipotent with those of papaveretum. Therapeutic doses cause minimal respiratory depression and cumulative doses exceeding 30 mg do not increase the degree of respiratory depression. Nalbuphine has no significant effects on the cardio-vascular system and causes less nausea and vomiting than morphine. The incidence of psychomimetic effects is low.

Burns

The incidence of thermal injury sustained in armed conflicts would appear to be increasing. Armoured fighting vehicles and, more recently, warships have been found to be highly flammable. The crews of both are issued with heat resistant anti-flash clothing, but this is not entirely appropriate to the infantry soldier despite the risk of exposure to phosphorus and other incendiary ordnance. Some protection of the torso and trunk could be expected from the heavier clothing worn by the infantry in cold climates: clearly, this would not be the case in a warm weather war where lightweight shirts and trousers would be worn.

The provision of analgesia and the initial treatment of burns casualties (who may also have sustained additional trauma) must follow clearly defined guide-lines.[9] Burns in excess of 25 per cent of the body surface area (BSA) and especially those with thermal injury to the respiratory tract, are at greatest risk. The pathophysiology of partial and full thickness burns in the first 72 hours post injury (the period of time during which the casualty would be usually treated by an FST) consists of capillary leakage, hypovolaemia, hypoxia and oliguria.[10] The casualty's condition on arrival at the FST will be related to the extent and thickness of the burn and the time for evacuation and may range from minimal systemic disturbance to complete peripheral circulatory failure.

The requirement for analgesia depends upon the area and depth of the burn. Intravenous increments of papaveretum 2 mg or morphine 1 mg will summate with any intramuscular opiate given en route to the FST. Respiratory depression must be avoided. Once analgesia is found to be adequate, it may be maintained by the continuous infusion of relatively low doses of opiates (papaveretum 2–3 mg/h). Alternatively, sub-anaesthetic doses of ketamine, a phencyclidene derivative, $0.5–1.0\,mg\,kg^{-1}\,h^{-1}$ by continuous infusion, has been found to be acceptable under these circumstances. Ketamine has the advantage over opiates because larger doses provide surgical anaesthesia should this become necessary for a tracheostomy to relieve laryngeal oedema, fasciotomy to improve tissue perfusion or simply for a change of dressing. A small dose of a benzodiazepine, midazolam or Diazemuls, will, in most cases, ensure a smooth recovery from anaesthesia without psychomimetic experiences.

Analgesia during evacuation from the FST to the field hospital can be tailored to suit an individual case; sublingual analgesia with buprenorphine has its most appropriate application at this point.

ANAESTHESIA IN THE FIELD

What follows has been written from the standpoint and perspective of a single-handed anaesthetist working with one surgeon in a self-contained and entirely self-supporting surgical unit equipped to receive, operate upon and nurse for up to 72 hours, a total of 50 severely wounded casualties plus as many less severely wounded as can be treated and accommodated.

It therefore behoves the anaesthetist to have familiarized himself with the drugs and equipment at his disposal and to have developed an anaesthetic technique which is simple, safe and relatively speedy both in induction and recovery from anaesthesia.

Given that an FST is furnished with a single operating table, a system for evaluation of the newly arrived casualties and their injuries must be exercised (triage). In a conventional war (non-nuclear, non-chemical, non-biological) normally the most seriously wounded casualties who are deemed likely to survive would receive attention first. This would not necessarily be the case in a mass casualty situation or in a thermonuclear conflict when it could become imperative to operate a reverse triage system.

Anaesthetic Apparatus

The anaesthetic apparatus (the Triservice Apparatus—TSA) currently available to the British military services is based upon the drawover principle and comprises two Oxford Miniature Vaporizers in series (*Fig.* 4.2).[11] The patient delivery system consists of a siliconized self-inflating bag, flexible plastic tubing and a T-piece for the addition of either 1 l/min or 4 l/min of supplemental oxygen to the normal carrier gas which is air. Manual compression of the self-inflating bag provides controlled respiration. Several mechanical ventilators have been used with the TSA to remove the tedium of manual compression and deliver a consistent tidal and minute volume. Many such ventilators have been found to be adequate, but it may be considered ill-advised under field conditions to rely completely upon a relatively sophisticated electro- or pneumatic mechanical device when electrical power or compressed gas may not be continuously available.

Also because of limitation of services, electrically operated cardiac oscilloscopes, defibrillators and coagulation monitors are not yet found on the normal equipment scales of an FST. The monitoring of the anaesthetized patient in the field, of necessity, rests with the unaided fingers, eyes and ears of the anaesthetist.

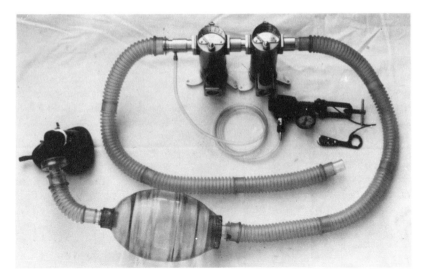

Fig. 4.2. The Tri-Service Anaesthetic Apparatus.
(Reproduced by courtesy of Major M. D. Jowitt, RAMC.)

The Anaesthetist

To be competent in a field environment, an anaesthetist needs to be relatively experienced. Personnel assigned to an FST or to a disaster support team should preferably be of senior registrar (resident) or junior consultant (staff member) status. These criteria are chosen in an attempt to combine experience with physical stamina; the latter requirement is dictated by the uncertain casualty case load, both in numbers and the extent of injury, and by the fact that the working and living conditions will be far removed from the ideal. The military anaesthetist has the same responsibilities of any anaesthetist during the surgical period; to keep the casualty alive, free from pain and in a fit condition for surgery.

Pre-anaesthetic Preparation

Some, but not all, casualties will require resuscitation prior to the induction of anaesthesia; intravenous fluids used before arrival at the FST will normally have been crystalloids, such as Ringer's lactate given via a peripheral vein.[12, 13] Further resuscitation may involve crystalloids, synthetic colloid solutions, 4·5 per cent human albumin, and group compatible blood, if donors ('blood on the hoof') are available. Venous pressure, as an indicator of intravascular volume, can be estimated from the extent of peripheral venous filling in a normothermic patient; this is then mentally integrated with the blood pressure, pulse rate, the pulse volume and character to estimate when sufficient volume has been replaced to optimize the casualty's cardiovascular system prior to surgery.

Whilst the use of fresh group compatible blood is clearly not ideal, two or three units have undoubtedly saved many lives in the field, not least because the active coagulation factors are sufficient to abort disseminated intravascular coagulation. The intraoperative scavenging and autotransfusion of autologous blood remains to be fully assessed for use in the field; similarly, it is doubtful if deep-frozen blood could be reconstituted in sufficient time for immediate use in a disaster situation or armed conflict occurring *de novo*. Nevertheless, the provision of stored blood to the battle field or to a civilian disaster in the developed world is ultimately a question of logistics. In the developing world it is doubtful whether the logistic back-up would be in place. Synthetic 'bloods' have been developed for use in disasters and war; the best known and most researched oxygen-carrying solution to date has been the perflurocarbon, Fluosol DA. At present this compound lacks a significant role in clinical practice in most countries and seems unlikely to fulfil its original expectations. An alternative to synthetic blood is stroma-free haemoglobin solution; this is retained within the circulation for 90 minutes and warrants consideration as an appropriate replacement fluid in the resuscitative period immediately before the surgical control of bleeding.

ANAESTHESIA

Induction of anaesthesia should commence only when the anaesthetist is sure that the casualty is in optimum condition given the facilities available. The surgeon and anaesthetist should be ever mindful of the 60 minutes of surgery rule and the likely nature and extent of the proposed surgery. This latter aspect can, in some cases, be little more than a guess as the extent of tissue trauma caused by a HVR within a body cavity is impossible to predict with any certainty.

All fresh battle casualties must be assumed to have a full stomach irrespective of the interval between the time of injury and the time of surgery. Consequently, they must be intubated and it is logical to ventilate them for the duration of the surgical procedure. An essential requirement for field anaesthesia is that the patients should recover quickly and be able to protect their own airway as soon as possible.

Premedication

The decision as to whether or not to order premedication for the casualty must be guided by the casualty's overall condition, by the elapsed time since the last dose of opiate received during his evacuation and the extent to which it has been absorbed, and by the likelihood of commencing his operation within 30–60 minutes of premedication. As a general rule, the authors have found it better practice to give an intravenous dose of an analgesic (e.g. fentanyl 50–100 μg) towards the end of the preoxygenation period, with a small dose of atropine (titrated against heart rate), rather than to attempt a formal intramuscular or oral premedication routine.

Oxygenation and Oxygen Supply

A period of preoxygenation is indicated in all but the lightly wounded casualty; an acceptable level of oxygenation can be achieved within two minutes by encouraging the casualty to breath deeply via the Triservice Apparatus, adding oxygen at a rate of 4 l/min, which results in an inspired oxygen concentration approaching 70 per cent ($FIO_2 = 0\cdot7$). A longer period of preoxygenation is required in patients with ventilation perfusion mismatch associated with trauma; however, the anaesthetist needs to balance clinical acceptability with the necessity to conserve oxygen, for resupply can be uncertain.

The provision of oxygen in the field is a major problem. The small portable cylinders contain only 340 litres of oxygen, are heavy to carry in any number, and are very difficult to refill. There is a real need for a suitable portable oxygen concentrator or oxygen generator.[15]

The oxygen concentrator uses a molecular sieve of zeolite, an hydrated double silicate with ion exchange properties, to produce nitrogen depleted air. Molecular sieve devices will deliver an oxygen concentration of up to 95 per cent, but the concentration varies inversely with the flow. Size and lack of reliability of the time cycling mechanism, which allows rejuvenation of the zeolite to take place, has prevented their extensive use until recently. A concentrator also requires maintenance.

The oxygen generator requires only electrical power and hydrogen peroxide as fuel. A precious metal catalyst is used to promote the dissociation of the fuel. The transportation of hydrogen peroxide in tanks or disposable containers is simple and safe, and the apparatus is light enough to be easily transported. The oxygen generator requires very little attention since the only moving part is a cooling fan, and operation of the apparatus is very simple.

Induction

Despite being over half a century old, sodium thiopentone remains the standard intravenous induction agent by which all others are judged; it is the induction agent favoured by one of the authors. Loss of consciousness is generally easily achieved with a dose of 2–3 mg/kg. The cardiorespiratory depression is both consistent and dose-dependent and must be allowed for when considering premedication for the casualty. The required dose of thiopentone can be minimized, as previously noted, by the injection of fentanyl 50–100 µg (or an equipotent dose of alfentanil) shortly before beginning the injection of the barbiturate. The exact weight of the casualty is seldom available to the anaesthetist; a best guess must therefore be used to estimate the induction dose of thiopentone. In recent years, the only competitors with thiopentone for the induction of anaesthesia in the field have been the opiates and ketamine. Enormous doses of opiates were used by Davidson and Cotev[16] in the Arab-Israeli war, using as much as 3 mg/kg of morphine reversed with naloxone. The technique was successful because the Israeli evacuation chain was extremely rapid and the facilities of a base hospital were immediately available to support the initial surgery and anaesthesia. Ketamine 2 mg/kg intravenously was used by Jowitt and Knight[17] during the 1982 Falklands campaign. Ketamine is an analgesic and simultaneously stimulates the cardiovascular system producing peripheral vasoconstriction and an increase in heart rate as a result of its action directly on the central nervous system.

Notwithstanding ketamine's proven success as an induction agent in hypovolaemic patients,[18] several other aspects of the drug's pharmacology warrant consideration. In critically ill patients ketamine may, unexpectedly, drop the blood pressure, produce vasodilation and depress the myocardium. Less dramatic but more frequently troublesome is the known propensity for ketamine to produce bizarre psychomimetic effects. One of the authors has seen an hallucinating postoperative casualty fighting and struggling to such an extent as to require restraint, disrupting his wounds, and his fellow patients' sleep. Ketamine should be used only in combination with the benzodiazepine, midazolam, which minimizes these psychomimetic effects.

Several new induction agents have recently become available and an extensive literature already exists relating to their properties. None, as yet, has reportedly been used on the battlefield casualty. The imidazole derivative, etomidate, offers rapid onset of action and recovery, with marked cardiovascular stability.[19] The substituted phenols (alkylphenols) of which propofol is the most successful to date, would appear capable of being compared favourably with thiopentone.[20] As no single induction agent currently available approaches the ideal, various drug combinations are becoming increasingly popular. A combination of drugs having similar pharmacokinetics, producing total intravenous anaesthesia, is perhaps the key to future successful anaesthesia in the field. Total intravenous anaesthesia, with its current and projected role in the field, is discussed separately.

Considerable emphasis has been placed upon the difficulties involved in evacuating casualties to surgical treatment; notwithstanding the evacuation interval (ideally less than 6 hours), the effects of analgesics, anticholinergics, fear and pain on gastric motility, it is deemed advisable to consider all casualties coming to surgery to have a full stomach, and to treat them accordingly. The authors have chosen to put their trust in the preoxygenation—cricoid pressure—sleep dose of thiopentone-depolarizing relaxant sequence rather than to attempt a pharmacological or nasogastric emptying of the stomach in the awake patient. The latter is avoided as convulsive retching in a patient with severe injury and a compromised cardiovascular system can only detract from a smooth induction of anaesthesia. Gastric intubation and aspiration may be attempted once anaesthesia is established and the airway protected with a cuffed endotracheal tube.

Red rubber endotracheal tubes, which are re-usable, are more appropriate to field anaesthesia than the disposable single-use plastic tubes which occupy a considerable volume of available storage space and do not withstand repeated sterilization in a cold water solution. A full range of endotracheal tubes should be carried as civilian casualties of any age may come to surgery.

Maintenance of Anaesthesia

Maintenance of anaesthesia is achieved by the vaporization of volatile agents in air, with or without additional oxygen as clinically indicated. A flow of additional oxygen of 1 l/min produces an FiO_2 of approximately 0·3. In the more severely injured it may be necessary to use the higher flow of additional oxygen until the patient's condition stabilizes.[21] For most operations, particularly body surface debridement, experience has shown that once a surgical plane of anaesthesia has been achieved, additional oxygen may be safely withdrawn and air alone used to vaporize the chosen volatile agents. The Oxford Miniature Vaporizer (OMV) can satisfactorily vaporize all the currently available agents, including diethyl ether. The combination of halothane and trichloroethylene has been the most commonly used to date, the former for its hypnotic and the latter for its analgesic effect. It is to be anticipated that ethrane or its isomer isoflurane may replace trichloroethylene but both are considerably more expensive and lack the analgesic property of the older agent.

The volatile agents are used in the lowest possible concentration compatible with reaching and retaining an acceptable surgical plane of anaesthesia. To ensure a rapid return to consciousness, it is normally necessary to withdraw trichloroethylene some 10–15 minutes before the operation ends. The different blood/gas solubility coefficients of halothane, ethrane and isoflurane require a modification of this timing.

The majority of patients will be electively intubated and the anaesthetist must decide whether to allow the patient to breathe unaided or to paralyse and ventilate. Spontaneous ventilation in casualties with modest peripheral wounds or body surface trauma can be considered as safe. Whichever technique is chosen, the anaesthetist must, on occasion, be free to leave the operating area to visit briefly both pre- and postoperative patients. To do this he must have absolute confidence in the skill of the operating room staff and, in particular, his anaesthetic assistant. The requirement for adequate training and flexibility within the team cannot be over-emphasized when considering surgical and anaesthetic aides. Similarly, the creation and maintenance of a high morale within a surgical team, particularly when working in a difficult situation, is of paramount importance to success.

Curare, introduced to clinical practice during the Second World War, was for many years the non-depolarizing relaxant of choice for field anaesthesia; however, the cardiovascular stability of the steroid based relaxants have proved them to be safer. Pancuronium bromide, the original member of this family, has been succeeded by vecuronium bromide.[22] This new relaxant does not cause tachycardia and has the major advantage, from the field anaesthetist's viewpoint, of being presented as a powder, so removing any temperature constraints on its storage or use world-wide in adverse climates. For a non-depolarizing relaxant with a shorter duration of action, alcuronium chloride seems unlikely to be replaced by atracurium besylate since the latter, despite the theoretical advantages of the Hoffman elimination pattern, needs to be refrigerated at 2°–8°C. Many differing factors need to be considered in determining the correct dose of relaxant for the individual casualty, such as the cardiovascular volume, the core temperature, the choice of inhalational agent and the dose and timing of preoperative analgesia. It is the authors' practice to estimate the weight of the patient, calculate the dose of relaxant (vecuronium 0·1 mg/kg) and to administer deliberately not more than 75 per cent of this dose. In casualties who are severely wounded, 50 per cent of the estimated dose will, in most cases, prove to be sufficient for a one hour procedure.

Intra-operative analgesia has, in the past, been produced by pethidine and morphine, the former being used only in small increments to circumvent hypotension. Pethidine is effective in attenuating the tachypnoea associated with tricholoroethylene. The same parameters as for relaxant dosage need to be considered when estimating the appropriate dose of analgesic; ideally, naloxone should not be required at the completion of a field anaesthetic. Fentanyl was the analgesic chosen by the authors during the Falklands campaign, principally for its haemodynamic stability. The newer, intensely analgesic, yet shorter acting derivatives of fentanyl may well prove to be yet more effective than the parent compound.

Regional Analgesia

There has been much speculation about the correct place of regional analgesia in war surgery; it is the authors' contention that, provided that the anaesthetist is confident of his skills, an appropriate block can be performed rapidly either immediately before, or after, surgery, preferably with bupivacaine. It should be performed principally to provide postoperative analgesia without the risk of nausea and respiratory depression. A satisfactory block benefits both patient and nursing team, and femoral nerve block may be considered as an example of this philosophy in patients with injuries to the thigh. However, there is no point in attempting a block for surgery, wasting 20 minutes to test its effectiveness or otherwise, and then having to resort to general anaesthesia. The sophisticated nursing techniques demanded for the correct postoperative management of intra- and extradural anaesthesia may not be available to a small surgical team. The near certainty of further evacuation, often with little warning, by road or air, tends to mitigate further against intradural anaesthesia. Caudally administered bupivacaine, as an alternative to intramuscular opiate has been found to be effective in relieving the pain of trench foot for as long as 6 hours. Intradural opiates might be considered for postoperative analgesia provided the situation was static and evacuation not anticipated for 24 hours; delayed respiratory arrest in a helicopter at night would be a difficult complication! A report of intrathecal ketamine appeared recently[23] but its role in military anaesthesia is unclear at present. The absence of hypotension or respiratory depression is attractive but central side-effects and short duration of surgical anaesthesia would appear to limit this application of the drug.

The field anaesthetist needs to preserve peripheral veins whenever possible, and to remain aware of the probability that the casualty will probably have one or more subsequent anaesthetics in the ensuing five to ten days. Clearly, sensitivity to halothane is a theoretical possibility in these circumstances. In assessing patients with postoperative jaundice, it should be taken into account that many of the casualties not only have had exposure to halothane, but also have been given units of unscreened and uncrossmatched blood during initial resuscitation.

Total Intravenous Anaesthesia

The use of total intravenous anaesthesia (TIVA) in the military context has been under a cloud ever since the fateful events of 7th December 1941 in Pearl Harbor. Lack of knowledge of the actions of thiopentone, particularly of its profound cardiovascular and respiratory depressant effects when used in large doses as the sole agent, led to disastrous consequences. At that time, all experience with the drug had been obtained in routine civilian practice and not with the injuries of war. This led Halford[24] to state that 'intravenous anaesthesia is an ideal method of euthanasia'.

The British Army Medical Services have had an interest for a long time in the use of TIVA and experience had been gained using Althesin and pentazocine by

Jago and Restall.[25] This was halted abruptly by the removal of Althesin from clinical availability by the manufacturers. The present interest in TIVA was stimulated by the problem of how to anaesthetize battle casualties in an operating theatre which was 'closed down' against a chemical weapon attack. The use of inhalational agents in a closed environment without a sophisticated extraction system leads rapidly to considerable pollution of the theatre, to the detriment of the personnel working in the area. Charcoal absorbers would provide a solution to the problem but they are bulky to carry and have to be regenerated or resupplied. Also, many patients will receive more than one anaesthetic and if halothane is not used on the first occasion the choice of anaesthetic method to be used at a later date will be much easier. The feasibility of using a mixture of ketamine, midazolam and vecuronium to fulfil the 'triad' of anaesthesia—namely hypnosis, suppression of unwanted reflexes and relaxation is currently being investigated by one of the authors (J.R.).

Ketamine has been available for use as an induction and maintenance drug since 1970. Its slow onset and relatively prolonged duration of action, together with the high incidence of adverse reactions during recovery have meant that ketamine has not been widely used for intravenous infusion. Cardiovascular stimulation and the production of reasonable analgesia make it an attractive drug in the treatment of hypovolaemic trauma patients. Patient acceptability of induction is very good; it produces bronchodilatation and the airway is not compromised postoperatively.

The combination of ketamine with a benzodiazepine has long been recognized as advantageous because of the complementary pharmacodynamic effects of benzodiazepines in producing muscle relaxation, anxiolysis, central sedation and in attenuating the emergence sequelae and cardio-stimulation of ketamine. Diazepam was used originally, but midazolam is better with a shorter half-life.

Vecuronium, a non-depolarizing muscle relaxant, is prepared as a buffered freeze-dried powder, which is easy to store at extremes of temperature and has a shelf life of at least three years. It has a stabilizing effect on the cardiovascular system and despite being a derivative of pancuronium it does not produce tachycardia. Minimal histamine release has been reported making it better than pancuronium and much better than atracurium and d-tubocurarine in this respect. It is non-cumulative and the breakdown products are innocuous. Reversal of the neuromuscular block by anticholinesterases is necessary.

After induction with midazolam 0·07 mg/kg, ketamine 1 mg/kg and vecuronium 0·1 mg/kg, the patients are intubated and ventilated. Anaesthesia is maintained with the following mixture:

Midazolam   5 mg ⎫
Ketamine   200 mg ⎬ made up to 50 ml with normal saline
Vecuronium   12 mg ⎭

This is infused, using a battery driven syringe pump, at an infusion rate of:

$$\frac{\text{Patient's weight in kg}}{2} \text{ in ml/h}$$

Ketamine, midazolam and vecuronium are all water soluble, have an approximate pH of 5 and mix without any precipitation or apparent diminution of their properties. The mixture is stable and can be used at least 24 hours after preparation. This means that if a heavy load of casualties is expected a litre bag of the infusate can be prepared at the beginning of the day. The technique is safe, cheap, flexible and non-polluting. When used with an air-entraining ventilator, the anaesthetist can have both hands free and, should the situation demand, the patient can be monitored by an assistant without any great difficulty.

Propofol (Diprivan), an oil-in-water emulsion, has recently been introduced as a short-acting intravenous anaesthetic suitable for both induction and maintenance of anaesthesia. It is prepared in 20 ml ampoules containing 1 per cent w/v of propofol. It must not be frozen and should not be mixed with other therapeutic agents or infusion fluids prior to administration. During induction there is a significant decrease in arterial blood pressure but little change in heart rate. A period of apnoea often occurs, and some patients will require controlled ventilation. Anaesthesia can be maintained with propofol by intermittent injection of incremental doses or by continuous infusion. Recovery after anaesthesia is very rapid and the patients are remarkably clear-headed.

CONCLUSIONS

There is a very considerable need for resuscitation, analgesia and general anaesthesia in the field. The standard must be of the highest and should not fall short of that expected in normal civilian life. There is a very real place for general, as opposed to regional, anaesthesia in the disaster or field situation. The Tri-Service Apparatus is a simple, easy to use, portable apparatus which can provide safe inhalation anaesthesia. We believe that the ketamine, midazolam, vecuronium mixture has provided a genuine and simple intravenous alternative.

Most importantly, any technique which is to be used in the field must be practised during cold surgical lists—the disaster situation is not the time for experimentation or the use of previously untried methods.

REFERENCES

1. Beecher H. K. (1955) The powerful placebo. *JAMA* **159**, 1602.
2. Beecher H. K. (1959) *Measurement of Subjective Response.* New York, Oxford University Press.
3. Kay B. and Cohen A. T. (1983) Postoperative pain relief (1): partial agonist/antagonist narcotic analgesics. *Hospital Update* **9**, 181–8.
4. Baskett P. J. F. and Withnell A. (1970) The use of Entonox in the ambulance service *Br. Med. J.* **2**, 41–3.
5. Stewart R. D. (1985) Nitrous oxide sedation/analgesia in emergency medicine. *Ann. Emerg. Med.* **14**, 139–48.
6. Derbyshire D. R., Bell A., Parry P. A. et al. (1985) Morphine sulphate for slow release. *Br. J. Anaesth.* **57**, 858–65.
7. Pert C. B. and Snyder S. H. (1973) Opiate receptor; its demonstration in nervous tissue. *Science* **179**, 1011–14.
8. Houde R. W. (1979) Analgesic effectiveness of the narcotic agonists–antagonists. *Br. J. Clin. Pharmacol.* **7**, 2975–3085.
9. Carson J. S. (1979) *Treatment of Burns.* London, Chapman and Hall.
10. Davies J. W. L. (1982) *Physiological Responses to Burning Injury.* London, Academic Press.
11. Houghton I. T. (1981) The Triservice Anaesthetic Apparatus. *Anaesthesia* **36**, 1094–1108.
12. Smith J. A. R. and Norman J. N. (1982) The fluid of choice for resuscitation of severe shock. *Br. J. Surg.* **69**, 702–5.

13. Williams J. G., Riley T. R. D. and Moody R. A. (1983) Resuscitation experience in the Falkland Islands campaign. *Br. Med. J.* **286**, 775.
14. Kirby N. G. and Blackburn G. (1981) *Field Surgery Pocket Book.* Her Majesty's Stationery Office, London.
15. Hall L. W., Kellagher R. E. B. and Fleet K. J. (1986) A portable oxygen generator. *Anaesthesia* **41**, 516–18.
16. Davidson J. T. and Cotev S. (1975) Anaesthesia in the Yom Kippur War. *Ann. R. Coll. Surg. Engl.* **56**, 304–11.
17. Jowitt M. D. and Knight R. J. (1983) Anaesthesia during the Falklands campaign. *Anaesthesia* **38**, 776–83.
18. Bond A. C. and Davis C. K. (1979) Ketamine and pancuronium for the shocked patient. *Anaesthesia* **39**, 1023–8.
19. Tarnow J., Hess W. and Klein W. (1980) Etomidate, Althesin and thiopentone as induction agents for coronary artery surgery. *Can. Anaesth. Soc. J.* **27**, 338–44.
20. Bahar M., Dundee J. W., O'Neill M. P. et al. (1983) Recovery from intravenous anaesthesia: comparison of disoprofol with thiopentone and methohexitone. *Anaesthesia* **37**, 1171–5.
21. Boulton T. B. (1978) Editorial. *Anaesthesia* **33**, 769–71.
22. Miller R. D., Rupp S. M., Fisher D. M. et al. (1984) Clinical pharmacology of vecuronium and atracurium. *Anesthesiology* **61**, 444–53.
23. Bion J. F. (1984) Intrathecal ketamine for war surgery. A preliminary study under field conditions. *Anaesthesia* **39**, 1023–8.
24. Halford F. J. (1943) A critique of intravenous anaesthesia in war surgery. *Anesthesiology* **4**, 67–9.
25. Jago R. H. and Restall J. (1977) Total intravenous anaesthesia. A technique based on alphaxalone/alphadolone and pentazocine. *Anaesthesia* **32**, 904–7.

Management Aspects

P. E. A. Savage

5

Disaster Planning in Developed Countries

INTRODUCTION

Over the past 30 years or so there has been a steady increase in the published literature on the management of casualties following natural and man-made disasters,[1-6] and a number of useful manuals have been produced to assist emergency service and hospital disaster planners.[7-13] The partial or complete failure of so many plans when a disaster occurs is not for the lack of information or guidance!

Developments in the science of disaster planning have been hindered somewhat by vagueness in terminology which has not yet been resolved. Even the word 'disaster' has not found universal acceptance although it is used in the *Index Medicus*. Planning for the care of a motorway pile-up involving 50 or so casualties differs in degree, if not in principle, from the management of thousands or hundreds of thousands of dead and injured following a natural disaster such as an earthquake or a typhoon. Attempts have been made to define the scale of disasters.[14] (*Table 5.1.*) As the world becomes more industrialized, the risk of national or international disasters following chemical or radiation incidents becomes more relevant to disaster planners. Another example where lack of standardization can cause confusion is the use of terminology in categorizing casualties according to the extent and nature of their injuries. This process of assessment or triage is fundamental to the management of mass casualties, yet there is often no national, let alone international, agreement on triage categories to be used in civilian disasters. Lack of agreement also applies to a system of casualty labelling at the disaster site and in the receiving hospital, where confusion can arise when a number of different labelling systems are in use at the

Table 5.1. Classification of disasters.

Category	No. of casualties dead or alive	No. of casualties admitted
Minor disaster	25–100	10–50
Moderate disaster	100–1000	50–250
Major disaster	>1000	>250

(Reproduced by courtesy of Rutherford and de Boer, 1983.)[14]

same time. Many authors have addressed this problem with little success in persuading others that their system has overwhelming advantages. A major difficulty in disaster planning is to know what stage a hospital or country has reached in its health care development. This was forcibly brought home to the author when he attended an international disaster conference held in a luxurious 5-star hotel at which the full range of disaster topics was thoroughly discussed. Yet a few miles away in the local town, all the ambulances were out of action and the hospital was incapable of providing basic health care for the local population, let alone an emergency capability for a disaster of whatever size. The concepts discussed in this chapter, and some of the proposals put forward may not be applicable to all hospitals and countries, yet they are current problems in disaster management that cannot be ignored.

TRIAGE

For some decades now, the word 'triage' has been used to describe the process of sorting casualties into various groups. However, the word triage implies two distinct processes. Not only are casualties sorted into categories depending on the severity of their injuries, but the categories will depend on what facilities can be provided at the time in terms of personnel and equipment. There are occasions when critically ill casualties have to be put to one side while the less severely injured, who have a greater chance of recovery, receive active treatment. Most modern triage classifications consist of four categories of casualty: those needing immediate resuscitation and life-saving measures; those needing urgent treatment; the 'walking wounded'; and the expectant or palliative group, the nature or extent of whose injuries are such as to make survival unlikely, regardless of the time and care taken in their treatment.[15, 16] The process of triage is a continuous one. At the disaster site the triage category influences the priority for evacuation, but needs to be interpreted sensibly. There is little point in keeping 50 or so non-urgent casualties in unsatisfactory conditions at the site, while the emergency services spend an hour or so extricating more seriously injured but trapped casualties. In most disasters it is the less seriously injured who are able to walk away from the site—and who will often enter the first available ambulance. At the emergency department entrance, the triage process is the key to effective mass casualty management. It is vital that resuscitation rooms and urgent treatment areas are reserved for those casualties who need these facilities.

Table 5.2. Standards of care

Optimum care	IDT completed within 12 h of injury.
Near optimum care	IDT completed within 24 h of injury.
	IDT delay beyond the optimum period of 12 h in non-threatening and low-morbidity injuries.
Delayed care	IDT cannot be completed for all casualties within 24 h from time of injury. Additional delay in IDT for selected low-morbidity injuries is accepted.
Temporary austere care	Mass casualty standards for 36–48 h with the expectation of reverting to better standards.
Extended austere care	The workload requires use of mass casualty standards for an extended period.

(**IDT** = initial definitive treatment.)
(Reproduced by courtesy of Berlin R. (1974) The role of the medical services. In: Sillar W. (ed.) *A Guide to Disaster Management*. Glasgow, Action For Disaster.)[17]

The non-urgent 'walking wounded' should be directed to another area altogether, and dead casualties taken to the mortuary.

Deciding on priorities for use of operating rooms is another key triage point, and requires decisions to be made by a designated senior member of the surgical staff. Here again, the facilities and medical and nursing staff available will influence the decision as to who should be operated on immediately, and who will have to wait. However, surgery for the less severely injured should not be unnecessarily delayed, while waiting for the critically injured who may never arrive. It is important to get on with the operative workload as soon as possible, provided that two operating rooms can be kept ready to receive casualties requiring life-saving surgery.

During World War II, 70 per cent of battle casualties received definitive surgical treatment of their injuries within 12 hours of being wounded. It was also possible for a well-trained and equipped surgical team to perform 7 emergency life-saving operations on severely wounded soldiers in a 12-hour session. These standards should be achievable by civilian hospitals in peace-time disasters. During any disaster it is important at an early stage to decide on what standards of care can be provided.[17] This relates very closely to the provision of initial definitive treatment of an individual casualty's injuries (*Table* 5.2). In order to reduce mortality and morbidity, it is obvious that the factor which limits an individual hospital's capability of providing ideal care for disaster victims is not the number of beds available, or the size of the emergency department, but the number of operating rooms that can be staffed and run continuously.

PRE-HOSPITAL MANAGEMENT

'Buddycare'

Following any serious accident, it is highly unlikely that skilled medical, paramedical or nursing attention will be immediately available, and a casualty's survival from a life-threatening event such as a blocked airway, respiratory or cardiac arrest, or exsanguinating external haemorrhage will depend on immediate assistance from a passer-by (or 'buddy') who is able to perform basic life support techniques.

The ABC of basic life support—airway, breathing and circulation—has been extensively documented and many excellent manuals are available for those interested in learning and teaching the techniques (*see* Chapter 3).[18] Studies in North America and Scandinavia have confirmed the value and safety of basic life support education programmes directed at secondary school children and adults. Although resuscitation skills decline rapidly if not used regularly, the quality of resuscitation attempts does not appear to affect the outcome significantly.

First Aid Societies

Organizations such as the Red Cross and St John Ambulance Brigade provide training courses and certificates of competence for those interested in learning first aid, and their members play a valuable part in society. Their skills are readily available at any time of night and day, in the home, at work or at sporting events. Following an accident in a country where these societies flourish, there is a good chance that a first aider will soon be on the scene. Following a disaster, the skills of these organized groups may be utilized to assist in dealing with casualties at the site, or in providing support for hard-pressed nursing staff in medical facilities.

Immediate Care Schemes

Family doctors, particularly in rural areas, have always been prepared to render immediate care to the victims of accidents while awaiting the arrival of an ambulance to transport the injured to hospital. During the past three decades or so, there has been an increase in the number of immediate care schemes in which a group of doctors have agreed to work together to provide a sophisticated rapid medical response, principally for road accident victims, but also for other kinds of accident.[19]

The essential elements of a successful immediate care scheme are that the practitioners should be well trained and equipped to deal with all life-threatening emergencies. They need a good communications system to be able to respond rapidly to emergency calls, and require the personality and communication skills to get on well with a wide variety of people, particularly members of the emergency services and with hospital-based colleagues. Above all they need to be enthusiasts!

Accident Flying Squads

In urban areas it is more usual to find accident flying squads based at hospitals with major accident units. Doctors may ride the ambulances as a matter of routine, but apart from training sessions, this is often a waste of skilled staff. More usually, trained and equipped doctors and nurses are taken to the scene of any significant accident, particularly if casualties are trapped and their extrication is likely to take some time.

Before embarking on setting up such a flying squad, hospital authorities need to reassure themselves that a number of criteria has been fulfilled. The experience and seniority of the medical and nursing team members must be appropriate to the tasks they will be expected to perform. Their equipment should be simple to use and suitably packed in easily transportable and accessible units. Their clothing needs to afford adequate protection from the weather and the hazards of the accident site, and be labelled for ease of identification. Following any incident in which the flying squad is dispatched, a full debriefing takes place within a reasonable period of time. In view of the risks involved in disaster site work, adequate personal insurance needs to be arranged for team members.[20, 21]

Paramedic: Advanced Trained Ambulance Crews

The training and experience of ambulance crews varies from country to country. In North America, particularly, the paramedic has become a highly-trained individual capable of carrying out resuscitation at the incident site using both basic and advanced life support techniques. There was a danger of some of these groups becoming almost autonomous in their professional activities, but it has generally been recognized that strict and continuous monitoring of their performance by doctors experienced in emergency medicine is necessary to prevent patient care being compromised by overzealous or inappropriate treatment.

Where the paramedic is an integrated member of the ambulance service, his or her skills may be invaluable in the care of disaster victims. Being familiar with the difficulties of carrying out resuscitation techniques in accident situations, the paramedic may be more skilled than a doctor who is used to working in a hospital environment.

SITE ORGANIZATION

Introduction

Disaster sites are chaotic and dangerous places, and not ones into which untrained or unsupervised individuals should venture. The objectives in bringing order out of this chaos is to save life, reduce or remove hazards and eventually to clear up the mess. The emergency services of fire and rescue, the police and the ambulance services are trained and equipped to achieve these objectives, each service working within the framework of its own organization and discipline. Optimum management of a disaster site requires that all emergency services work closely together with a pre-agreed system of mutual consultation and a multidisciplinary system of communication and command (*Fig.* 5.1). First aid and medical services are integrated into this system, usually in association with the ambulance service. Whenever an accident of any significance occurs, an initial response by units of the fire, police and ambulance services occurs. Depending on the size of the incident and the number of likely casualties, a 'disaster' may be declared which automatically leads to a more extensive

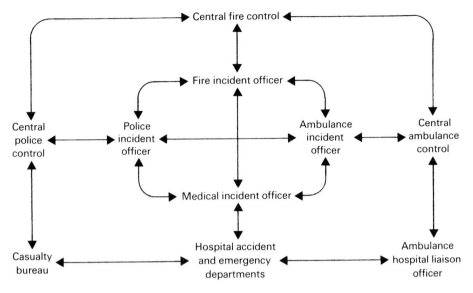

Fig. 5.1. Interservice communications at a disaster site.
(Reproduced by courtesy of Hines K. C. (1985) The medical incident officer and the mobile medical team. In: Robertson B. (ed.) *Guide to Major Incident Management.* Ipswich, British Association for Immediate Care.)[13]

mobilization of the emergency services, the alerting of appropriate medical facilities and the setting up of the agreed chain of emergency service command.

The Fire Service[22]

Historically, the first fire brigades were introduced to save life and to protect property resulting from major fires. This role has been extended in the modern fire service to the saving of life in any emergency situation, and in many countries has been combined with the job of extrication and rescue of victims, tasks that often require special knowledge, expertise and equipment. The main feature of a modern fire service is that each fire appliance is manned by a resourceful and disciplined group of men who have been trained not only to use the equipment available but to work together as a team. At a disaster site, most fire services have at their disposal a control vehicle which provides the commanding officers with additional communications facilities as well as reference files of data relevant to the incident and its locality. All officers in charge of an incident, whatever its size, are aware of the importance of control and co-ordination of manpower and resources, so that an appropriate response to a rapidly changing situation may be made.

The Police Service[23]

Following an incident of any size, police officers will arrive at an early stage. Like their colleagues in the fire service, their prime objectives are to preserve life and to protect property, but once the fire service is dealing with this aspect of the disaster, the responsibility of securing the site and establishing priority routes of access, including routes to hospitals, falls to the police. Identification of injured and dead victims and the provision of casualty lists have urgent priority with the setting up of a casualty bureau. Sightseers and volunteers will often need firm but tactful directions, property must be protected from criminal elements who may take advantage of the confusion, and evidence sought and recorded of factors that may have contributed to the disaster. The police are usually the only emergency service which has the legal authority to give an order to citizens of a country, and this includes members of other emergency services. The senior police officer, therefore, co-ordinates the activities of the other two emergency services, the 'incident officers' conferring together on plans of action of their individual services.

The Ambulance Service[24]

The primary objectives of the ambulance service during a disaster are to provide sufficient ambulances, manpower and equipment to deal with all casualty needs at the site while maintaining an adequate emergency service for the rest of the community. The principles of on-site management are much the same as for the fire and police services. Once the magnitude of the incident is recognized by the crew of the first attending ambulance, they must immediately 'think big'. Their task is no longer to aid the injured, but to make as complete an assessment of the situation as circumstances permit, and to pass the message back to ambulance control. Whenever a disaster is reported, or sometimes merely suspected, the senior controlling officer opens a specially prepared major incident sub-control which is equipped with all necessary task sheets, check lists, maps and special plans for particular disaster sites such as airports, dockyards, oil installations, petrochemical works, conventional and nuclear power stations. The opening of a reserved emergency radio channel is an important step in maintaining lines of communication between ambulance control, the site and medical facilities, while allowing everyday radio traffic to continue uninterrupted. The ambulance incident officer has a key role in the organization of the management of casualties. An experienced officer with knowledge of the resources at his disposal and the capabilities of nearby hospitals, he is able to make appropriate arrangements for the extrication, assessment, stabilization and transport of casualties to medical facilities.

Extrication of trapped casualties is usually possible by fire or rescue teams without the intervention of medical personnel, as modern powered equipment enables the rapid and safe removal of any metal or other material from around the casualty. However, there is no doubt that if extrication is going to be difficult or prolonged, or if the casualty is unconscious or suffering from severe injuries, the presence of a doctor trained and experienced in this type of work is invaluable. Even when medical intervention is not indicated, rescue workers are often reassured by a medical presence to whom they can turn immediately for advice should a problem arise that would risk further injury to the trapped casualty. An assessment of the likelihood of casualties being trapped and the need to summon medical assistance is an urgent task of the ambulance incident officer. After any disaster, the dazed and shocked victims and those suffering from minor injuries (the 'walking wounded') are the first to leave the immediate disaster area. Casualty collection stations are identified in a safe area, preferably under cover, where an initial triage is carried out by an experienced casualty selection officer. It is this officer who decides on priority for transportation. Stretcher bearers are mustered at assembly points and are sent forward as required to carry out victims. Four men per stretcher are required for anything but the shortest distance over easy territory.

The ambulance incident officer arranges with the police incident officer for ambulance parking points to be sited and identified, and from here ambulances are called forward to casualty loading points adjacent to the casualty collecting stations. Routes to and from the site and medical facilities are arranged and kept clear by the police force.

Although every disaster is likely to be unique in some respects, the characteristic feature of nearly every disaster is that a general organizational plan of management can be applied to each one. One of the difficulties at the site is for one individual, however experienced, to be able to grasp all the changing facets and make appropriate decisions on all aspects of casualty management. The casualty evacuation plan is a key measure in site disaster management and one to which considerable thought and planning should have been devoted before any disaster occurs. The elements of the plan take into account the size and location of the disaster; the number and type of casualties, particularly the likely number of trapped casualties or difficulties in entering or leaving the site; the proximity of medical facilities and the travelling time both during the day and night; and the resources of medical facilities in terms of skilled personnel, beds and operating rooms. In some situations, the ambulance incident officer can formulate and execute the casualty evacuation plan from the site ambulance control; in others, this may be done centrally from ambulance control. However, on many occasions a more central command involving ambulance and medical participation is appropriate. This becomes part of a community disaster plan.

The confirmation of death by a medical practitioner is a legal requirement which must be complied with before corpses can be removed to an official mortuary. This is often an unpleasant and gruesome task with which to burden doctors who have already spent time and energy in treating the injured. Arrangements whereby pathologists attend the temporary mortuary officially to certify death overcome this problem.

All the incident officers need to be easily identified by labelled jackets, and their control posts or vehicles suitably sited and clearly identified by an appropriate flag or notice during the day, or by a flashing emergency light at night. An order should be made that the emergency flashing lights of all other emergency vehicles are turned off.

The Medical Incident Officer

The role of doctors at disaster sites remains controversial. Untrained and inexperienced doctors often cause more problems than they solve. In situations where there is a well co-ordinated ambulance service response, the ambulance incident officer may well have the experience and confidence to direct the process of triage, resuscitation and stabilization of casualties by paramedics, and to decide on priorities of evacuation to medical facilities. On other occasions the advice of a medical incident officer may be invaluable, particularly if he or she takes an active role in community disaster planning. Special medical and nursing teams may be required to perform tasks such as amputations, triage, resuscitation, or to provide medical aid for members of the emergency services.

Spreading the Casualty Load: Triage Hospitals

A key component of effective disaster management is to spread the casualty load to available health facilities in such a way that the injured receive prompt and appropriate treatment and that individual hospitals are not overwhelmed. The factors influencing the ability of ambulance or medical incident officers to spread the casualty load include the number of casualties and the type of injuries sustained; the proximity, size and facilities of local hospitals; and the ease and speed with which casualties can be evacuated from the disaster site.

Casualties with major burns or requiring cardiothoracic or neurosurgical treatment are candidates for direct transfer to specialized units, although it may not be possible for these units to accept a large number of injured. The 'walking wounded' with relatively minor injuries may be transported by bus or truck to a less well staffed or equipped hospital, while the more severely injured are taken to a hospital capable of dealing with major trauma.

In some circumstances, a community hospital or even a large building such as a school or church may be used as a 'triage hospital'. Casualties are brought here from the disaster site for further assessment and initial treatment of their injuries. After a period of observation and stabilization, they are then either sent home or transported to a more appropriate hospital. Triage hospitals may be staffed by local doctors and first aiders, reinforced by special triage and resuscitation teams from major hospitals.

Community Disaster Planning

The emergency service disaster plans need co-ordinating with those of the medical services and local and regional government. In large-scale community disasters involving a very large number of casualties, disruption of community services or an on-going disaster of uncertain duration (historically famine, pestilence or war, but now widespread chemical or radioactive pollution), local, regional, national or even international disaster planning becomes essential.

HOSPITAL DISASTER MANAGEMENT

Primary Treatment Areas

On arrival at a hospital, each casualty is identified with a unique disaster number, usually incorporated in a disaster tag, and his injuries are rapidly assessed so that he can be put into an appropriate triage category.

Those needing *immediate care* are taken to areas where life-saving resuscitation can be performed. The severely but less critically injured are taken to an *urgent treatment area* where they are further assessed and initial treatment commenced. The walking injured are directed to a *non-urgent* treatment area. The location of all these primary treatment areas needs to be identified in each health facility and, equally important, the areas into which expansion can take place need to be identified should the casualty load exceed the available space in the first site. Although in some disasters it may be necessary to convert halls and gymnasia for casualty treatment purposes, it is usually more efficient to use existing clinical areas, and to move the casualties through them as fast as is safely possible.

A *resuscitation team* of two doctors and two nurses may care for 8 casualties an hour, but should not be responsible for more than 2 casualties at any one time. The utilization of an existing hospital trauma team would fill this role. An *urgent care team* of one doctor, two nurses and two aides may care for 15 casualties an hour, but should not be expected to look after more than 5 casualties at any one time. *Non-urgent* casualties are supervised by one doctor, two nurses and two aides until extra staff become available. Standards of casualty care in a disaster should be identified at an early stage using the concept of *initial definitive treatment* for the various injuries.

Secondary Treatment Areas

After the initial assessment, resuscitation and possible stabilization have been carried out as quickly as possible, the casualty is moved by trolley, stretcher or chair to a secondary treatment area accompanied wherever possible by the nurse who has been looking after him. Here, the injuries are further assessed and documented and the initial plan of definitive management is decided upon and treatment of specific injuries commenced. Management of a large number of casualties requiring secondary treatment is most successfully achieved if all casualties, regardless of age, sex or type of injury, are sent to one area. In hospitals this is best achieved by the early designation of *receiving wards*. Rather than use existing available empty beds, it is more efficient to clear one or more wards and arrange for staff and pre-arranged supplies of linen, drugs and dressings to be brought to these areas. Here, the process of triage is repeated by experienced staff whose principal aim is to determine orders of priority for operating room time. Casualties are further stabilized and resuscitation continued if necessary.

Casualties admitted to receiving wards are cared for by *casualty teams*. Each team consists of one doctor, four trained nurses, four student nurses and two aides responsible for the care of 20 casualties. A senior doctor acts as *receiving ward surgeon*, supervising the work of the casualty teams, revising the triage category of casualties as necessary, and preparing lists of casualties requiring surgery, together with an estimate of the time required for each operation. Those casualties who are critically injured, but who are considered salvageable, will require more intensive resuscitation and are sent to a *preoperative ward*. This area requires all the facilities of a modern intensive therapy unit (ITU), but in many hospitals such facilities may not be available, either because an ITU does not exist, or because it is already full of ill patients. The saving of life and the reduction of morbidity in critically ill casualties require *operating rooms*. The number of such rooms that can be staffed is the main limiting factor in the provision of ideal definitive care for a large number of severely injured casualties.

Supervision of the operating rooms is the responsibility of the *operating room controller,* an experienced surgeon who, working closely with the senior operating room nurse, decides on priorities for operating room time and assigns medical and nursing staff to the care of individual casualties. Only by having regular discussions with senior medical staff in primary and secondary treatment areas is the operating room controller able to obtain an accurate overall picture of the casualty load. Individual surgeons must not be permitted to take their 'personal' patients to the operating room without the agreement of the operating room controller. The operating room controller should spend most of his time in the operating area being available to advise more junior surgeons on aspects of surgical management, redeploying members of surgical teams as necessary, and making sure that teams have adequate periods of rest. An operating team working continuously under stress for longer than 8–12 hours, depending on the severity of the case, is unlikely to continue performing in the most efficient way.

Each *surgical team* consists of one anaesthetist, one surgeon, an assistant surgeon, one scrub nurse and one circulating nurse (shared between two theatres if necessary). A trained assistant should be assigned to assist the anaesthetist during induction of anaesthesia and in the postoperative recovery phase of the procedure. Extra help is particularly required between cases as it is during this phase that time is so often lost.

Casualties recovering from anaesthesia are supervised by a *recovery team* consisting of an anaesthetist, two nurses and two aides. The recovery area may be an existing facility in the operating department or a special ward or part of a receiving ward.

One of the recurring difficulties in operating room management during disasters is to assess accurately the total operating time required to deal with a large casualty load. There is often a tendency during the early stages of a disaster, when the demand on operating room time is unknown, to delay all operations while awaiting the casualty with critical injuries that require immediate life-saving surgery. All too often, however, the initial wave of casualties arriving at hospital is those with the less severe injuries who have been able to leave the disaster site without too much difficulty. The more severely injured, who often need extricating from the wreckage, arrive at a later stage. Provided there are enough operating rooms available, it is often wise to start less urgent surgery earlier rather than later.[25] One of the duties of the operating room controller is to consider the triage categories for surgery. There will be those whose injuries require the most rapid emergency surgery; those with injuries which can wait from 6 to 12 hours without serious risk, and who can be operated on within the 12 hour period; while in a third group the risks involved in transferring a patient to another hospital are less than the risks of waiting more than 12 hours for a free operating room.

Some types of injuries, particularly thermal burns, require the continuing use of operating room time over a period of days or weeks for dressings and skin grafting. Estimates of this demand need to be made once the problem has been identified, and arrangements made not only to provide sufficient operating room time, but also sufficient numbers of surgeons and anaesthetists skilled in the management of such cases.[26]

Support Departments

All departments of a modern hospital have a part to play in the disaster plan.

Clinical departments such as radiology, pathology and pharmacy will need to adapt their procedures to provide a rapid and reliable service for a large number of casualties. The linen room, stores, central sterile supplies department and catering respond to specific demands from the treatment areas. Medical records, physiotherapy, domestic staff and porters, social workers and the clergy all have a part to play.

Radiology

Radiology is essential for the evaluation of a casualty with major injuries, and for the assessment of any possible fracture or dislocation. It is not possible to fill all these needs during the early stages of a disaster, and personnel and radiology equipment should be concentrated on the severely injured. If diagnostic radiology machines are not a permanent feature of the resuscitation rooms, there is still some discussion on whether it is better to move a critically injured casualty to the radiology department, or to move a portable radiology machine to the bedside. The advantages of high quality films obtained with more powerful equipment in the department, has to be weighed against possible delay, aggravation of injuries or unrecognized deterioration in clinical condition while the casualty is in the radiology department. With the aim of rapid assessment and resuscitation in the primary treatment areas, there is no place for X-rays in the initial evaluation of clinical status. However, they will be required for the secondary treatment areas, particularly the preoperative area, the receiving wards and the operating rooms. Casualties in the minor treatment area requiring X-rays for suspected fractures or dislocations should either be held back in a radiology waiting area until the more urgent cases have been dealt with or, where the radiology department has a number of rooms, should be examined in small batches. It is important that the department is not swamped with a large number of distressed casualties. Senior radiologists review each X-ray as it is developed and provide an immediate report, handwritten if necessary. A wax pencil report written on the film itself is better than no report at all. To avoid the unrecognized deterioration of a casualty's condition while in the radiology department, it is wise to assign a *radiology department medical team* consisting of one doctor and one nurse to the department if a large number of casualties are being referred for diagnostic radiology.

Blood Transfusion

Although whole blood is still required for the resuscitation of the exsanguinated casualty, a strict code of practice should be applied in a disaster to prevent blood and blood products from being wasted. In the primary treatment areas with the rapid throughput of a large number of casualties, there is not time to administer typed blood, and circulating fluid volume can be restored with crystalloid or colloid solutions. A more detailed evaluation of each casualty in the secondary treatment areas by an experienced doctor allows blood requirements to be calculated to avoid overtransfusion or waste. A foolproof system of labelling casualties, blood samples and cross-matched blood is mandatory. Appeals for blood donors during a disaster often cause more problems than they solve, and reliance on a screened pool of regular blood donors, or on a local or national blood transfusion service is safer and more satisfactory.

Communication, Control and Command

Communication

Good communication, control and command are essential in successful disaster management. The emergency services responsible for site management recognize their importance, and in their daily operational plans have a system which has been regularly put to the test. Most civilian hospitals in peacetime, however, have not found it necessary to do so and the introduction of a military style of command structure is often difficult at short notice.

Many hospital plans fail right at the start with the alert. Usually, two alerting systems are required, one during the working day when wards and departments are fully staffed, and another for the silent hours of nights, weekends and holidays. To avoid overloading the hospital telephonists with a large number of alerting calls, a fan-out or cascade notification system should be used whereby a limited number of alerting messages are made, the recipients being responsible for passing the message further down the line. The majority of hospital staff report to their usual place of work or head of department when a disaster alert is declared. Some staff are assigned to key roles or to perform important tasks by being given action or task cards. Only a few senior members of the hospital staff need to know all the details of the hospital and community disaster plan. At varying stages of the disaster, information will be required about hospital departments, their staffing, level of preparedness and stock levels of supplies and equipment; bed availability and location; staff availability and deployment; casualty identification, location and clinical status. All this information requires continuous updating and is processed through a hospital information centre. Information may be passed by word of mouth, by telephone or intercom, by written message, or by computer or radio. Hospital secretaries have a vital role to play.

Communication with the disaster site, with ambulance and medical incident officers, medical teams and ambulance dispatchers requires reliable telephone and radio links, sometimes using communication satellites.[27]

Command

A number of functional sites where command is important may be identified. The emergency receiving area is the first part of a hospital to receive the influx of casualties. Whereas most plans specify a 'senior and experienced doctor' to take on the task of triage and initial casualty management, in many hospitals such an individual is not immediately available. In these circumstances the senior departmental nurse should take command until the senior doctor arrives. Clinical supervision in the secondary treatment areas is the responsibility of designated senior medical staff who are deployed to the receiving wards, preoperative ward, operating department and minor treatment area. The normal care of inpatients must continue, and a senior doctor should supervise this.

All disasters are different, and individual hospitals' circumstances vary so much from place to place and country to country. In every institution a senior doctor, nurse and administrator must work together from a control centre where they can not only co-ordinate the hospital's response to the casualty load, but also adjust and modify the hospital plan.

REFERENCES

1. *Readings in Disaster Planning for Hospitals.* (1966) Chicago, American Hospital Association.
2. Savage P. E. A. (1971) Disaster planning: a review. *Injury* 3, 49–55.
3. Frey R. and Safar P. (eds.) (1980) *Disaster Medicine.* Heidelberg and New York, Springer-Verlag.
4. Cowley R. A. (ed.) (1982) *Mass Casualties.* Washington, US Dept. of Transportation.
5. Safar P. (ed.) (1985) Disaster resuscitology. *J. Wld. Assoc. Emerg. Disaster Med.* Vol. II, Suppl. I.
6. Manni C. and Magalini S. I. (eds.) (1985) *Emergency and Disaster Medicine.* Heidelberg and New York, Springer-Verlag.
7. Garb S., Eng E. (1969) *Disaster Handbook.* Heidelberg and New York, Springer-Verlag.
8. *Principles of Disaster Preparedness for Hospitals.* (1971) Chicago, American Hospital Association.
9. Richardson J. W. (ed.) (1975) *Disaster Planning.* Bristol, Wright.
10. Savage P. E. A. (1979) *Disasters – Hospital Planning.* Oxford, Pergamon.
11. Spirgi E. H. (1979) *Disaster Management.* Bern, Huber.
12. de Boer J. and Baillie T. W. (1980) *Disasters – Medical Organization.* Oxford, Pergamon.
13. Robertson B. (ed.) (1985) *Guide to Major Incident Management.* Ipswich, British Association For Immediate Care.
14. Rutherford W. H. and de Boer J. (1983) The definition and classification of disasters. *Injury* 15, 10–12.
15. Kirby N. G. and Ellis H. (1981) *Field Surgery Pocket Book.* London, HMSO.
16. Haywood I. R. (1984) Triage. *J. Br. Assoc. Immed. Care* 7, 31–5.
17. Berlin R. (1974) The role of the medical services. In: Sillar W. (ed.) *A Guide to Disaster Management.* Glasgow, Action For Disaster.
18. Safar P. (1987) *Cardiopulmonary Cerebral Resuscitation.* Third edition. Stavanger, Laerdal.
19. Easton K. (1977) Immediate care. In: Easton K. (ed.) *Rescue Emergency Care.* London, Heinemann.
20. Snook R. (1975) *Medical Aid at Accidents.* London, Update Publications.
21. Savage P. E. A. (1976) Disaster planning – protective clothing for medical team members. *Injury* 7, 286–7.
22. MacKenzie W. J. (1985) The fire service in major incidents. In: Robertson B. (ed.) *Guide to Major Incident Management.* Ipswich, British Association For Immediate Care.
23. Matthews P. (1985) The police role in major incidents. In: Robertson B. (ed.) *Guide to Major Incident Management.* Ipswich, British Association For Immediate Care.
24. Moss J. (1985) The role of the ambulance service. In: Robertson B. (ed.) *Guide to Major Incident Management.* Ipswich, British Association For Immediate Care.
25. Bliss A. R. (1984) Major disaster planning. *Br. Med. J.* 288, 1433–4.
26. Sharpe D. T., Roberts K. H. N., Barclay T. L. et al. (1985) Treatment of burns casualties after fire at Bradford City Football Ground. *Br. Med. J.* 291, 945–8.
27. Cowley R. A. (1985) The use of communication satellite systems in major disaster situations. In: Manni C. and Magalini S. I. (eds.) *Emergency and Disaster Medicine.* Heidelberg and New York, Springer-Verlag.

6

Disaster Planning in Developing Countries

INTRODUCTION

The impact of catastrophic destruction of human lives and property upon a nation which is in mid-phase of political, industrial and agricultural development is cruel and heart-rending. Repeated or episodic disasters tumble the building blocks of a society which, however deep lie its foundations in history, has not solidified its institutions and its role in the family of nations.

Developing nations and regions present a general commonality in that they have been either deprived of or otherwise have been unable to develop a national socio-economic structure during the time of the first industrial revolution. In many cases their major or only role was the supply of raw materials to the nations presently regarded as developed. They are currently energetically engaged in crash programmes for the emplacement of heavy industry and/or attempts to participate fully in the second industrial revolution, the Information Revolution, associated with the development of computer telecommunications. In this socio-economic milieu, epitomized by the emergence of a national ethos, experimentation in forms of government and the management of expanding populations within the perimeters of a finite supply of food, shelter and energy is typical. In the developed nations, it is not often recalled that the first industrial revolution was accompanied by a concomitant evolution of a sophisticated medical science and medical care systems for individual patients and mass casualties.

The fact that the later developing countries tend to lie in the path of natural disasters is probably significant. Moreover, the accelerated catch-up programmes designed to use formerly exported raw materials and build heavy industry are associated with industrial accidents which were common in Western Europe and the United States during their formative phases. Efforts to find the optimum national political structure often lead to conflict and bloodshed. Thus, the developing nations can be expected to have a large number and variety of disasters. For much the same historical reasons, their traditional medical capability is likely to be insufficient to cope with such disasters so increasing the vulnerability of their people and formative institutions to catastrophic events.

Disaster management, medical and otherwise, is a large scale societal activity. Organizing for any single disaster within a setting of episodic natural catastrophes, incomplete industrialization, and political instability or open conflict is a monumental problem. Professional disaster managers, international disaster organizations and prosperous nations must recognize the nature and complexity of the difficulties. Humane and ethical behaviour require global advance planning and the response should take into account the special situations, cultures and resources of the developing countries. The Hippocratic Oath and the other accepted ethics of medical care demand no less. The donor physician and allied professionals who engage in international medical disaster care do well to remember that they are guests in the stricken host nation. Assuredly, the magnitude and complexity of the developing countries' disaster problems cannot excuse inadequate response on the part of those who should provide adequate aid. Nor should the developing countries, themselves, fail to prepare their societies and their citizens on the basis of expediency, growth or political metamorphosis.

OVERVIEW OF HAZARD ASSESSMENT AND MEASURES OF DISASTER PRE-PLANNING

As a background to aid medical planners and providers, 58 countries in 6 different areas of the world were examined to provide the rudiments of understanding. Personal observation was augmented by information obtained from the United Nations Disaster Relief Organization (UNDRO), a number of international charitable organizations, the files of the United States Office of Foreign Disaster Assistance and past and recent interviews with medical disaster experts in the Pan American Health Organization, the World Health Organization, and others.

To provide the reader with a quick reference guide, a simplistic Preparedness Index based on national disaster planning and organization was designed. The author begs the indulgence of the reader and the nations involved for any errors and misconceptions. The countries studied represent a major portion of the earth's surface and people. They have been subjected to an extraordinarily numerous and diverse set of disasters.

Within 6 extensive geographical areas selected, recent catastrophes and their consequences were examined to provide indicators of the magnitude of disasters which strike those regions and countries. The hazard assessment included the significant medical indices and socio-economic estimates. The population estimates, annual growth rates, infant mortality rates and gross national product per capita were recorded. National pre-planning data and implementation systems were examined as far as possible. The availability of international sources of disaster aid was recorded at sample disasters. A resumé of the findings is presented in the Appendix (p. 452). The results of the degree of preparedness for disasters is recorded in *Table* 6.1.

Nations providing no evidence of significant pre-planning are indicated by an '0' rating. Where available information pointed to a set of procedures rather than a formal plan, the preparedness index of '1' was awarded. The presence of a formal plan, but one which appeared limited or inadequate, provided an index of '2'. The existence of solid pre-planning, which appeared satisfactory to mitigate damage, rated an index of '3'. When a formal disaster response plan appeared strong and provided a model, an index rating of '4' was applied.

Disaster preparedness and response systems were evaluated and indexed in an

Table 6.1. Disaster Preparedness Index

	Country	Plan	Structure
Africa	Mauritania	4+	4−
	Ghana	4	4
	Gambia	2	0
	Chad	0	2
	Mali	0	2
	Zambia	0	2
	Burkina-Faso	1	1
	Cape Verde	0	1
	Niger	0	1
	Zaire	0	1
	Senegal	0	1
East Africa	Ethiopia	0	2
	Kenya	0	2
	Somalia	0	2
	Sudan	0	2
	Djibouti	1	1
	Tanzania	1	1
	Uganda	0	1
Asia	Pakistan	4	4
	Philippines	4	4
	Nepal	0	4
	India	0	4−
	Bangladesh	2	3−
	Turkey	2	2
	Indonesia	0	2
	Burma	0	2−
	Sri Lanka	0	1+
Caribbean	Jamaica	4+	4+
	Antigua/Barbados	4	4
	Belize	4	4
	Dominica	4	4
	Dominican Republic	4	4−
	Montserrat	3	4
	Grenada	0	4

	Country	Plan	Structure
	Trinidad/Tobago	3+	3+
	St Kitts/Nevis/Anguilla	3	3+
	St Lucia	3	3+
	Haiti	2	2+
	Guyana	0	1+
Oceana	Mauritius	4	4
	Madagascar	3	2
	Maldives	2	2
	Reunion	2	2
	Seychelles	1	1
South/Central America	Chile	4−	4+
	El Salvador	3	4
	Honduras	3−	3
	Nicaragua	3	2−
	Guatemala	1+	3+
	Peru	1	3
	Ecuador	2−	2−
	Costa Rica	0	2
South Pacific	Papua New Guinea	4	4+
	Fiji	3	4
	Tonga	0	2−
	Western Samoa	0	1+

RATING SCALE

0 = No national disaster plan or existing structure

1 = Set of procedures and ad hoc or event basis structures

2 = Formal plan that seemed to be limited or permanent structure with apparent limited capacity

3 = Formal, satisfactory plan or structure

4 = Formal, above average plan with relative strength; or permanent, above average structure with an apparently wide reach and/or development relationship.

analagous manner. An index rating of '0' was applied when no existing organization designed to address disaster could be elicited. An index rating of '1' indicates that an organization had been set in place in that nation on an ad hoc basis. Organizational arrangements which existed but appeared limited in capacity or reach were indexed at '2'. Apparently satisfactory permanent systems were rated as '3'. Where national plans and organization appear permanent and above average, an index rating of '4' was applied.

In addition to the numerical ratings, from time to time a plus (+) or a minus (−) was also assigned, indicating that while a country's plan or structure met the criteria of the rating category, there was either a clear indication of some added sophistication (+) or of some particular problems (−), e.g. a plan *appears* to be well-developed, but is constrained by inadequate implementing funds.

While there is frequently detailed descriptive matter on countries' disaster plans and organization, anecdotal information also surfaces describing disaster response effectiveness as adequate or inadequate. Regardless of detailed planning documents and elaborate systems, the best of plans and preparedness can only be expected to mitigate damage. Consequently, in almost no case has it been possible to make a definitive assessment of the effectiveness of the plan or the system but lessons derived from actual catastrophes will be presented in the third part of this analysis.

Finally, an examination was made of the resources provided for disaster planning, prevention, assistance and mitigation during the past several years by the US Agency for International Development, by the myriad non-profit US organizations supporting assistance programmes in developing countries through international relief organizations and, overall, by the family of United Nations Organizations.

There is obviously considerable variation in the hazards faced by the developing world and its capacity to address the disaster. In addition to the sudden catastrophes, developing countries are more prone to and less able to absorb the effects of the slow, insidious disasters, such as drought, famine, epidemics of infectious disease, endemic water contamination, soil erosion, deforestation, pest infestations and the demands created by large numbers of tragically displaced persons. Civil strife arising during the formative phases of government development seriously interferes with both internal and external disaster management and exacerbates problems in many directions. For countries like Chad, Ethiopia or Nicaragua, the impact of continuous fighting and displacement of populations has created multiple, simultaneous, sudden and slow disasters. Economic, political and civil strife overlayed by climatic conditions can induce rapid urbanization where the resources are unable to sustain the new population. The flight from farms diminishes national planting and harvesting activity. Further, the resource draining effects of civil strife militate against development efforts which, in themselves, often act as disaster deterrents or as avenues of control and mitigation, and place constraints on the contribution of external assistance.

Many developing countries put inadequate resources into disaster planning because so many other priorities compete for the same money and services. Paradoxically, countries that have moved successfully toward development are also faced with the down side of new kinds of disasters, for example, chemical and pesticide poisoning, as has occurred in El Salvador and Jamaica. Indeed, as countries become increasingly developed, preparation for great natural disasters must be modified and expanded to include the risks of growing technical industrialization. Fortunately, there are common elements in coping with all forms of disaster and a strong programme for all disasters allows a degree of cost-effectiveness in disaster management. This is particularly true of disaster medicine as the human body has a limited set of pathophysiological defences.

THE SIX REGIONS SURVEYED

Africa and East Africa

Eleven Central and West African countries were examined: Burkina-Faso, Cape Verde, Chad, Gambia, Ghana, Mali, Mauritania, Niger, Senegal, Zaire and Zambia. Seven countries in East Africa were studied as a separate unit, although they presented with many similar patterns: Djibouti, Ethiopia, Kenya, Somalia, Sudan, Tanzania and Uganda.

Most of these countries have a low gross national product per capita, although several do have growing economies. With few exceptions, they have had severe droughts resulting in famine or food shortages affecting tens of millions over the past two decades. Further, many of these countries also have had experience of having to cope with large masses of refugees (movements either to find food or escape from war), which has severely overextended their existing resources.

For many of the African countries, malnutrition underlies other disease and injury. Correction of malnutrition and the treatment of infectious disease is the foundation block of disaster medicine. While large portions of the African soil are known to be poor, with substantial land degradation, the intricacies of the relationship between agricultural stagnation and environmental deterioration have reached levels of complexity beyond the planning capacity of many governments. Poor sanitation is endemic in Burkina-Faso, Chad, Gambia, Ghana, Niger, Sudan and Tanzania; transportation and supply system inadequacies are the rule in Chad, Gambia, Mali, Zaire, Djibouti, Somalia, Sudan and Uganda; high disease levels and low health care access prevail in Burkina-Faso, Chad, Gambia, Mali, Mauritania, Niger, Zaire, Djibouti, Somalia, Sudan and Uganda. Low density rural populations, labour shortages, erratic distribution and provision of resources, and unfortunate political intervention, all come together to present an overwhelming complex of disasters—all clearly linked to a historical development phase.

The consequence of these factors is that disaster preparedness and planning on a national scale, and the establishment of national disaster systems, become virtually impossible in many cases. Disaster assistance and disaster medicine must frequently come from beyond the border.

Of the eleven Central and West African countries, seven have no national disaster plans and one has no system at all. Another five appear to respond to disasters on only an ad hoc basis. And yet, some countries have developed exemplary responses. Gambia has an existing national disaster plan, although its detail and effectiveness are unclear. Mauritania, among the eleven countries in this area, has indications of intricate national disaster plans and systems with initial efforts to tie disaster prevention to development. Ghana, too, is notable for its self-reliance. Ghana has in place a national mobilization task force with a reputation for some very effective work. The Ghanaian government's clear commitment to disaster planning and preparedness provides lessons for the entire world. Chad and Mali have made some beginnings in structuring emergency response organizations.

In East Africa, Kenya and Tanzania possess sufficient significant assets to enable them to be relatively self-reliant in a disaster. However, drought, famine and refugee problems affect Djibouti, Ethiopia and Somalia. Of the seven East African countries, five have no comprehensive national plans; two, Djibouti and Tanzania, appear to have limited emergency operating procedures. Ethiopia, Kenya, Somalia and Sudan have permanent disaster-emergency systems, but are plagued with a host of accompanying difficulties. Inadequate data collection and major logistic problems are, for these nations, underlying obstacles to internal and external assistance.

Asia

The nine Asian countries examined (Bangladesh, Burma, India, Indonesia, Nepal, Pakistan, Philippines, Sri Lanka and Turkey) greatly contrast with the background profiles of the African countries.

Among the considerations are larger populations, more experience in responding to disasters and longer histories of working with regional international organizations. Key medical indicators such as infant mortality rates are generally improving. While each country in the Asian group studied has its share of disaster response and other system problems, each also has a good share of system assets, some of which are at very sophisticated levels of development. While the absolute effect of any disaster in the Asian countries is often quite substantial, disasters tend not to have the long-term, far-reaching effects that massive drought, famine and refugee problems bring to much of Africa.

Asia and the Indian subcontinent share with Africa a general disproportion of population to land, food and other essential supplies. These elements, along with poor sanitation and limited portable water, result in endemic malnutrition, infection, dehydration and populations which are prone to impaired immune systems.

On the asset side, many countries, such as Burma, India, Indonesia, Nepal, Pakistan, the Philippines, and in Asia Minor and Turkey, have excellent energy sources. Elements of the first Industrial Revolution and the Information Revolution are being rapidly assembled in various degrees in India, Nepal, Bangladesh, Pakistan and Sri Lanka. This technological spurt has brought with it both disaster management potential and the threat of technological and industrial hazards. Thus, India and its neighbours benefit from an ingenious disaster warning system based on satellite communications. INSAT and future companion satellite systems, along with a growing computer capability, have been used in a brilliant manner to provide an early storm warning system. Since lethal weather catastrophies occur with cyclones and floods, an early warning system, based on high technology, is a very high priority.

The increase in technical capacity in itself brings with it the threat of disaster. The area has been stricken by the sinking of large commuter vessels and the escape of lethal inhalants. The incident at Bhopal may be the first example of such a disaster.

The Caribbean

The fourteen countries of the Caribbean area are clearly striving for effective disaster preparedness.

Nearly all the countries are considerably smaller than most of the Asian and African nations. With one exception (Haiti), infant mortality rates are many times lower—some approaching those of highly industrialized countries, e.g. Antigua and Barbuda at 24/1000 births; Trinidad and Tobago at 23·9; and Jamaica and Grenada at 15. Most growth rates are fairly low, but in many Caribbean countries, the GNP per capita is relatively high, e.g. St Kitts-Nevis-Anguilla, $920; Dominican Republic, $1072; and Trinidad and Tobago, $4800—fourth highest in the hemisphere. Literacy rates also tend to be high. While there are a variety of system problems, there are also many viable working systems in most of the Caribbean countries.

The Caribbean arc is subject to hurricanes, floods, some drought, volcanoes and earthquake activity. With increasing technical and political change, several of the countries are also affected by chemical hazards and incidents of civil strife.

With the Caribbean group, 14 countries were evaluated. Six, Antigua and Barbuda, Barbados, Belize, Dominica, Dominican Republic and Jamaica, have developed what appear to be strong, above average national disaster plans. The same countries also have good, permanent, detailed disaster organizations in place. Jamaica has demonstrated serious mitigation projects and research in the field of disaster scholarship. Grenada, without evidence of a national planning document, nevertheless seems to have a well organized structure to cope with disasters.

Five other countries (Montserrat, St Kitts-Nevis-Anguilla, St Lucia, St Vincent, and Trinidad and Tobago) each appear to have growing national disaster plans supported by good organization and effective systems.

Only Guyana and Haiti have disaster implementation organizations that appear to be less than satisfactory and only Haiti, apparently, has no planning arrangements at all.

The relative success of disaster planning and organization in the Caribbean can be attributed to a number of factors within each country. However, what appears to be the primary influence is each nation's participation in the Pan Caribbean Disaster Preparedness and Prevention Project (PCDPPP) which provides data collection and a wide range of information to member countries.

Oceana

These six relatively small island countries (Comoros, Madagascar, the Maldives, Mauritius, Reunion and the Seychelles) may be among the more overlooked countries when disaster and disaster assistance issues are considered. There appears to be limited external donor involvement for these nations, despite the fact that most of them are subject to a series of disasters, including cyclones, droughts and food shortages, floods, volcanic activity, deforestation and erosion, and some epidemics. The difference among them in terms of their disaster planning and response capacities is fairly wide. The Comoros, Madagascar, the Maldives and Reunion are beset by a rather substantial number of basic deficits ranging from weak economies and poor health to food, transportation and sanitation problems. By contrast, Mauritius and the Seychelles, each with relatively high GNP per capita of $1300 and $1800, respectively, have a number of systems strengths in their favour, including well-developed communications facilities and good transport and health-care systems. Mauritius has a comprehensive crop insurance programme and the Seychelles has strong tourism and construction industries.

Of the six countries, four have national disaster plans. Mauritius and Madagascar seem to have solid, national, well co-ordinated arrangements for addressing disasters, including aspects of prevention and mitigation. Only the Comoros and the Seychelles appear to have no known, formalized structures. Each, however, appears to address problems on an event basis, and participates in a relevant regional organization.

South and Central America

The eight countries assessed in South and Central America (Chile, Costa Rica, Ecuador, El Salvador, Guatemala, Honduras, Nicaragua and Peru) present, overall, a broad, mid-level picture of disaster planning and preparedness. Their disaster history of the past 25 years includes earthquakes, volcanic eruptions, droughts, hurricanes, floods, landslides, El Niño, epidemics and, more recently, escalating armed conflicts as well as an increased incidence of exposure to hazardous materials such as pesticide poisoning, etc.

El Salvador, Ecuador, Guatemala, Honduras and Peru comprise at least half the countries and suffer from inadequate health care. Water safety and sanitation problems affect Ecuador, Guatemala, Honduras and Nicaragua. The countries most affected by guerilla warfare and terrorism at present are El Salvador, Guatemala, Nicaragua and, to some extent, Peru, and this has powerful effects upon their economies.

By contrast, Chile has a fairly effective set of systems, including a health status approaching that of the most heavily industrialized countries, a multi-faceted health care delivery system, growing power capacity and extensive telecommunications. Costa Rica has the advantages of a good transportation system, a high level of health care as indicated by an infant mortality rate of 28/1000 births, a strong agricultural sector, a diverse energy capacity and a very high literacy rate. Peru's assets include rich mineral deposits, some good initial efforts at disease control and a high literacy rate.

In planning and disaster organization Chile stands out as the one country with both an elaborate, extensive organization and national disaster planning system. While there is evidence that disaster funding may be insufficient, there is also testimony to good stockpile strategy and capacity, and the integrated involvement of many donor groups with the governmental efforts.

Even with its many immediate problems, El Salvador seems to have the next best disaster planning and appropriate organization. It has placed disaster planning in the context of improving both the economic and political sectors of the country, and has established long-range goals.

The other countries that seem to have national plans are Honduras and Nicaragua. Guatemala, Honduras and Peru have established satisfactory disaster organizations. Oddly, Costa Rica, with a solid array of reasonably well functioning socio-political systems and a high level civil defence organization, has no formal national disaster plan—in spite of a 13-year-old national emergency law.

South Pacific

Four relatively small countries represent the South Pacific area—Fiji, Papua New Guinea, Tonga and Western Samoa. These countries are affected by hurricanes, some volcanic and earthquake activity as well as by landslides, tsunamis, floods and drought.

These nations are characterized by relatively low to medium growth, but frequently high dependency rates. Most have respectable infant mortality rates. Two of the countries, Fiji and Papua New Guinea, enjoy fairly high GNP per capita—respectively, $1150 and $800. Early warning systems seem rather effective for all but Tonga. All have areas of isolated population served by less than adequate road systems.

Fiji appears to have the widest range of socio-economic assets, including its own medical school. It is a prime service area for refuelling on Pacific airline flights and acts as a South Pacific communications centre and is developing its power resources. Papua New Guinea has the advantages of good telecommunications and long-range economic planning by the government. Western Samoa enjoys relatively good health status, high literacy, a strong telecommunications system and considerable hydro-electric power.

Only Fiji and Papua New Guinea have known satisfactory national disaster plans supported by effective organizations. Though Tonga and Western Samoa seem not to have national disaster plans or comprehensive disaster organizations, each has some response mechanism directed toward disaster, e.g. a central hurricane committee in Tonga and an early warning observatory and seismology station in Western Samoa.

INTERNATIONAL RESOURCES FOR DISASTER-STRICKEN DEVELOPING COUNTRIES

Donor assistance in response to disasters and emergencies—especially in the less developed countries—has expanded and become increasingly realistic. Estimates made from information of the United Nations Disaster Relief Co-ordinator's Office (UNDRO) indicate that for the 1984 fiscal year, relief contributions amounted to over US $1 billion to the countries under discussion (*Table* 6.2). Of this, approximately US $968 million went to alleviate severe drought problems in six African countries. Funds were contributed by five major public sources: UNDRO itself, the large UN system of agencies, inter-governmental organizations, individual governments, and trans-national non-governmental philanthropies.

Individual governments have provided money, manpower and equipment directly and through international channels. The United States makes major contributions through the UN system. In addition, between 1964 and 1984, the

Table 6.2. International disaster relief: April 1984–March 1985*

Country	Disaster type(s)	$ millions
1. Bangladesh	Cyclone	0·03
2. Burkina-Faso	Floods, drought	14·30
3. Burma/Mandalay	Fire	0·30
4. Cape Verde	Floods	0·50
5. Chad	Drought, civil strife	87·75
6. Cormoros	Storm	0·02
7. Ecuador/Galapagos	Fire	0·02
8. Ethiopia	Drought, famine, refugees	520·00
9. Fiji	Cyclone	3·21
10. Ghana	Drought	11·33
11. India	Bhopal gas leak	0·21
12. Madagascar	Cyclones	2·23
13. Mali	Drought, cholera	74·90
14. Mauritania	Drought	42·49
15. Niger	Drought	108·00
16. Philippines	Typhoons	11·16
17. Somalia	Drought	4·07
18. Sudan	Drought	134·66
TOTAL		$1 015·26

* (Report of the Office of the United Nations Disaster Relief Co-ordinator.)

US Office of Federal Disaster Assistance (OFDA) responded to approximately 672 disasters in the areas of the world covered by this report, donating US $162 million (US $32 million each for relief in droughts and food shortages and US $32 million for assistance after cyclones, hurricanes and typhoons). While the average support in dollars per disaster was higher for the Caribbean and Latin American countries, the largest proportion of funds—over 40 per cent—was allocated to African countries who also bore the largest share of all disasters— over one-third of the total number. The Asian countries were the second largest recipients of US aid (OFDA) dollars during the 20-year period—benefiting from 26 per cent of the total, or US $42·1 million.

The cost of disaster and developmental assistance is high. While only a limited effort has been made to compare national contributions through the UN system, it can be pointed out that for 1984 the ten largest donor countries—the United States, Italy, West Germany, Canada, Saudi Arabia, the United Kingdom, the Netherlands, Australia, Bulgaria and Sweden—gave a total of US $623·6 million, according to calculations drawn from UNDRO data. (*See Table* 6.3.)

Another major source of funding is the group of US non-profit, private and voluntary organizations. These groups working in lesser developed countries are providing more than US $430 million annually in a combination of development and specific disaster aid. Four of the five largest of the private voluntary organizations—CARE, Catholic Relief Services, the International Rescue Committee and Church World Services—are contributing over US $215 million per year in response to disaster and development needs. World Vision Relief alone has donated close to US $70 million to lesser developed countries.

Table 6.3   Ten largest disaster donor countries, 1984–5 (UNDRO Reports)

Country	$ millions
1. United States	323·7
2. Italy	93·3
3. West Germany	43·8
4. Canada	38·6
5. Saudi Arabia	38·4
6. United Kingdom and Northern Ireland	25·2
7. Netherlands	21·6
8. Australia	17·6
9. Bulgaria	12·6
10. Sweden	8·8
TOTAL	$623·6

With the vast sums of money being directed and applied to disaster assistance, it is appropriate to examine the extent of donor effectiveness. Donor involvement has not always been smooth, and continues to be beset by a number of problems. While many ad hoc UN groups are appointed to look into specific major disasters, UNDRO is the primary vehicle for international disaster assistance. It serves as a clearing house, is a prime source of training and information and plays a very important co-ordinating role in disasters. It works with at least two dozen UN and regional agencies. In the Caribbean, UNDRO has been especially effective in guiding a regional preparedness programme (PCDPPP) and in establishing an effective early warning network for hurricanes. In the African famine, it has worked extremely well with many competing agencies. As occurs with many public agencies, UNDRO also sometimes suffers from a degree of bureaucratic inertia.

This problem is compounded by the fact that UNDRO has no clear policy authority. While many countries work closely with UNDRO, others may not necessarily work through it in an emergency. Although UNDRO efforts are extensive and generally effective, it cannot be regarded as the universal international disaster umbrella.

Many donor governments tend to help with disasters in terms of 'quick-fix' policies, particularly in the areas of drought and famine relief. The traditional approach is one of crisis orientation supported by short-term projects, often without adequate follow-up. Often, too, the assistance may lead to large policy conflicts within the donor nation. For example, the United States is a major agricultural exporter to lesser developed countries. Any long-term interest in helping these countries to solve their very serious food problems would ultimately lead to changes in good import/export ratios.

Problems are caused by the length of time that may elapse in international circles between an appeal for disaster assistance and the delivery of relief because of delays in governmental decisions. Ten to twelve months are sometimes required to analyse the need and actually deliver help. It is sometimes expedient to use development dollars for disaster relief and/or prevention. However, in the United States, it can frequently take so long to clear development funds that the acute phase of a particular disaster may already be over before funds arrive.

Host country and donor country relationships often present difficulties not anticipated by disaster managers, which can put very substantial strains on aid co-ordination and logistics. For example, some countries are unwilling to accept assistance from former colonizers, political opponents or a country's leader may be reluctant to ask for help in an emergency until it is too late. At other times disorganization, inefficiency and dishonesty are encountered at the point of delivery of assistance.

Nevertheless, difficulties are usually overcome by humane considerations. The extensive, long-term work of the private voluntary organizations has been especially laudable. Of nearly 500 donors listed in the 1983 Technical Assistance Information Clearing House (TAICH) Directory, 190 are voluntary organizations, more than 200 are religious groups and another 100 represent businesses, professional organizations and foundations. The private voluntary organizations have many objectives and most pursue a spectrum of development and project aid. However, 13 per cent have disaster only missions. Private voluntary organizations have, however, shown themselves to be extremely helpful to host governments in society-disrupting disasters where the existing infrastructure and long-term relationships can readily be used. Pre-eminent among these is the vast network of Red Cross and Red Crescent agencies which, in many developing countries, are key sources of leadership, organization, supplies, and overall assistance. The Red Cross and Red Crescent organizations have been virtually indispensable to government disaster relief efforts in such nations as Bangladesh, Pakistan, Turkey, Belize, Haiti, Trinidad and Tobago, El Salvador and Nicaragua. In a few areas, such as Nepal, they may even operate with the informal authority of an official government body.

In spite of significant growth in sophistication over the years, private voluntary organization effectiveness is still hampered at times by some of the same problems suffered by public organizations. For some, policy limits flexibility and only short-term projects are supported rather than the vital long-term issues to assure continued aid and self-reliance.

Though many private voluntary organizations are far more responsive to countries' needs than they were in years past and have been able to help improve policies as well as guiding direct aid projects, at times these organizations suffer from inadequate staffing; and frequently find themselves jointly involved in major relief efforts with other groups but experience difficulty with co-ordination of objectives, strategies and operations.

Disaster response needs sometimes compete with normal, on-going development programmes. Emergencies may be viewed as a disturbing deviation in development activities which can be compounded by the outside organization having established working relationships with host agencies other than with those set up specifically to address disasters.

Religious constraints may affect the availability of disaster aid. Several years ago (1979 earthquake) the Catholic Relief Services was the only religious organization the Turkish government would allow in the country. Certain religious volunteer organizations, which may be construed as being more concerned with prosyletizing, may be anathema in Moslem countries. The providers of disaster medicine have an obligation to function within the religious beliefs of a nation.

LESSONS

Many lessons may be appreciated from a background study of the developing nations of the world. These nations cover a large portion of the earth's land mass. Their collective populations are enormous; their political systems vary greatly and are in a state of flux. Their degree of entry into the first and second industrial revolutions represents a wide spectrum. In their justifiable race to attain immediate political and economic goals they are exceedingly vulnerable to all forms of disaster. Disaster management systems which unfortunately bring no immediate return on either human or financial investment often receive considerably less attention. Rapid development was a gamble in the history of the now developed nations; it is also a high stakes game for the developing nations of today.

Increasing populations encroach on arable land and forests. The luxury of bypassing occupation and utilization of non-arable lands exercised by the developing nations of another era is not necessarily available to many newly developing nations.

However, emerging nations do have some advantages. The Information Revolution provides an opportunity for rapid, satellite-mediated communications, computer modelling, education and warning systems. There are few disaster configurations—simply an increased number—and an increased number of victims. Satellite and other sensing systems provide individual nations, and those groups concerned with worldwide disasters, with an opportunity for the study of the behaviour of disasters which was denied to the earth-bound populations of the last century. An international agency is sorely needed to co-ordinate and distribute this information so that the available data could be used by both national governments and by the international organizations. The African hunger disaster has certainly demonstrated the willingness of the world's public to respond if appropriately informed.

Disaster management should not commence when the dying begins. A region's potential hazards, existing disaster response systems, supplies of energy and the status of both local and traditional medicine are essential data for those who would provide assistance. International support should be prepared to reinforce local preparedness systems already in place. Local authorities have the first and primary opportunity for providing medical care and imported physicians and other health professions must be knowledgeable about the countries and the people whom they expect to serve. Emergency medical techniques are not necessarily transferrable from nation to nation. Disaster medical task forces should, under no circumstances, impinge on the resources of the already victimized country's energy, transport, food, shelter and interpreters.

The Industrial Accident at Bhopal, India

On 3 December, 1984, a cloud containing methyl isocyanate escaped rapidly into the atmosphere and reached surrounding villagers. A concentration of 0·05 mg/ml of air has toxic effects, attacks the sclera and, when inhaled, produces destruction of the epithelium and alveoli of the pulmonary system. The chemical escaped from a storage tank into the surrounding air at night when its unpleasant and irritating odour was less likely to be detected and the majority of victims were sleeping. Bhopal's victims suffered blindness and pulmonary oedema causing at least 2000 deaths and an equal or greater number of permanent injuries. The Indian medical authorities were prompt in applying symptomatic management of these injuries. They mobilized a large number of health workers in a remarkably short span of time. However, the capabilities for treating mass casualties in the field are obviously less than equal to those of a critical care hospital unit. Only an adequate warning system and implementation of an appropriate evacuation plan on the night of 3 December might have lessened the mortality and the morbidity materially.

Disasters should not come as a surprise. They tend to have a prodrome. Five weeks before the escape of methyl isocyanate from the Union Carbide pesticide plant, the authors discussed with Indian scientists the imminency of an industrial disaster, at a UNESCO meeting in Madras. The evident hazards noted were the rapid completion of industrial plans, substandard maintenance and the close proximity of plant workers' families and other villagers to factory boundaries— the 'danger zone'. Industries producing pesticides, plastics and other chemical-based products have toxic intermediate and waste products. In both the developed and lesser developed nations workers and, perhaps more importantly, adjacent resident populations, are at risk.

The lessons to be learned from this tragedy include the need for:
1. An acceptance of the possibility of disaster and its consequences by plant managers and nearby residents.
2. Education of workers and potentially exposed populace in specific survival methods.
3. Education of all regional health personnel in the pathogenesis and emergency treatment of injuries likely to result from the industrial mishap. Medical treatment regimens should be printed in advance and distributed with the first warning. Appropriate antidotes should be stockpiled by both industrial and governmental agencies.
4. A distinctive and adequate warning system practised routinely and including distribution of simple instructions to the endangered populace.
5. The establishment of an uninhabited safety zone between such plants and land available for residence. (At Bhopal, Union Carbide paid an annual rent of less than US $40/acre including taxes because of governmental subsidies.)
6. Independent periodic plant inspections with the probability of a hazardous material disaster reported to all relevant governmental officials. (There is evidence that a series of economic misfortunes reduced the expected sales of the Bhopal plant, requiring excessive storage of toxic materials at the plant site.)
7. Rapidly deployable regional medical facilities designed to support local health teams and health care facilities.
8. Precautions associated with the transport of hazardous materials. Local authorities should know what hazards are being moved through their area. Local physicians and hospitals should be appraised of the best supportive and specific treatment.

Mexico City Earthquake
At 7.10 a.m., on 20 September, 1985, a relatively small portion of the Pacific Plate System, the Cocos Plate, struck and slid under the massive North American

tectonic plate, 250 miles west of populous Mexico City. Seven thousand people died; 3000 buildings were devastated and, for a long period, 40000 people were homeless. Medical, engineering and governmental lessons were learned:

1. Engineers learned that the layers of soft clay which underlie portions of the city transmit much more ground movement than had been calculated. The significance of the architectural design of buildings was brought vividly to the fore and the vulnerabilities and avoidance methods have been described by Christopher Arnold of Building Systems Development, Inc. The US National Science Foundation is now supporting the development of a video disc instruction manual on how to alleviate this problem.

2. The Surgeon General of the Mexican Army rapidly deployed 7000 men in an effort to remove victims from fallen buildings and then sought to bull-doze down the ruins 48 hours after the earthquake in order 'to prevent epidemics'. The people of the city resisted violently and insisted on a prolonged search. Living victims were presented to the medical authorities after more than a week's entrapment, and no epidemics occurred. The demonstration of the value of prolonged rescue efforts, and the durability of trapped victims, is a lesson for disaster medicine which rivals our understanding of survival for long periods after immersion in frigid waters.

The INSAT Weather Warning System

Each year cyclones occur on the West and East Coast of the Indian subcontinent. In the decade preceding 1980 at least 400 storms crossed the Bay of Bengal. Death and injury levels ranged upwards to the hundreds of thousands. For the fishing fleets and the residents of the coastal plain survival is dependent on early warning systems. The mobilization of medical facilities for traumatic injuries is similarly dependent on an appropriate lead time. In this decade, India has deployed one satellite and is in the process of deploying a second. The simple, and generally reliable, remote sensing provided by geostationary satellites relays information to governmental executives and police stations along the coastal plains about these massive storms and offers an opportunity to evacuate the population to preconstructed shelters. Coastal shipping, including the major fishing fleet, requires earlier warnings than do land residents. Simple radio receiver systems have been advocated and are being installed on board these ships.

Rehydration of Infants

Prior to the Korean War, Rosenthal of the United States Public Health Service pointed out that burn shock could be treated by the oral ingestion (with or without gastric intubation) of water containing sodium bicarbonate and sodium chloride. In 1953, Fox, Silverstein and others advocated this treatment, adding potassium chloride to the solution.

Physicians from the developed nations, not realizing the scope of the problem, advocated the intravenous route of rehydration and realimentation.

Fortunately, the impossibility of intravenous alimentation and hydration for large numbers of infants suffering from diarrheal syndromes became evident to the World Health Organization, and perhaps the most brilliant advance in treating such cases has been the advocacy and promulgation of Oral Replacement Therapy (ORT). In its simplest form this can be accomplished by a primitive mother adding a pinch of salt and three fingers of sugar to a litre of water. This is perhaps the most successful approach to mass casualties since the medical world developed an understanding of the pathology and treatment for shock due to many causes.

CONCLUSION

There are many lessons to be learned by disaster medical personnel who operate in developing nations. The lessons range from the need for pre-disaster understanding of the individual countries to the search for ingenious use of simple, but effective, remedies.

J. Adler

7

Assessment of Disasters in the Developing World

PHASES OF DISASTERS

The continuing phase of disasters begins immediately after the acute or impact phase, which, in the majority of events, lasts 1–2 days. In some prolonged natural disasters, like famine, floodings or extensive fires, or in 'man-made' disasters such as industrial or nuclear accidents or civil strife, the acute phase may last for weeks or even months. The 'acute' phase may also be defined as the time span during which the affected community has to cope with its own resources, before outside help can arrive.

The continuing phase can be subdivided into two periods (*see Fig.* 7.1)

—the *consolidation* phase—following the acute phase and lasting 2–3 weeks.

—the *rehabilitation* phase, which may begin in the middle of the consolidation phase.

As most natural disasters tend to occur and recur in the same geographical areas on the globe, reactions and mechanisms for coping by the affected populations will influence the outcome of the event more than external help, which will usually arrive too late.

It is therefore important that external aid agencies should adapt their actions to the abilities of the stricken population—without causing dependency and a feeling of helplessness.

A disaster may be triggered by a sudden and unexpected event of nature, such as by earthquakes, volcanic eruption or tidal waves, but an extensive loss of life or material damage is also caused by man himself. By constantly changing his environment man can make it more hazardous. Thus deforestation will increase flooding and drought, and the size of deserts.

Also, by constantly expanding, his habitat will stretch into ever more hazardous areas. For example, the continuously growing populations of the Third World live on the seashores of Pacific islands exposed to sudden tidal waves (tsunami), or on the slopes of mountainous ridges in Asia or Southern America, prone to sudden flooding and landslides. In California and the Near East they are threatened by sudden earthquakes or by active volcanoes. As the vast majority of people, especially in the Third World, do not have the choice to move from these dangerous areas and live elsewhere, they tend to return to their damaged houses and villages, as soon as the emergency phase has terminated.

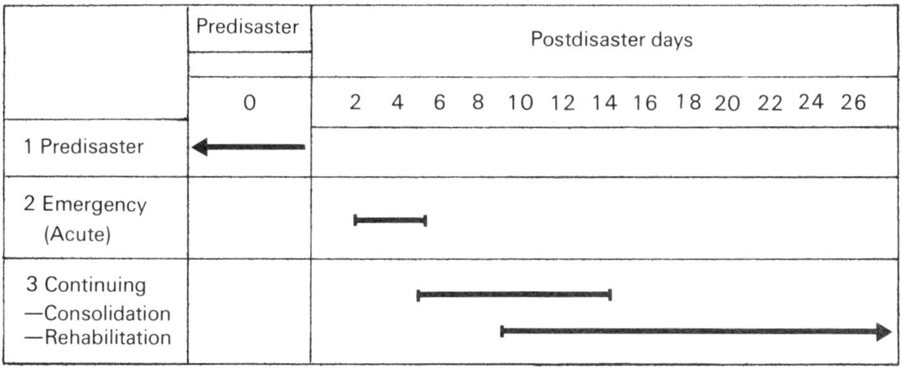

	Predisaster	Postdisaster days													
	0	2	4	6	8	10	12	14	16	18	20	22	24	26	
1 Predisaster	◄────────														
2 Emergency (Acute)		┣━━━┫													
3 Continuing —Consolidation —Rehabilitation				┣━━━━━━━┫											

Fig. 7.1. The phases of the disaster process.
(Modified from: *Environmental Health Management After Natural Disasters,* PAHO, 1982.)

THE EFFECTS OF DISASTERS

Disasters may have both similar and different effects on the population and its infrastructure. The main events and their effects are summarized in *Table* 7.1.

In disasters causing substantial damage to the infrastructure of dwellings, roads, communication, power and water supply and health services, people will be at least forced to evacuate the disaster area temporarily. This movement will be to a 'safer' place, perhaps to high grounds after flooding, to an open area after an earthquake, or to a more fertile part of the country during a drought.

Only in very unusual circumstances will populations have to be evacuated permanently. This happened in Seveso in northern Italy where the contamination from a chemical plant with only a few kilograms of dioxine has made part of the village uninhabitable for more than 10 years.

Table 7.1. Effects of disasters

Effect	Earthquakes	Storms	Floods Tidal waves	Drought Famine	Civil strife	Industrial nuclear accidents
Death	Many	Few	Many	Many	Moderate	Moderate
Injuries	Many	Moderate	Few	None	Many	Many
Damage to infrastructure	Often	Some	Often	None	Often	None
Population movements	Rare	Rare	Common	Common	Common	Rare
Increased incidence of communicable disease	Rare	Rare	Common	Common	Common	Rare

(Modified from: *Emergency Health Management after Natural Disaster.* Available from PAHO.)

In the recent accident in April 1986 in the nuclear power plant in Chernobyl in the Soviet Ukraine, an explosion occurred in the fourth unit of the plant causing a fire which damaged the reactor and its core and caused the release of a large amount of radioactive substances. More than 200 persons were directly affected by radiation and about 20 people died in the months following the disaster, in spite of intensive care including bone marrow transplantation. A population of about 150000 people had to be temporarily evacuated and an area within the radius of 30 km is presently contaminated and uninhabitable.

The direct and indirect effects of such an extensive contamination spreading widely beyond the borders of the affected country are not yet fully appreciated.

SECONDARY HEALTH RISKS

In continuing disasters, such as drought, people will converge on communities less affected by famine in search of food and support. Those who are stronger will trek along main roads to more fertile parts of the country. This was observed in northern Ethiopia during the famine of 1984–5. In order to provide necessary relief and protect the surrounding population from looting, responsible government agencies assemble these refugees in camps. The number of people in these camps may increase very rapidly if a crisis continues, as in 1979–80 when hundreds of thousands of refugees crossed the border from Kampuchea into Thailand as a result of civil war.

In one of these camps, in Sakei, more than 30000 Kampuchean refugees were crowded in a camp in an area of less than 20000 sq m, allowing a net area of $2/3$ sq m for each person. The hot and humid climate, the compromised sanitary conditions in the camp and the lowered resistance of the emaciated victims due to longstanding malnutrition and malaria caused a sharp increase in morbidity, as shown in *Table 7.2.*

Table 7.2. Admissions to the camp hospital in Sakei-Thailand during one week in November, 1979. (No. of hospital beds—1000)

Disease	No. of patients	%
Fever/malaria	112	39
Pneumonia	63	22
Anaemia	28	10
Malnutrition	24	8
Meningitis	20	7
Diarrhoea	20	7
Others (inc. T.B.)	23	8
	290	100

N.B. About 75% of all patients were infested with parasites.

(Reproduced by courtesy of Adler et al. (1981) Medical mission to a refugee camp in Thailand. *Disasters* 5, No. 1.)

Often epidemics break out in refugee camps, but especially among the susceptible part of the population. During a measles epidemic in the camp of Khao I Dang on the Thai-Kampuchean border, complications of measles accounted for about 18 per cent of all hospitalizations between December 1979 and the end of February 1980.

An epidemic of cholera which struck Ethiopia in late 1984 and early 1985 involved 800 cases and caused 150 deaths among 5000 refugees in a camp in the province of Wollo, in just two weeks.

Summary

The risk factors causing a deterioration in the health status among displaced persons will be as follows:

—Disruption of family and social structure with accompanying psychological stress.
—Crowding in camps and temporary settlements.
—Deficient sanitary conditions, vector and pest control.
—Lack of epidemiological surveillance.
—Malnutrition.
—Decreased resistance to communicable diseases.
—Discontinuation of medical care for chronic diseases.

REFUGEE CAMPS AND SANITARY REQUIREMENTS

If possible, the establishment of camps should be avoided because of the increased risk of the spread of communicable diseases. Nevertheless, in conditions prevailing in continuing disasters, when large numbers of the population will have to move from the affected area, camps may have to be constructed to provide a safe and sheltered environment.

A camp should be planned for a limited number of people on an adequate site on elevated ground to prevent inundation in the rainy season. It should be adequately ventilated but protected from storms, floods and tidal waves. The camp should be easily accessible to vehicles through a paved road with an internal net of paved roads and walk ways.

Public areas, administration offices, communal kitchens and hospitals should be constructed near the entrance to the camp and its main road of access. In the majority of areas the camps must be fenced to prevent unauthorized access and mixing with the surrounding population. The fence should not be of barbed wire, to prevent both injuries at night and a feeling of forced imprisonment. Shelters should preferably be built with locally available building material, like bamboo, or by erecting tents of adequate size to allow for the accommodation of entire families. Ample space should be available between the shelters and tents for family cooking, washing and playgrounds for children. Drainage ditches should be dug for the rainy season. The floors of shelters should be covered with plastic sheets or bamboo mats, or elevated on wooden pallets if the ground is wet. Each person should receive a bamboo mat or a mattress and at least two blankets.

Water Supply

In the majority of cases, a safe public water supply will not be available and water will have to be pumped from local water holes or wells. Because of the risk of contamination, water will have to be purified in large containers or tanks with chlorine tablets. Daily examination of the chlorine content at the water faucets should be performed by trained personnel with the aid of a simple 'Chlorine assessment kit'. Water should be supplied from the containers through a closed pipe system to faucets, evenly distributed throughout the camp. Absorption pits for the drainage of spilled water have to be dug at each distribution point. In hot climates the daily minimum requirement is 30–40 litres of water for each person.

Latrines

The disposal of human excrement presents a difficult problem, especially in crowded camps with many sick people suffering from diarrhoea. Many will be too sick and weak to walk without help to a distant latrine and therefore will defaecate between the shelters. In such cases sanitary teams appointed by the camp administration must immediately cover the excrements with soil or sand mixed with lime and chlorine powder for disinfection. Pit latrines should be dug at a minimum distance of 75–100 m from the nearest shelter, in a down-wind direction. The distance of latrines from the communal kitchen, feeding centre and storage areas should be even greater.

The main problem in warm climates is to prevent flies from multiplying on human excreta in the latrines. In all open latrines the contents should be covered with earth, lime and chlorine powder several times a day. The minimum requirement is one pit latrine per 20 persons.

Insect and Pest Control

Flies and mosquitoes spread disease, specially in warm and humid climates. Rats and mice are attracted by human settlements and by inadequate protection of food stores.

The control of insects and pests can best be achieved by meticulous sanitary measures in the camp area. In addition, insecticides and pesticides may be needed, but should only be used by trained personnel, taking the utmost precautions to prevent accidental poisoning.

ASSESSMENT OF HEALTH NEEDS

During and immediately after the acute phase of a disaster, an assessment of the most urgent needs of the stricken community has to be performed. Assessment is a continuous process of gathering new information, reviewing it in reaction to previous information and forming updated policies. Graphically it may be represented by a circle with several segments for each disaster phase (*Fig.* 7.2).

The assessment of health needs is usually performed by the remaining local health personnel, e.g. public health nurses, community health workers, sanitary personnel, physicians and administrators. These workers are most familiar with the local population, its structure and needs. It is a well known fact that disasters

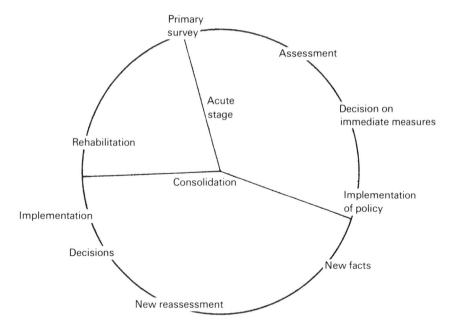

Fig. 7.2. The circle of assessment in disasters.

that disrupt local government and the social framework produce individuals who take the initiative, becoming the 'self-appointed leaders' of the community. It is of vital importance that outside agencies recognize these individuals, have them participate in decisions and the implementation of policy. The anticipated needs for the affected community will be:

1. Search and rescue teams to save trapped victims.
2. Emergency medical services to stabilize the injured.
3. Prevention of secondary health hazards from fires, gas leaks, flooding or the spillage of dangerous substances, by evacuation of the population in danger.
4. Providing shelter, water, food and clothing.
5. Providing information about relatives' dead, hospitalized or evacuated.

The objective of assessment is to accumulate relevant facts from the disaster area based on objective observation and surveys. If the stricken area is large, an aerial survey, preferably by photography, may be the most efficient and expedient way to acquire the necessary information. This information should include a demographic profile, including the location of the affected population, its immediate needs for survival, epidemiological facts and the inventory of the remaining health services. (*See Table* 7.3, for a comprehensive example of how much of the information can be collected and tabulated.)

The information, gathered in a systematic and objective manner, should be immediately forwarded to government and other relevant health or relief agencies who plan to support the affected area.

Table 7.3. Survey form on population and health needs in a disaster area

---

A. DEMOGRAPHIC PROFILE

(Country, Province, Town): _____

Location: _____

Languages: _____

Nature of Disaster: _____

Time of Impact: _____ No. of People Affected: _____

Refugee Camps; Location and No. of people in each camp: _____

People Without Shelters (Location): _____

B. ESSENTIAL SERVICES

Water Supply (including Wells, Pumps, Containers, Purification, Distribution): _____

Food Supply (Source, Baby Food, Cooking, Distribution): _____

Intensive Feeding (No. of people in programme): _____

Specify Needs for Water and Food: _____

Sanitary Services (Specify Latrines, Water Requirements for Personal Hygiene, Soap, Toilet
   Paper, etc.): _____

Blankets and Mattresses needed: _____

Clothing and Footware needed: _____

C. BURIAL SERVICES (Specify needs)

D. EPIDEMIOLOGY

Specify Endemic Diseases in Area: _____

Communicable Diseases Presently in Area : _____

Immunization Programmes, Existing and Ongoing: _____

Malnutrition Existing: (Specify Approx. Percentage in Age Groups): _____

Secondary Risks to Population (Flooding, Fires, Toxic Material, etc.) _____

Mortality Rate in Age Groups (per 1000): _____

E. PRIMARY HEALTH SERVICES

Clinics (No. of Population Served by each Clinic): _____

Other Services (First Aid, Ambulance, Visiting Mobile Teams, etc.): _____

Mother and Well Baby Clinics (Nos. and Population Served): _____

Personnel Required (Specify Nurses, Doctors, Auxiliary Personnel): _____

Drugs and Other Equipment Needed: _____

Vaccinations Needed (Specify Types, Amounts): _____

No. of Ambulances Needed: _____

Table 7.3. (*continued*)

F. HOSPITALIZATION

General Hospitals in Area (Nos. Distance from Disaster Site, No. of Beds Each): _____

Special Hospitals in Area (Psychiatric, Maternity, Geriatric, etc.): _____

Needs for Additional Facilities (Field Hospitals, Specify Services and Required Beds): _____

Supporting Services (Specify Needs for Lab. X-Ray and other Services): _____

Needs for Drugs and Other Equipment (incl. Generators and Transportation): _____

G.

Information Gathered By: _____

Sources (Personal Survey, Local Health Services, or other Sources): _____

Date: _____ Signature: _____

THE CONSOLIDATION PHASE

This period follows the emergency phase of the disaster and continues for about two weeks in the continuing phase. It is characterized by the end of the 'isolation' period—by which time outside help will usually have arrived. During this period local leadership will have emerged and local government, aided and supported by regional and national administrations, will begin to function again.

The first step will be to reconvene a local 'Disaster Management Committee' which should preferably have been established in the pre-disaster period. This committee should include senior representatives of all vital services, including health services. *Fig.* 7.3 depicts a possible chart of organization.

The director of the Committee should be a leader of the local community, such as the mayor, the senior police officer or the chief of fire services.

In several countries the Civil Defence Services are responsible for disaster management and the senior officials of these organizations may lead the Committee. If a state of national emergency is proclaimed, the Armed Forces may be in command of the disaster area and the commanding officer will be responsible.

The tasks of the Committee will be as follows:

—Assess the immediate and continuing neeeds of the population.

—State priorities for re-establishing vital services—including health services.

—Mobilize all available manpower and material resources to repair the damaged infrastructure including water and power supplies, communication and transportation services.

—Plan the reconstruction of permanent housing and public buildings (schools, hospitals, etc.).

—Restore production, commerce, education and the return to a normal pattern of life.

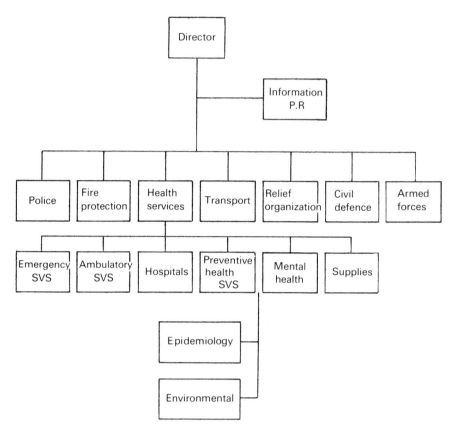

Fig. 7.3. The structure of a disaster committee. (SVS = services)

HEALTH SERVICES

Public health services will be restored in stages with the priority of meeting the most essential needs of the population first.

Primary Care and Nutrition

These are the most important services and should, therefore, be restored immediately after the emergency phase. The displaced population, dwelling in temporary shelters or refugee camps, will be exposed to intercurrent diseases, like upper respiratory tract infections, diarrhoea and other communicable diseases.

Infants and children, in particular, will need special attention to prevent dehydration and deterioration in their nutrition. In some areas where famine is prevalent, supervised feeding programmes will have to be established, either as part of an existing medical facility or as an ambulatory service.

If the famine is widespread, there will be parts of the population who will not be able to attend the feeding programmes or distribution centres regularly, because of transportation and communication problems. In such a situation which occurred in northern Ethiopia in 1984–5, food has to be brought to the most remote places by ground transport, aircraft or even helicopter.

Any feeding programme will have to receive constant medical support as malnutrition is almost always concomitant with infections and parasitic diseases. This problem arose in a refugee camp on the Thai-Kampuchean border in 1979 when many infants and children on intensive feeding had to be hospitalized intermittently because of bouts of malaria, bacillary dysentery and hook-worm infestation. Some of the children suffered from severe iron-deficiency anaemia, which did not respond to parenteral iron and folic acid treatment, because of severe hypo-albuminemia. A programme of whole blood transfusions was initiated with immediate beneficial results.

Rehydration can usually be obtained with supervised drinking of *Oral Rehydration Salt* solutions. In cases where oral fluids cannot be given, because of vomiting or lack of response, isotonic electrolyte solutions with glucose may be administered intraperitoneally. A 19-gauge needle or intravenous cannula is connected to the tubing of the i.v. set and introduced obliquely at an angle of 45° about 2·45 cm below the umbilicus in the abdominal midline (*Fig.* 7.4).

This method is applicable to small children and infants in whom the introduction of intravenous lines is difficult and fluid overloading common. In the most severe cases of dehydration and in adults, i.v. lines have to be used to restore fluid depletion quickly.

Public Health Clinics

Ambulatory services should be established in camps or areas where large numbers of refugees are assembled. The clinic should be centrally located, easily accessible to the population and clearly marked with a red cross sign or flag.

Ample space, protected against sun and rain, has to be provided for patients waiting to be attended. Medical triage should be performed by an experienced nurse or doctor to ensure prompt attention to all severe cases.

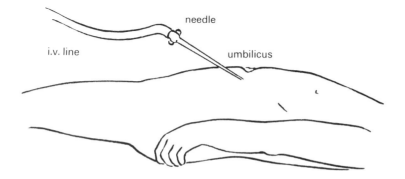

Fig. 7.4. The introduction of intraperitoneal fluids in children.

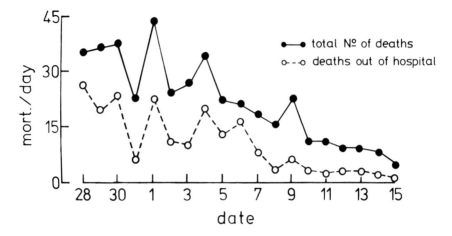

Fig. 7.5. Mortality rate (from 28 October to 15 November, 1979) in a refugee camp in Thailand.

Follow-up cases should receive treatment and drugs in a separate section. If necessary, the clinic may be expanded to become a day-care centre where intensive feeding or rehydration may be performed.

In crowded conditions with compromised sanitary arrangements, measles, meningococcal meningitis, typhoid fever, hepatitis and cholera may assume epidemic proportions and immunization has to be considered. Mass vaccination can be performed by mobile teams in camps or at distribution centres.

Recording of all patients attending the clinic is important to monitor the incidence of disease, and any unusual occurrence has to be reported immediately to the responsible health authorities.

All camps and temporary dwellings should be screened regularly by health teams, so as to locate sick people and bring them to medical attention. Experience in refugee camps in Thailand in 1979–80 and in Ethiopia during the recent famine has shown that about 50–60 per cent of all deaths occurred outside the local hospitals (*Fig.* 7.5). Most of these patients were too weak to go to the clinic or the hospital on their own, and their relatives and neighbours left them to die in their tents.

Hospitalization

Hospitals in the disaster area will be fully occupied for several weeks after an extensive disaster has occurred. In some instances, where evacuation of casualties to local hospitals is difficult or prolonged, 'field hospitals' may be deployed in the disaster area itself, usually provided by the armed forces or by foreign aid agencies. A field hospital may provide specialized surgical care to casualties in the immediate post-disaster phase and stabilize them for further transportation. During the 'continuing' phase they may provide regular hospitalization to the affected population. A hospital may be located in a refugee camp and operated by the organization administering the camp, or it may be established near an existing medical facility. In most cases the field hospital will

contain a limited number of beds and only the basic medical specialities.
    It should include the following services and departments (*see Fig.* 7.6).
    —*admission*—for the triage, diagnosis and stabilization of patients who then
        will be transferred to the proper ward;
    —*general medical ward*—for adult care;
    —*paediatric ward*—for infants and children up to the age of 15.
    —*obstetric/gynaecological ward;*

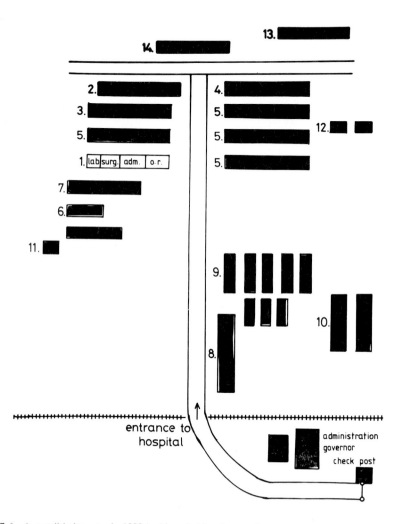

Fig. 7.6. A possible layout of a 1000-bed hospital in a large refugee camp.

Legend: (1) Admission, Laboratory, X-Ray and Operating theatre; (2) Gynaecology and obstetrics;
(3) Paediatric ward; (4) Infectious diseases; (5) General medicine; (6) Rehabilitation; (7) Kitchen
(hospital); (8) Kitchen (camp); (9) Feeding unit; (10) Orphanage; (11) Morgue; (12) Administration;
(13) Medical store; (14) Staff latrines.

—*isolation ward*—for the infectious diseases which may spread throughout the camp;

—*surgical and orthopaedic ward;*

—*an operation theatre*—in which minor surgery may be performed under local, inhalational or intravenous anaesthesia. Major cases should be transferred to a fixed local hospital;

—*a laboratory*—for basic analyses of urine, blood counts, blood smears for malaria, stains for acid-fast bacilli and gram stains. Stools should be examined for parasites and ova;

—*a radiology facility*—preferably with a lightweight and mobile machine equipped with polaroid films;

—also the hospital should include a kitchen, a storage area, a morgue, an administration area and sanitary facilities.

A medical director, preferably a physician with administrative skills, experienced in disaster situations, has to be appointed, supported by a limited staff—including a chief nurse, administrator and pharmacist. His tasks will be to decide admission and treatment policies and to ensure co-ordination between the various medical teams, the camp administration, health officials in the affected country and voluntary relief organizations.

Daily meetings should be held with the representatives of all teams and agencies operating in the camp and hospital to discuss medical and management problems.

REHABILITATION

The objective of this phase, which may continue for months or years, is to re-establish pre-disaster medical services for the affected population. The services should be improved and incorporate the lessons learned during the previous phases. Very often policy-makers argue that medical services provided during the continuing and rehabilitation phases should not exceed services regularly provided for the population in the predisaster phase. Doubtless, the ratio of doctors and nurses will increase substantially during the disaster situation, because of the greater health risks which threaten the exposed population.

Farmers, living in the widely spread rural dwellings and villages in the northern provinces of Ethiopia, were certainly less exposed to epidemics of measles, cholera and other communicable diseases than the thousands of refugees incarcerated in camps.

The return to 'normality' is vital for the affected population, to avoid dependence on outside nutritional and medical support. To diminish this dependence, the local population and their leaders should actively participate in their own rehabilitation. Construction workers, and even the unskilled must be employed by both the local government and by the relief agencies to rebuild their homes and the damaged infrastructure of their own community. Local politicians and administrators should be encouraged to participate in the planning of reconstruction from the earliest possible stage.

S. W. A. Gunn

8

The Co-ordination of Governments and the Relief Agencies

Drought, famine, war, refugees, epidemics, mass casualties and technological catastrophes, whether happening singly or, worse still, in conjunction, are events and risks that are increasingly threatening or striking large populations. A single disaster can destroy laboriously constructed services and instantly annihilate costly health systems and facilities. Even a technologically advanced and financially sound government will have difficulty in facing such an emergency. Worse still, there is at present a 'disaster belt' of earthquakes, cyclones, volcanic eruptions and desertification that extends over most of the non-industrialized world, affecting over 90 developing countries which hardly have the financial possibility, human resources, technical knowledge or planning capacity to cope with such disabling situations. Hence the need for concerted action by governments, relief agencies, and the international community in general.

By 'international community' is meant not only the usually solicited donor governments and the classic organizations such as the United Nations and the Red Cross, but also the vast network of relief agencies and institutions, official or benevolent, large or small, governmental, inter-governmental or non-governmental, lay or religious, each founded for a definite purpose, each with resources large or small, all pursuing humanitarian assistance of different kinds.

It must be stressed, and be realized from the outset of any relief operation that, whatever the nature of the disaster or the emergency circumstances, the primary responsibility for managing the disaster and caring for the victims rests with the government concerned. It is also important for the in-coming helper to realize that whatever the magnitude of outside assistance, it is the stricken country that bears most of the brunt—up to 80 per cent or more—of the efforts of relief and reconstruction.

INTERNATIONAL AID

Emergency assistance during a disaster will involve planning, mobilization and co-ordination both at the national and the international levels. Increasingly, however, international assistance is also being extended in the preventive field, in the form of training and preparedness for disasters, especially in countries known to be at risk.

ACTION OF THE
INTERNATIONAL COMMUNITY
IN DISASTER

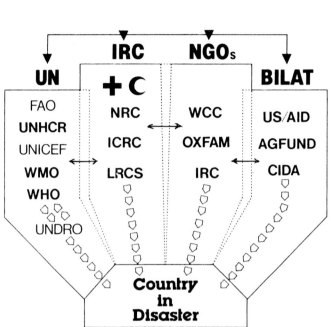

Fig. 8.1. Diagram showing the 4 principal mechanisms of co-ordinated international action in disasters.

Following a disaster, assistance by governments and relief agencies is expected and often provided generously. Mechanisms therefore must exist or be put into motion to organize this international effort and to co-ordinate it to ensure maximum effectiveness.

Four principal systems are involved in international aid, historically most of them born of a disaster, to alleviate disaster. The ICRC was founded more than a century ago on the battlefield of Solferino, the League of Red Cross Societies as a result of the First World War, the United Nations after the Second World War, and Oxfam after the troubles and famines in Bangladesh. This chapter does not deal with wartime assistance or conflict situations, where of course the Geneva Conventions come into play.

In disasters, international aid by governments and relief agencies, and their co-ordination, can be represented by the diagram in *Fig.* 8.1. This shows the 4 principal mechanisms: (1) the United Nations, (2) the International Red Cross, (3) the Non-Governmental Organizations (NGO) and (4) bilateral direct assistance by governments.

The United Nations

The UN is the supreme assembly of all nations and has general co-ordinating as well as specific roles to play in disasters. Each Specialized Agency of the UN system has a task of its own: FAO deals with agricultural emergencies, WFP with food supplies, UNHCR with refugees and mass migrations, UNEP with environmental disasters, UNICEF with children's welfare, and WHO steps in whenever the health of a population is endangered. The activities of these organizations are not limited to emergencies, and indeed long-term development is their constant concern.

To take an example of a refugee disaster, the UN High Commissioner for Refugees will have overall responsibility; the World Health Organization will be responsible for the health aspects of the camps; food will not be its concern. This is the responsibility of the Food and Agriculture Organization and of the World Food Programme, but if food shortages create malnutrition and, say, Vitamin A deficiency, then WHO will be involved. Logistical problems and supplies will probably fall under the Representative of the United Nations Development Programme. *Fig.* 8.2. shows the flowchart of contributions in an emergency through UNHCR.

These are many and diverse elements and call for proper co-ordination. Within the UN this task is carried out by UNDRO, the Office of the UN Disaster Relief Co-ordinator.

Naturally, co-ordination is needed not only within the United Nations, as outlined above, but also, and especially, among all the other participants in the concerted relief action. This usually is an ad hoc arrangement, like the 1985–6 Office of Emergency Operations for Africa against the drought and famine disaster in that continent.

The International Red Cross

There is sometimes confusion about the various Red Cross organizations. The International Red Cross is made up of three components:

    a. the International Committee of the Red Cross (ICRC)
    b. the League of Red Cross and Red Crescent Societies
    c. the National Societies.

The ICRC is an entirely Swiss organization and intervenes principally in conflictual disasters and wars and in matters of humanitarian law.

The League is the international federation of all the National Societies and is concerned above all with natural disasters.

The third element is the *National Societies*, such as the British Red Cross or the Egyptian Red Crescent, whose activities are primarily geared to the needs of their own countries.

It is important to realize that although the Red Cross is a non-governmental organization it enjoys official status in every country. This distinguishes it from the general run of NGOs and gives it special importance.

The Non-Governmental Organizations (NGOs)

There is a host of voluntary humanitarian organizations doing good work in disasters. The World Council of Churches, Caritas Internationalis, Terre des

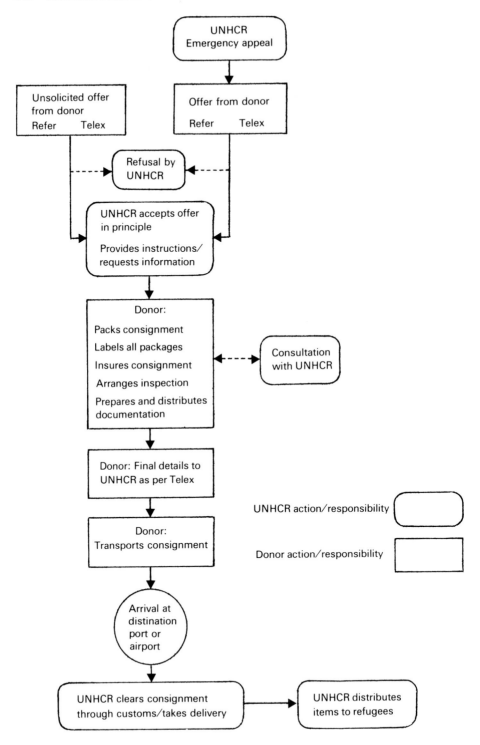

Hommes, Médecins sans Frontière and Oxfam are just a few of the better-known examples out of the several thousand relief agencies. Some specialize in specific fields, such as nutrition or the provision of artificial limbs, while others cover a wider field.

The overall agency that brings all these relief organizations together is ICVA, the International Council of Voluntary Agencies.

The proficiency of and need for these agencies is acknowledged by governments and by the UN and mechanisms exist for many of them to have official relations with such governmental bodies.

Bilateral Aid

This is direct assistance negotiated between a donor government, e.g. the United Kingdom, or group of governments, e.g. the European Economic Community, with a beneficiary government, e.g. Ghana.

Some countries have a permanent machinery for such aid; for example ODA (the Overseas Development Administration) in the UK, the Swedish International Development Agency (SIDA), the Canadian International Development Authority (CIDA), etc.

As will be seen from *Fig.* 8.1, the systems overlap and arrows show a constant inter-relationship between the various organizations. This is intentional and real, and provides a reasonable measure of co-ordination.

NON-EMERGENCY INTERNATIONAL WORK FOR DISASTERS

While the above-mentioned facts mainly concern the co-ordination of international action in emergencies, governments and relief agencies are also becoming increasingly involved in non-emergency, preventive and preparedness programmes of different kinds.

Thus, studies on the nature and disease profile of disasters have already shed light on the needs following each kind of disaster. University courses in London, France, USA and elsewhere are producing better trained disaster managers. The World Health Organization has (*see* p. 169) devised an Emergency Health Kit that responds to most of the immediate requirements of 10 000 people for 3 months. The Council of Europe has established a Centre for the Study of Disaster Medicine in San Marino, while several periodicals specialize in emergency and disaster medicine. An extensive bilingual dictionary has been published to expedite urgent action and facilitate co-ordination. Several national and international associations exist for the study and promotion of scientific disaster management. All this enhances preparedness and action.

In present-day disaster response, governments, inter-governmental bodies and relief agencies work together for the populations stricken by mass emergency

Fig. 8.2. Example of the sequence of co-ordinated action in mobilizing contributions for a refugee emergency.
(Reproduced by courtesy of UNHCR.)

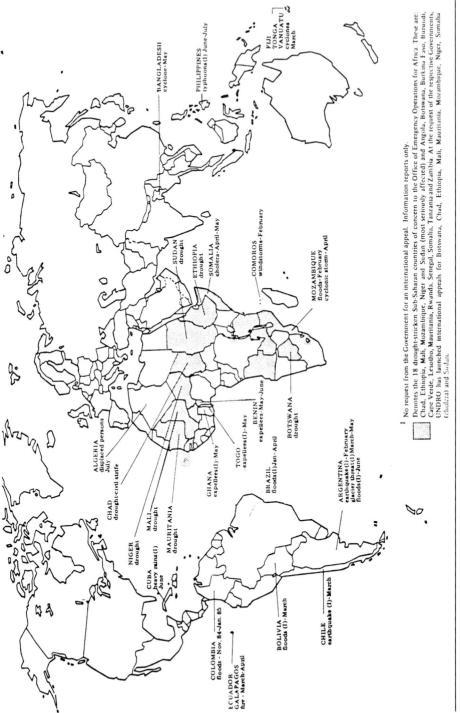

Fig. 8.3. World map showing United Nations assistance in a variety of disasters in many countries during the first half of 1985. (Reproduced by courtesy of UNDRO.)

(*see Fig.* 8.3). Management is so complex that co-ordinated action is indispensable, and the international community has set up co-ordinating mechanisms that work reasonably well. Their absence would mean an operational disaster on top of a natural disaster.

FURTHER READING

Assar M. M. (1971) *Guide to Sanitation in Natural Disasters.* Geneva, World Health Organization.
Clarke R., Ehrlich A., Gunn S. W. A. et al. (1986) *London Under Attack—Report of the GLAWARS Commission.* Oxford, Blackwell.
Gunn S. W. A. Disaster medicine and the international response to major emergencies (1987) (In press) *J. R. Coll. Surg. Ireland.*
Gunn S. W. A. (1985) La médecine des catastrophes: une nouvelle discipline médico-chirurgicale. *Helv. Chir. Acta* **52**, 11–13.
Gunn S. W. A., Murcia C. and Parakatil F. (1984) *Dictionnaire des Secours d'Urgence en Cas de Catastrophe.* Paris, Conseil International de la Langue Francaise.
Jeannet E. (1985) *Catastrophes et Médecine.* Lausanne, Payot.
Prevention and mitigation of disaster: sanitary aspects, Vol. 8 (1982) Office of the United Nations Disaster Relief Co-ordinator, UN, Geneva.
United Nations High Commissioner for Refugees (1986) *UNCHR Guide to In-kind Contribution in Refugee Emergencies.* Geneva, UNHCR.
WHO Emergency Health Kit: Standard Drugs and Clinic Equipment for 10 000 Persons for 3 Months. (1984) Geneva, World Health Organization.

Training for Disaster Medicine

INTRODUCTION

To provide good medical care for the victims of a disaster the doctor, nurse or paramedic requires astute clinical judgement, skills in acute medicine, familiarity with the arrangements and plans for such a disaster, a high degree of flexibility, firm decision making, a sturdy personality and, above all, compassion.

To follow the classification adopted in this book, the training requirements can broadly be considered under two headings, although there is extensive overlap between them.

1. Disasters Occurring in the So-called 'Sophisticated World'

These are usually related to some form of man-made disaster such as transport accidents, terrorism or war, or chemical or nuclear contamination on a large scale, but then also may be due to upheavals of nature such as volcano, earthquake, hurricane or tidal wave in regions where these are prone to happen.

2. Disasters Occurring in the Developing World

These are frequently due to a cruel freak of nature such as flood, earthquake, volcano, famine or drought. Because of poor resources, infrastructure and planning there is often an unnecessary massive mortality and morbidity. The disaster may be an acute event on top of a chronic state of ill health and deprivation among the population—'the straw which broke the camel's back'.

DISASTERS IN THE 'SOPHISTICATED WORLD'

Most areas of the sophisticated world are provided with a reasonable service for coping with day-to-day small scale emergencies. There are well trained professional ambulance and rescue services and a widespread network of hospitals offering an extensive range of specialist skills and facilities. With flexibility and co-operation across the routine but artificial boundaries, the majority of disasters can be catered for without major disruption. In many ways guidance must take the form of 'Do what you normally do only more of it'. However, certain extra principles, training and skills must be added to provide the optimal care for a large number of patients under disaster conditions.

The Prehospital Phase

The skills of the paramedic ambulanceman and the immediate care doctor include basic and advanced trauma life support, the early management of spinal and limb fractures, chest, abdominal and head injuries, and burns.

The acquisition of such skills requires training both in the field and in the hospital. Field training is needed to be aware of the limitations and constrictions imposed by the relatively hostile environment and to determine the suitability of techniques and equipment for use under much less than ideal circumstances. Hospital training is needed to acquire the theory of trauma management and practical skills such as endotracheal intubation, cricothyrotomy, intravenous cannulation and infusion, drug therapy, the insertion of chest drains, the application and use of pneumatic counter pressure devices (MAST) suits, the immediate treatment of fractures and burns, and the relief of pain.

It has been the authors' experience with student paramedic ambulancemen in Bristol that such hospital training requires approximately 400 hours of theoretical and practical tuition over and above the skills of the basic ambulanceman. The training should preferably be acquired by secondment in one block of 3–4 months. To become reliably proficient at endotracheal intubation and intravenous cannulation requires on average 50 attempts at each procedure.

During this period the student paramedic is also taught advanced cardiac life support which will stand him or her in good stead in everyday practice. As far as possible, the equipment used for training in hospital should be the same as that used by the paramedic in his field environment. Refresher courses of a few days each year are required to maintain the expertise and achieve recertification. Training to at least similar standards should also be acquired by doctors who may be asked to work in the field. These skills are paramount in the majority of disasters as well as the everyday accident and emergency but must be added to and modified for the multicasualty incident.

Additional Skills Required for Multicasualty Incidents

Triage

Triage skills are not normally required in day-to-day incidents as the number of patients is small and all are catered for virtually simultaneously. Where mass casualties are concerned, however, the first health care professional (usually an ambulanceman) must quickly assess the casualties to ascertain those with life-threatening injuries requiring immediate treatment and evacuation. Experience has shown that, until doctors arrive, well trained paramedics are quite capable of this task although they may perhaps be somewhat pessimistic in their allocation of patients to the various categories.[1] In this rapid assessment it is well to remember the words of Dr Ronald Stewart of Pittsburgh who reminds us that 'patients have fronts and backs and lefts and rights'. The obvious injury may not necessarily be the one that is a threat to life.

Another feature characteristic of the mass casualty incident is that those with mortal wounds may well have to be left on one side and made as comfortable as possible until such time as those with survivable injuries have been attended to. This agonizing decision is not usually faced in the field under normal conditions and it takes balanced clinical judgement and a sturdy personality to get the priorities right.

Training in triage skills can be acquired through disaster exercises, particularly in conjunction with the military services who are especially practised in this field. Those deciding on the casualties' 'injuries' for such an exercise would do well to take their examples from the actual casualty list of a real disaster in similar circumstances, e.g. an aircraft crash or terrorist incident.

Triage skills can also be taught economically by paper exercises. The students are provided with a list of the injuries occurring in a number of casualties and, having been told the facilities and personnel available, are asked to allocate priorities to the casualties giving their reasons for doing so. An important part of this exercise is the debriefing and discussion which occurs afterwards. An example list of casualties for such an exercise is given in the appendix at the end of this chapter.

Triage training should include familiarity with the documentation used locally for disaster incidents (e.g. triage cards, *see* Chapter 2). Every effort should be made to integrate and standardize such documentation on at least a regional, if not a national, scale.

'Working out of a Box'

Hospital doctors, as a rule, have little experience of working outside their own cosy and ordered environment. Practice at a disaster incident is the converse of this situation. Equipment must be scaled down to the minimum that is portable. Working surfaces do not exist, and assistance may be unavailable or unskilled. Self-reliance and a ruthless determination of priorities are essential.

Practice using a minimum of equipment can be obtained by the far-sighted practitioner by working with the local ambulance service in a 'ride along' capacity, attendance in a professional capacity at dangerous sporting events, such as motor racing and rallying, powerboat racing, marathon running and massive crowd events such as Papal visits. Part-time military service also involves regular drills using the minimum of equipment under field conditions.

The Command System

Management of the major incident requires an effective command system. The health care professional, while retaining his clinical freedom in the care of his individual patients, must be prepared to subject him or herself to command from other disciplines such as the fire brigade, demolition experts, military or political authorities. Usually, the ultimate authority rests with the police and this will be particularly applicable in the terrorist incident or violent political demonstration which are becoming one of the most common reasons for disaster alerts.

Strict security will be required in many major incidents and medical personnel will be required to carry identification cards. Training in disaster exercises should always include security checks and involvement of the command system so that all disciplines are made aware of the need to integrate with the priorities of others.

Flexibility in Practice

Medical personnel must be prepared to be flexible under disaster conditions. Every doctor should ensure that he is trained in basic resuscitative measures such as airway care, artificial ventilation, control of haemorrhage and intra-venous cannulation. Those designated to attend the actual incident outside hospital should undertake the equivalent of the advanced trauma life support course promulgated by the American College of Surgeons, which includes cannulation of central veins for rapid transfusion, the insertion of chest drains, and the management of limb and spinal fractures and burns. Experience can be gained in routine hospital practice or by using cadaveric animal preparations. It is essential that doctors should be prepared to work outside the normal scope of their own specialty—anaesthetists must be able to insert chest drains and manage fractures; surgeons should ensure that they are trained in airway care and central venous cannulation. The intensive care unit, operating room and the emergency department are ideal venues to gain such experience.

It must be remembered that a disaster may be 'compound'—that is, the medical facilities themselves may be affected by the incident such as an earth-quake[2] or a terrorist bomb explosion. In this case flexibility in practice is of the essence, and plans and action will have to be quickly redrawn to evacuate patients to hospitals outside the area or use tented field hospitals provided by the military or similar source.

Environmental Hazards

Many disaster incidents are associated with environmental hazards such as contamination from nuclear (*see* Chapter 30) or chemical (*see* Chapter 27) sources. There may well be dangers from unusual infections and medical personnel may be required to work in extremely unpleasant climatic conditions. Suitable protective clothing is required and training should be provided in its use particularly for exposure to nuclear or chemical agents. Familiarity with decontamination procedures should be acquired. All should be aware of the symptoms in relief workers, including their medical colleagues, who may be affected by over-exposure to any of these environmental hazards and be prepared to direct them to a place of rest and revival and decontamination.

Communications

Most disaster incidents are afflicted by relative communication failures. There is a great risk of those in the field not communicating effectively with those in the hospital, and those in the hospital not communicating with each other. Experience has shown that mobile radios are essential within the hospital for key personnel and that both mobile telephones and mobile radios are required in the field. Doctors and nurses require training in radio operation and discipline and in the use of the internationally agreed phrases and words to denote letters of the alphabet. Training can be acquired from the local ambulance service, coastguard or air training school.

Communication with the media is essential (*see* Chapter 12) and information should be channelled through agreed sources. Discipline and training is required to ensure that each and every one in the field does not grant interviews on their own special viewpoint of the incident and that individual patient confidentiality is not infringed. Nevertheless, given authoritative information, the media can be helpful, and usually will gladly make available their own communications expertise and equipment.

Psychological Factors
Even medical personnel will need to be warned that they will often experience the 'horror' factor at an incident which may impair their judgement and expertise. Little training can be offered as few of us will know how we will react until faced with the actual situation. It is also essential to be reminded that no individual is indispensible and that fatigue occurs in us all so that no-one should expect to be 'on duty' for longer than eight hours at the site. There is no room for the 'pride' factor in a major incident and everyone must be prepared to hand over to a colleague at the appropriate time.

Who should be Trained

The Ambulance Service
Clearly, the major provision of care for the disaster victims will be undertaken by the ambulance service. More and more are being trained to paramedic level which ensures a high degree of general education in the subject and the availability of practical expertise in the management of severely injured individual patients. Nevertheless, in the majority of incidents with large numbers of survivors, a substantial proportion will have minor or intermediate injuries only which can be very adequately catered for by the ambulanceman or Emergency Medical Technician (EMT) with basic training.

Particular training in triage and awareness of the 'horror', 'fatigue' and 'environmental' factors are required for the mass casualty incident.

The Doctors
Most disaster plans involve the provision of medical teams at the site of the incident who may be drawn from a nearby hospital (preferably not the hospital designated to receive patients), or from immediate care family practitioners.[3] Hospital teams usually consist of anaesthetists and emergency physicians. They will require training in triage, the command system, the constrictions of working in the field, in ambulances, in helicopters, environmental conditions, and a realization of their own limitations.

The Nurses
Many centres in the UK, Europe and Australia incorporate nurses as part of the mobile hospital team, and there is little doubt that they have made an invaluable contribution in many incidents. Apart from their role as expert medical assistants, their universal image as a caring profession brings considerable relief to the distressed casualties and their friends and relatives. Nurses will require special training emphasis in the command system, field medicine and environmental hazards.

The Other Rescue Services
Members of the police force, the fire brigade, aircraft and ships' crews, airport staff, factory and hotel personnel, etc. should all be given training in basic life support and first aid. They should be aware of the relevant disaster plans and be taught accurate reporting so that vital information concerning the imminent

dangers, approximate number of casualties, principal types of injuries and so forth can be transmitted effectively to the appropriate authorities.

In Hospital

Again, the principles of care of patients involved in a multicasualty incident will, by and large, follow the principles of normal clinical practice. There are, however, a number of extra skills which will be needed and some deviations from normal practice which may be required to achieve the greatest good for the greatest number. All hospital personnel must be acquainted with the hospital disaster plan and regular drills must be arranged to take account of different disaster scenarios and the regular turnover of staff which takes place within any large institution.

Additional Skills Required for the Multicasualty Incident

Many of the additional skills required in the prehospital phase will be needed at the hospital. These will include dynamic triage, communication, liaison and awareness of the command system and security arrangements. Certain personnel will need to be designated and trained, in so far as it is possible, to care for grieving relatives. Administrators should be trained in press and police liaison and be capable of interpreting medical reports.

Surgery

The old military adage that 'the minimum is plenty' applies particularly to the multicasualty incidents. Operating rooms and teams are likely to be at a premium and surgeons must resist the temptation to embark on extensive, prolonged surgery in one particular patient at the expense of denying treatment to several other potential survivors. Many surgeons in the UK and Europe have, fortunately, little experience of penetrating gunshot and shrapnel wounds and will, with advantage, take cognisance of their military colleagues' advice to follow the technique of debridement and delayed primary suture. Two operating tables may need to be used simultaneously in a single theatre and anaesthetists may supervise two patients at once with the help of a trained nurse or operating department assistant. These variations should be incorporated during training of surgeons, anaesthetists and operating room staff.

DISASTERS IN THE DEVELOPING WORLD

Disasters have always been prevalent in the developing world with a loss of life that is almost beyond comprehension on very many occasions. Frequently the situation is on-going and assistance is required over a prolonged period. Advances in media technology and presentation have resulted in the stark details of many such disasters being brought into the homes of millions through newspapers, periodicals, radio and television. Compassion is aroused, and there is no shortage of volunteers wishing to help their fellow man in his miserable plight in the wake of a disaster. However, to be of any value at all, even the most gifted nurse or doctor requires special training and guidance before jumping on the first plane after a news broadcast.

Basic Talents

The basic talents required are diplomacy, tolerance and compassion, combined with administration and leadership qualities, a gift for teaching and skills which are relevant to the particular problem and a knowledge of the facilities which may be available. Details of the types of skill needed are given in several chapters in this book. A command of the appropriate language is a valuable extra asset but the barriers can be overcome by interpreters.

Self-Protection

Volunteers should ensure that they themselves are in good health and be prepared to live in relatively primitive conditions. They should ensure that they are protected against infections which may be prevalent in the area, in so far as that is possible, and should receive guidance in taking their own personal supply of appropriate medication. A sick volunteer merely serves to compound the problem for others and may not have the natural immunity to disease which has been acquired by the local population.

Public Health

All who contemplate serving in the developing world in a disaster situation should ensure that they revise their knowledge of public health and basic sanitation principles. They should ensure that they are familiar with immunization and vaccination procedures and reinforce earlier protection programmes (*see* Chapter 18) as well as providing cover for outbreaks of new infections.

Nutrition

Clearly, chronic malnutrition is frequently a major problem in many developing countries and health workers all require basic training in this aspect of care (*see* Chapter 19). Parenteral rehydration and nutrition may be required in severe cases if there are suitable facilities but this route should only be used if it is possible to ensure that the intravenous line will not become infected.

Resuscitation

Help from outside rarely arrives in time for classical resuscitation procedures involving airway care and ventilation to be of any value. However, Safar's experience of the earthquake in Peru in 1970 has led him to the conclusion that intravenous volume replacement may often be of significant value as late as two or three days after the event.[4] There were reports of similar experiences after the earthquake in Mexico City in 1985.

Therefore, those attending such disasters as earthquakes and volcanic eruptions should ensure that they have training in advanced trauma life support techniques in readiness.

The Aftermath

The effective volunteer should be able to leave the scene of a disaster bequeathing certain talents and skills. Teaching and training the resident population on site is a more valuable contribution than individual clinical practice, though the two are inevitably intertwined.

On return to the sophisticated world, the doctor, nurse and paramedic will be armed with an increased knowledge and experience which should be imparted to others. He or she will also have an assessment of the needs of the incident and the area, and will be able to advise on the most valuable equipment and supplies that are required. With charisma, they will be able to enlist further training support and assistance which, in the long term, must be aimed at a self-sufficiency able to withstand better the disaster event which, sadly for many, is inevitable due to nature's upheavals.

REFERENCES

1. Baskett P. J. F. (1986) Experiences gained for the anaesthetist in disaster exercises. *Anaethesia Points West* **19.2**, 69–72.
2. Romo R. C. (1986) The Mexico City earthquake—An international disaster overview. *J. Wld. Assoc. Emerg. Disaster Med.* **1–4**, 4–8.
3. Zorab J. S. M. and Baskett P. J. F. (1977) In: *Immediate Care*. London, Saunders, p. 213.
4. Safar P. (1986) Resuscitation potentials in mass disasters. *J. Wld. Assoc. Emerg. Disaster Med.* **1–4**, 34–47.

FURTHER READING

Adler J. (1986) Experience of a medical team at the Harbo Refugee Camp in Ethiopia. *J. Wld. Assoc. Emerg. Disaster Med.* **1–4**, 224–7.
Baskett P. J. F. and Durner P. (eds.) (1985) Airport and aircraft disasters. *J. Wld. Assoc. Emerg. Disaster Med.* **1**(2).
Burkle F. M. (ed.) (1984) *Disaster Medicine*. New York, Medical Examination Publishing House.
Cowley R. A. and Baskett P. J. F. (eds.) (1986) Vols. 1–4. *Contributions for the Second International Assembly on Emergency Medical Services—Focus on Disaster Baltimore Md. USA 1986 and the 4th World Congress on Emergency and Disaster Medicine, Brighton, UK, 1986*. R. A. Cowley, MIEMSS, 22 S. Greene Street, Baltimore Md. 21201, USA.
Manni C. and Magalini S. I. (eds.) (1985) *Emergency and Disaster Medicine*. Heidelberg and New York, Springer-Verlag.
Safar P. (ed.) (1985) *Journal of the World Association for Emergency and Disaster Medicine*. Supplement 1, Disaster resuscitology. Pittsburgh, Resuscitation Research Centre, University of Pittsburgh.
Safar P. (ed.) (1985) Military and disaster medicine. *J. Wld. Assoc. Emerg. Disaster Med.* **1**(1).
Spirgi E. H. (1979) *Disaster Management*. Bern, Hans Huber.
Tachakra S. S. (1986) The Bhopal disaster. *J. Wld. Assoc. Emerg. Disaster Med.* **1–4**, 217–20.
WHO Emergency Health Kit (1984) *Standard Drugs and Clinic Equipment for 10000 Persons for 3 Months*. Geneva, World Health Organization.

APPENDIX TO CHAPTER 9

TRAINING IN TRIAGE BY PAPER EXERCISES

Substantial training in triage can be gained easily and inexpensively by paper exercises. The student is given brief details of the incident and the casualties and asked to place them in order of priority for assessment and immediate treatment and allocate a triage category. An example is given below of one such exercise, with acknowledgement to Lt. Col. Ian Haywood RAMC.

Background Details

It is 15.15 hours on a sunny public holiday. You are the only doctor on duty in a small hospital. It would take about 50 minutes to obtain the assistance of another doctor.

You receive a message from the ambulance control centre that ambulance crews have just extricated 6 casualties from a serious road accident and will be with you in about 10 minutes. They give you the following resumé of the patients:

Patient A is a 23-year-old male who is 'shocked', complaining of a tight constricting pain in left chest and probably has fractured ribs. He is crying out that he thinks he will die if something is not done to help him breathe. There is a fracture of the left wrist.

    Pulse 120   BP 90/60   Resp. rate 34

Patient B is a woman in labour at term who was on her way to hospital at the time of the accident. She has multiple bruises and is now having uterine contractions every 5 minutes.

    Pulse 80   BP 110/70   Resp. rate 22

Patient C is a 26-year-old woman. She is crying hysterically and complains of pain in the neck and lower back. Her neck has been immobilized in a collar. She has a compound fracture of the left tibia, a swollen right foot and, possibly, a fracture of the left forearm.

    Pulse 90   BP 140/100   Resp. rate 24

Patient D is a man who appears to be in his sixties. He was pulseless when found and cardio-pulmonary resuscitation was commenced immediately but, so far, no spontaneous pulse has been felt.

Patient E is a man in his mid-forties who is unconscious, but responding to painful stimuli, and apparently moving his legs. He is cyanosed and bleeding from the mouth and nose. There is a laceration of scalp, a deformity of the left ankle and abrasions across the lower abdomen compatible with a seat belt lesion.

    Pulse 120   BP 104/80   Resp. rate 3(+)

Patient F is a female teenager who is conscious but 'shocked'. She is complaining of severe left upper abdominal pain with abrasions at this site. She has a broken right wrist.

Pulse 120   BP 90/50   Resp. rate 26

QUESTION PAPER

Write Only on this Sheet

Read the background scenario and patient synopsis. Then answer the questions below **IN ORDER:**

1. List the order in which you would examine and carry out immediate treatment of the patients described.
2. Now turn to the individual case sheets in the order you have answered in Question 1. If it appears from them that your answer in 1 was wrong, think again, but **DO NOT** alter your original answer.

PATIENT . . . . (i)
                          (ii)
PATIENT . . . . (i)
                          (ii)
PATIENT . . . . (i)
                          (ii)
PATIENT . . . . (i)
                          (ii)
PATIENT . . . . (i)
                          (ii)
PATIENT . . . . (i)
                          (ii)
PATIENT . . . . (i)
                          (ii)
PATIENT . . . . (i)
                          (ii)

3. Now give an evacuation triage priority to each patient:
   A   B   C   D   E   F   G   H

INDIVIDUAL CASE SHEETS

Patient A

You should have seen this patient second. If you did, proceed with Questions (i) and (ii) below and then proceed to the next patient; if not, return to Question 1.

i. List which (if any) of the procedures below you will initiate in the order you would do so:
   a. Pass endotracheal tube
   b. Perform cricothyroidotomy
   c. Insert needle left chest
   d. Insert chest drain left chest

   e. Set up i.v. line
   f. Give morphine intramuscularly
   g. Give morphine intravenously
 ii. List your instructions to nurses:
   a. Nurse on left side
   b. Nurse semi-prone
   c. Check resp. rate quarter-hourly
   d. Keep i.v. running to keep BP above 120 systolic
   e. Take blood for cross-matching

Patient B

You should have seen this patient fifth. If you did, proceed with Questions (i) and (ii) below and then proceed to the next patient; if not, return to Question 1.

 i. List which (if any) of the procedures below you will initiate in the order you would do so:
   a. Carry out vaginal examination immediately to assess cervical dilation
   b. Take blood for cross-matching
   c. Send patient to obstetric unit
   d. Give morphine intravenously
 ii. List your instructions to nurses:
   a. Check foetal heart rate every 5 minutes
   b. Hand patient's case over to nurses
   c. Check urine for albumen
   d. Get patient to sign consent for elective Caesarean section
   e. Check pulse and blood pressure every 15 minutes

Patient C

You should have seen this patient fourth. If you did, proceed with Questions (i) and (ii) below and then proceed to the next patient; if not, return to Question 1.

 i. List which (if any) of the procedures below you will initiate in the order you would do so:
   a. Immobilize left leg
   b. Set up i.v. fluids
   c. Immobilize right ankle
   d. Apply plaster of Paris to right forearm
   e. Take blood for cross-matching
   f. X-ray cervical spine
   g. Give morphine intravenously
   h. X-ray left leg, right foot and left arm
   i. Assess neurological status
 ii. List your instructions to nurses:
   a. Keep patient lying down
   b. Reassure patient
   c. Watch colour of toes
   d. Measure abdominal girth every 30 minutes
   e. Measure pulse and BP every 15 minutes

Patient D

You should have seen this patient sixth. If you did, proceed with Question (i)
below; if not, return to Question 1.

   i. List which (if any) of the procedures below you will initiate in the order
you would do so:
- *a.* Order immediate ECG
- *b.* Give adrenaline i.v.
- *c.* Defibrillate if in ventricular fibrillation
- *d.* Give sodium bicarbonate
- *e.* Ventilate with oxygen rich mixture
- *f.* Pass endotracheal tube

Patient E

You should have seen this patient first. If you did, proceed with Questions (i)
and (ii) below and then proceed to the next patient; if not, return to Question 1.

   i. List which (if any) of the procedures below you will initiate in the order
you would do so:
- *a.* Take blood for cross-matching
- *b.* Set up i.v.
- *c.* Pass endotracheal tube
- *d.* Perform cricothyroidotomy
- *e.* Apply pressure dressing to scalp
- *f.* Give i.v. diazepam
- *g.* Secure airway with oropharyngeal airway
- *h.* Ventilate with self-inflating bag/valve/mask

  ii. List your instructions to nurses:
- *a.* Nurse patient on back
- *b.* Prepare for peritoneal lavage
- *c.* X-ray cervical spine
- *d.* Check pupils every 30 minutes
- *e.* Nurse in recovery position

Patient F

You should have seen this patient third. If you did, proceed with Questions (i)
and (ii) below and then proceed to the next patient; if not, return to Question 1.

   i. List which (if any) of the procedures below you will initiate in the order
you would do so:
- *a.* Apply plaster of Paris to right wrist
- *b.* Give i.v. morphine
- *c.* Take blood for cross-match
- *d.* Set up i.v.
- *e.* X-ray cervical spine
- *f.* Check haemoglobin level
- *g.* Prepare for peritoneal lavage

  ii. List your instructions to nurses:
- *a.* Pass urinary catheter

b. Pass nasogastric tube
c. Give metronidazole
d. Check pulse and BP every 15 minutes
e. Check abdominal girth every 15 minutes

THE CONTINUING PHASE

S. W. A. Gunn

10

Emergency Supplies for Disasters in Developing Countries

Disasters and large-scale emergencies have been increasing in frequency and magnitude, a trend that has been particularly devastating to the developing countries that can least cope with them. International assistance has been growing in parallel, and although a sign of generosity and solidarity, it too has created problems, particularly in the provision of emergency supplies, medicines and equipment. In disaster situations a great number of governments, relief organizations, the United Nations system, the World Health Organization and others respond to the immediate needs both by assisting the stricken country and

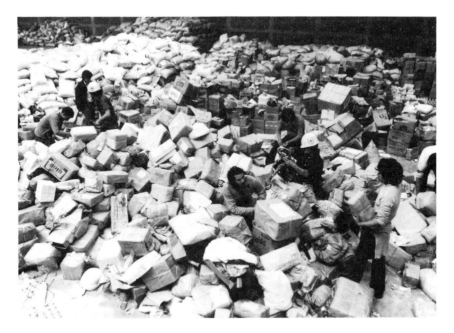

Fig. 10.1. The disorganized, unmarked and irrelevant contributions sent without co-ordination create a logistical disaster.
(Reproduced by courtesy of UNDRO/SYGMA/Laffont.)

by co-ordinating the work—in this case the health and sanitation work—of the international community (*see* Chapter 8).

An important proportion of the aid provided in emergencies almost invariably consists of medicaments and essential dispensary equipment. Quantities of requested (necessary) or non-requested (unnecessary) supplies are despached by donor agencies, governments, the UN, the Red Cross and many voluntary agencies or even individuals. The effectiveness and usefulness of such aid are often seriously hampered by donor and recipient alike through lack of assessment of the real needs, unrealistic requests, inappropriate equipment, non-essential pharmaceuticals, diversity of supplies, unsorted shipments, unintelligible labelling, expensive machinery, expired products, late arrival, customs restrictions, etc. *Fig.* 10.1 shows the chaos this can create.

Following several years of study, field testing and trials, the international community now has at its disposal lists of standard drugs and clinic equipment that significantly obviate the above-mentioned difficulties and maximize emergency response. Only three major recommended lists or pre-packed material will be mentioned here, those of the World Health Organization, Oxfam and the International Committee of the Red Cross.

WHO EMERGENCY HEALTH KIT

This has been prepared by the WHO Emergency Relief Operations office in conjunction with the UN High Commissioner for Refugees, the London University School of Hygiene and Tropical Medicine and the League of Red Cross. It has been adopted quasi-universally by national authorities, donor governments and relief organizations as the reliable, standardized, inexpensive, appropriate and quickly available source of the required pharmaceuticals and essential laboratory equipment in any disaster situation. The material is pre-packed by UNICEF and a few other supply firms, ready for despatch anywhere in the world. The contents are calculated for the needs of 10000 persons over 3 months.

Although the kit's main objective is to respond to *emergency relief* needs, stockpiling it in sufficient quantities can also serve as a measure of *disaster preparedness*. The advantages are summarized in *Table* 10.9. The overall purposes are to encourage standardization of the drugs and equipment for emergencies, to permit swift initial supply, to rationalize urgent requests and responses, to have a corpus of material that is familiar to all relief workers everywhere, and to encourage preparedness.

Any country may, of course, assemble similar kits through its own facilities, either for its own use or for assistance to others, in which case it is wise not to alter the standard specifications.

Lists A, B and C of WHO

The WHO Emergency Health Kit is made up of two lists of pharmaceuticals (A and B) and one list of clinic equipment (C). Together they make up a complete, prepackaged set of parcels ready for immediate use.

Table 10.1. List A, WHO Emergency Health Kit:* Basic drug requirements for 10 000 persons for 3 months

LIST A

BASIC DRUG REQUIREMENTS FOR 10 000 PERSONS FOR 3 MONTHS

Refer- ence No.	Drug [group in Essential Drugs list[a]]	Pharmaceutical form and strength	Total required for 3 months (rounded up)
A.1	**Analgesics** [2.1]		
	A.1.1 acetylsalicylic acid	tab. 300 mg	17 000 tab.
	A.1.2 paracetamol	tab. 500 mg	4 500 tab.
A.2	**Anthelmintics** [6.1]		
	A.2.1 mebendazole ☐	tab. 100 mg	2 100 tab.
	A.2.2 piperazine	syrup 500 mg/5 ml (30-ml bottles)	5 litres
A.3	**Antibacterials** [6.3]		
	A.3.1 ampicillin ☐	pulv. susp. 125 mg/5 ml	420 bottles of 60 ml
	A.3.2 benzylpenicillin	pulv. inj. 0.6 g (1 million IU)	500 vials
	A.3.3 phenoxymethylpenicillin	tab. 250 mg	9 500 tab.
	A.3.4 procaine benzylpenicillin	pulv. inj. 3.0 g (3 million IU)	375 vials

[a]The figures in square brackets refer to the categories and subcategories in the Model List of Essential Drugs contained in the report of the WHO Expert Committee on the Use of Essential Drugs (WHO Technical Report Series, No. 685, 1983).

☐ Square symbol indicates that alternative drugs could be used. See page 7, under Explanatory note 1.

Abbreviations used:

amp.	=	ampoule(s)
cap.	=	capsule(s)
oint.	=	ointment
pulv. inj.	=	powder for injection
pulv. susp.	=	powder for suspension
tab.	=	tablet(s)

Table 10.1. (*cont.*)

List A

Refer-ence No.	Drug [group in Essential Drugs list[a]]	Pharmaceutical form and strength	Total required for 3 months (rounded up)
	A.3.5 sulfamethoxazole + trimethoprim ☐	tab. 400 mg + 80 mg	7 500 tab.
	A.3.6 tetracycline ☐	tab. 250 mg	9 000 tab.
A.4	**Antimalarials** [6.7][b]		
	A.4.1 chloroquine ☐	tab. 150 mg	8 000 tab.
	A.4.2 chloroquine ☐	syrup 50 mg/5 ml	3 litres
A.5	**Antianaemia** [10.1]		
	A.5.1 ferrous salt + folic acid (for use during pregnancy only)	tab. 60 mg + 0.2 mg	15 000 tab.
	A.5.2 ferrous salt	tab. 60 mg	30 000 tab.
A.6	**Dermatologicals** [13]		
	A.6.1 benzoic acid + salicylic acid	oint. 6% + 3%, 25-g tube	100 tubes
	A.6.2 neomycin + bacitracin ☐	oint. 5 mg + 500 IU/g, 25-g tube	50 tubes
	A.6.3 calamine lotion ☐	lotion	5 litres
	A.6.4 benzyl benzoate	lotion 25%	35 litres
	A.6.5 gentian violet [not in Essential Drugs list]	crystals	200 g (8 bottles)

[a]The figures in square brackets refer to the categories and subcategories in the Model List of Essential Drugs contained in the report of the WHO Expert Committee on the Use of Essential Drugs (WHO Technical Report Series, No. 685, 1983).

[b]For treatment of chloroquine-resistant malaria, see List B—item B.6.2.

☐ Square symbol indicates that alternative drugs could be used. See page 7, under Explanatory note 1.

Abbreviations used:	
amp.	= ampoule(s)
cap.	= capsule(s)
oint.	= ointment
pulv. inj.	= powder for injection
pulv. susp.	= powder for suspension
tab.	= tablet(s)

Table 10.1. (*cont.*)

			List A
Refer- ence No.	Drug [group in Essential Drugs list[a]]	Pharmaceutical form and strength	Total required for 3 months (rounded up)
A.7	**Disinfectants** [15]		
	A.7.1 chlorhexidine ☐	solution 20%	5 litres
A.8	**Antacids** [17.1]		
	A.8.1 aluminium hydroxide	tab. 500 mg	5 000 tab.
A.9	**Cathartics** [17.5]		
	A.9.1 senna ☐	tab. 7.5 mg	400 tab.
A.10	**Diarrhoea (replacement solution)** [17.6]		
	A.10.1 oral rehydration salts	sachet 27.5 g/litre	6 000 sachets
A.11	**Ophthalmologicals** [21.1]		
	A.11.1 tetracycline ☐	eye oint. 1%, 5-g tube	750 tubes
A.12	**Solutions** [26.2]		
	A.12.1 water for injection	amp. 2 ml	500 amp.
	A.12.2 water for injection	amp. 10 ml	500 amp.
A.13	**Vitamins** [27]		
	A.13.1 retinol (vitamin A)	cap. 60 mg (200 000 IU)	500 cap.
	A.13.2 retinol (vitamin A)	cap. 7.5 mg (25 000 IU)	400 cap.

[a]The figures in square brackets refer to the categories and subcategories in the Model List of Essential Drugs contained in the report of the WHO Expert Committee on the Use of Essential Drugs (WHO Technical Report Series, No. 685, 1983).

☐ Square symbol indicates that alternative drugs could be used. See page 7, under Explanatory note 1.

Abbreviations used:	
amp.	= ampoule(s)
cap.	= capsule(s)
oint.	= ointment
pulv. inj.	= powder for injection
pulv. susp.	= powder for suspension
tab.	= tablet(s)

* Reproduced by courtesy of the World Health Organization. Slight modifications may be introduced in later revisions.

Table 10.2. List B, WHO Emergency Health Kit:* Drugs for use by doctors and senior health workers (in addition to List A)

LIST B

DRUGS FOR USE BY DOCTORS AND SENIOR HEALTH WORKERS
(in addition to List A)

Reference No.	Drug [group in Essential Drugs list[a]]	Pharmaceutical form and strength	Total amount
B.1	**Local anaesthetics** [1.2]		
	B.1.1 lidocaine☐	inj. 1% vial of 50 ml	10 vials
B.2	**Analgesics** [2.2]		
	[B.2.1 pethidine☐[b]	inj. 50 mg in 1-ml amp.	10 amp.]
B.3	**Antiallergics** [3]		
	B.3.1 chlorphenamine☐	tab. 4 mg	100 tab.
B.4	**Antiepileptics** [5]		
	B.4.1 diazepam	inj. 5 mg/ml, 2-ml amp.	10 amp.

[a]The figures in square brackets refer to the categories and subcategories in the Model List of Essential Drugs contained in the report of the WHO Expert Committee on the Use of Essential Drugs (WHO Technical Report Series, No. 685, 1983).

[b]This substance is subject to international control under the Single Convention on Narcotic Drugs (1961) and the Convention on Psychotropic Substances (1971). *NOT* supplied with the Emergency Health Kit: to be obtained locally in accordance with approved national procedures.

☐ Square symbol indicates that alternative drugs could be used. See page 7, under Explanatory note 1.

Abbreviations used:

amp.	=	ampoule(s)
cap.	=	capsule(s)
inj.	=	injection
inj. sol.	=	injectable solution
oint.	=	ointment
pulv. inj.	=	powder for injection
tab.	=	tablet(s)

Table 10.2. (*cont.*)

List B

Refer-ence No.	Drug [group in Essential Drugs list[a]]	Pharmaceutical form and strength	Total amount
B.5	**Antiinfectives** [6]		
	B.5.1 metronidazole☐	tab. 250 mg	1 500 tab. (2 tds 5/7 for 50 patients)
	B.5.2 benzylpenicillin	pulv. inj. 3.0 g	100 vials
	B.5.3 chloramphenicol☐	cap. 250 mg	2 000 cap. (2 qds 5/7 for 50 patients)
	B.5.4 cloxacillin☐	cap. 500 mg	3 000 cap. (1 qds 7/7 for 35 adults) (1 bd 7/7 for 30 children)
B.6	**Antimalarials** [6.7]		
	B.6.1 quinine	inj. 300 mg/ml	20 amp. of 2 ml (average of 4 ml per patient)
	B.6.2 sulfadoxine + pyrimethamine	tab. 500 mg + 25 mg	150 tab. (2-3 stat. for 50 patients)

[a]The figures in square brackets refer to the categories and subcategories in the Model List of Essential Drugs contained in the report of the WHO Expert Committee on the Use of Essential Drugs (WHO Technical Report Series, No. 685, 1983).

☐ Square symbol indicates that alternative drugs could be used. See page 7, under Explanatory note 1.

Abbreviations used:	
amp.	= ampoule(s)
bd	= take twice a day
cap.	= capsule(s)
inj.	= injection
inj. sol.	= injectable solution
oint.	= ointment
pulv. inj.	= powder for injection
qds	= take 4 times a day
stat.	= at once
tab.	= tablet(s)
tds	= take 3 times a day
x/7	= x number of days per week

Table 10.2. (*cont.*)

List B

Refer-ence No.	Drug [group in Essential Drugs list[a]]	Pharmaceutical form and strength	Total amount
B.7	**Plasma substitute [11.1]**		
	B.7.1 dextran 70	inj. sol. 6%/500 ml with 10 giving sets	5 litres
	(or Polygelatin, e.g. Haemaccel	500 ml with 10 giving sets	10 litres Eds.)
B.8	**Cardiovascular [12]**		
	B.8.1 glyceryl trinitrate	tab. 0.5 mg	100 tab.
	B.8.2 propranolol☐	tab. 40 mg	100 tab.
	B.8.3 digoxin	tab. 0.25 mg	100 tab.
	B.8.4 digoxin	inj. 0.25 mg/ml in 2-ml amp.	10 amp.
	B.8.5 epinephrine	inj. 1 mg/ml in 1-ml amp.	10 amp.
B.9	**Dermatologicals [13]**		
	B.9.1 nystatin	cream 100 000 IU/g, 30-g tube	10 tubes
	B.9.2 hydrocortisone	cream 1%, 30-g tube	10 tubes
B.10	**Diuretics [16]**		
	B.10.1 furosemide☐	tab. 40 mg	100 tab.
	B.10.2 furosemide☐	inj. 10 mg/ml in 2-ml amp.	10 amp.

[a]The figures in square brackets refer to the categories and subcategories in the Model List of Essential Drugs contained in the report of the WHO Expert Committee on the Use of Essential Drugs (WHO Technical Report Series, No. 685, 1983).

☐ Square symbol indicates that alternative drugs could be used. See page 7, under Explanatory note 1.

Abbreviations used:

amp.	=	ampoule(s)
cap.	=	capsule(s)
inj.	=	injection
inj. sol.	=	injectable solution
oint.	=	ointment
pulv. inj.	=	powder for injection
tab.	=	tablet(s)

Table 10.2. (*cont.*)

List B

Refer-ence No.	Drug [group in Essential Drugs list[a]]	Pharmaceutical form and strength	Total amount
B.11	**Gastrointestinals** [17]		
	B.11.1 promethazine☐	tab. 25 mg	100 tab.
	B.11.2 promethazine☐	syrup 5 mg/5ml, bottle of 250 ml	10 bottles
	[B.11.3 codeine☐[b]	tab. 30 mg	100 tab.]
B.12	**Hormones** [18]		
	B.12.1 hydrocortisone	pulv. inj. 100 mg	10 vials
B.13	**Opthalmologicals** [21.1]		
	B.13.1 sulfacetamide	eye oint. 10%, 5-g tube	250 tubes
B.14	**Oxytocics** [22]		
	B.14.1 ergometrine☐	tab. 0.2 mg	100 tab.
	B.14.2 ergometrine☐	inj. 0.2 mg/ml in 1-ml amp.	10 amp.
B.15	**Psychotherapeutics** [24]		
	B.15.1 diazepam☐	tab. 5 mg	100 tab.

[a] The figures in square brackets refer to the categories and subcategories in the Model List of Essential Drugs contained in the report of the WHO Expert Committee on the Use of Essential Drugs (WHO Technical Report Series, No. 685, 1983).

[b] This substance is subject to international control under the Single Convention on Narcotic Drugs (1961) and the Convention on Psychotropic Substances (1971). *NOT* supplied with the Emergency Health Kit: to be obtained locally in accordance with approved national procedures.

☐ Square symbol indicates that alternative drugs could be used. See page 7, under Explanatory note 1.

Abbreviations used:	
amp.	= ampoule(s)
cap.	= capsule(s)
inj.	= injection
inj. sol.	= injectable solution
oint.	= ointment
pulv. inj.	= powder for injection
tab.	= tablet(s)

Table 10.2. (*cont.*)

			List B
Refer- ence No.	Drug [group in Essential Drugs list[a]]	Pharmaceutical form and strength	Total amount
B.16	**Respiratory** [25]		
	B.16.1 aminophylline☐	inj. 25 mg/ml in 10-ml amp.	10 amp.
	B.16.2 salbutamol☐	oral inhalation, 0.1 mg per dose	5 aerosols
	B.16.3 beclometasone	oral inhalation, 0.05 mg per dose	5 aerosols
B.17	**Solutions** [26.2]		
	B.17.1 compound solution of sodium lactate☐	inj. sol., 500 ml	10 litres
	B.17.2 glucose	inj. sol. 50% hypertonic, 10-ml amp.	10 amp.
	B.17.3 sodium chloride	inj. sol. 0.9% isotonic, 500 ml with 10 giving sets	5 litres
	B.17.4 water for injection	10-ml amp.	100 amp.

[a]The figures in square brackets refer to the categories and subcategories in the Model List of Essential Drugs contained in the report of the WHO Expert Committee on the Use of Essential Drugs (WHO Technical Report Series, No. 685, 1983).

☐ Square symbol indicates that alternative drugs could be used. See page 7, under Explanatory note 1.

Abbreviations used:	
amp.	= ampoule(s)
cap.	= capsule(s)
inj.	= injection
inj. sol.	= injectable solution
oint.	= ointment
pulv. inj.	= powder for injection
tab.	= tablet(s)

Table 10.3. List C, WHO Emergency Health Kit:* Basic medical equipment for a clinic (items marked with an asterisk (*) may need replacing every 3 months)

LIST C

BASIC MEDICAL EQUIPMENT FOR A CLINIC
(Items marked with an asterisk (*) may need replacing every 3 months)

Refer-ence No.	Description	Quantity
C.1	Sterile disposable syringes, Luer 2 ml	4 000*
C.2	Sterile disposable syringes, Luer 10 ml	1 000*
C.3	Sterile disposable needles 0.8 × 40 mm/G21 × 1½″ (0.8 × 38 mm)	2 500*
C.4	Sterile disposable needles 0.5 × 16 mm/G25 × 5/8″ (0.5 × 15 mm)	2 500*
C.5	Interchangeable glass syringes, Luer 2 ml	5
C.6	Interchangeable glass syringes, Luer 10 ml	5
C.7	Interchangeable needles, 144 assorted, Luer	2 packets
C.8	Sterile swabs	5 000
C.9	Emergency suture sets with needles, packet of 12	15 packets*
C.10	Needle-holder	1
C.11	Scalpel handle, No. 3 size	2
C.12	Artery forceps	2
C.13	Dissecting forceps	2
C.14	Blades, disposable, size 10	100*
C.15	Scissors, straight	6
C.16	Scissors, suture	1
C.17	Thermometers, clinical	10
C.18	Stethoscopes, standard and fetal	2 of each
C.19	Sphygmomanometer, anaeroid	1
C.20	Diagnostic set (auroscope, ophthalmoscope)	1
C.21	Batteries, alkaline, dry-cell, "D" type, 1.5 V, for item C.20	4*
C.22	Vaginal speculum, Graves	2
C.23	Metal syringe for ear-washing, 90 ml	1
C.24	Tongue depressor, metal	1
C.25	Nasogastric tubes, size Ch. 5 (premature), polyethylene	5*

Table 10.3. (*cont.*)

List C		
Refer-ence No.	Description	Quantity
C.26	Nasogastric tubes, size Ch. 8 (infant), polyethylene	10
C.27	Nasogastric tubes, size 12, polyethylene	5*
C.28	Scalp vein needles	50
C.29	Gloves, reusable, small	100
C.30	Gloves, reusable, medium	100
C.31	Gloves, reusable, large	100
C.32	Dressing trays with lid, stainless steel	4
C.33	Basins, kidney, 350 ml, stainless steel	2
C.34	Bowls, round with lid, 240 ml, stainless steel	4
C.35	Bowls, round, 600 ml, stainless steel	4
C.36	Gauze swabs, 5 × 5 cm, packets of 100	10 packets
C.37	Gauze swabs, 10 × 10 cm, packets of 100	10 packets*
C.38	Sterile gauze swabs, 10 × 10 cm, packets of 5	50 packets*
C.39	Eye pads (sterile)	6 packets*
C.40	Paraffin gauze dressings, 10 × 10 cm, tins of 36	3 tins*
C.41	Sanitary towels	200*
C.42	White cotton wool, rolls of 500 g	2 rolls*
C.43	Zinc oxide plaster, 25 mm × 0.9 m roll	120 rolls*
C.44	Gauze bandages, 25 mm × 9 m	50*
C.45	Gauze bandages, 50 mm × 9 m	50*
C.46	Gauze bandages, 75 mm × 9 m	50*
C.47	Plaster of Paris bandages 3″ × 3 yds (7.5 cm × 2.7 m), packet of 1 dozen	1 packet
C.48	Pneumatic splint set, multipurpose	1*
C.49	Safety pins, 40 mm	500*
C.50	Hand towels	2*
C.51	Soap, cleansing	60 bars*
C.52	Nail brushes, surgeon's	5*
C.53	Health cards with plastic envelopes	10 000*
C.54	Plastic envelopes for drugs	10 000*
C.55	Plastic sheeting 910 mm wide	2 m
C.56	Aprons, plastic	2
C.57	Tape measures, 2 m (6 ft)	2
C.58	Weighing scale, adult, 140 kg × 100 g	1
C.59	Weighing scale, infant, 25 kg × 20 g	1
C.60	Height measuring board	1
C.61	Sterilizer, dressing, pressure type, 350 mm diameter × 380 mm	1
C.62	Stove for C.61, kerosene, single-burner, pressure	1

Table 10.3. (*cont.*)

Refer-ence No.	Description	List C Quantity
C.63	Basic laboratory kit and spares	1
C.64	Filter, water-candle, aluminium, 9 litres	1
C.65	Rapid reagent tablets (Clinitest or similar)	5 bottles*
C.66	Rapid reagent strips (Multistix or similar)	5 bottles*
C.67	Airway (children's set)	1
C.68	Book: *WHO Emergency Health Kit*	1

* Reproduced by courtesy of the World Health Organization.

List A contains 25 simple medicines for use by auxiliary and minimally trained health workers for symptomatic treatment (*Table* 10.1). List B provides 31 additional medicines for use by doctors or senior health workers for diseases that have been clinically diagnosed (*Table* 10.2). List C is the equipment section and comprises generally available simple, robust, standard clinic and laboratory equipment (*Table* 10.3). A copy of the book detailing the kit is included, and it contains standardized treatment schedules for the disease conditions most likely to be encountered.

The material is intended *to cover the initial needs only,* pending a proper assessment of the specific emergency and of longer-term requirements.

The WHO Lists do not include vaccines and accordingly no refrigeration equipment is provided. No sophisticated laboratory items are foreseen; if necessary, cold-chain and other facilities should be discussed with the national health and disaster management authorities.

OXFAM NUTRITIONAL KITS

Oxfam, which has a remarkable record of assistance in emergencies and for development, has produced useful guides and lists, of which the three nutritional kits are particularly recommended for emergency feeding problems. Nutritional Kit No. 1 is for nutritional assessment and surveillance, No. 2 is for supplementary feeding, and No. 3 for therapeutic feeding.

Only Kit No. 1 is detailed here (*Table* 10.4). This nutritional assessment and surveillance kit enables relief workers to measure the nutritional status of children in disaster situations and villages at risk. In case of need for nutritional intervention, it can be used to identify the recipients for feeding programmes and monitor the ongoing situation. It can be the basis of decision for using the other kits or not.

Table 10.4. OXFAM Nutrition Kit No. 1

Equipment
For nutritional surveys and ongoing monitoring:

1 height stick (150 cm) and 1 'read off' marker ⎱ wooden
1 length board (100 cm)   ⎰
1 Salter spring scales: 25 kg
1 Salter spring scales: 50 kg
10 fibreglass tape measures
2 instruction leaflets for shakir strips
2 registers
10 exercise books
2 pairs scissors
10 pens, 10 pencils, 2 rubbers, 2 pencil sharpeners
2 rulers, 2 clip boards, 1 box drawing pins
1 packet of graph paper
1500 identity bracelets
2 dymo machines
2 boxes dymo tape (red) ⎱ for insertion into identity bracelets
2 boxes dymo tape (blue) ⎰
50 height for weight graph sheets
1 holdall (heavy duty nylon)

Books

Control of Communicable Diseases, by the US Public Health
   Association (×2)

Management of Nutritional Emergencies in Large Populations,
   by WHO (×2)

Nutrition for Developing Countries, by M. King (×2)

Selective Feeding, by S. Peel (×2)

RED CROSS EMERGENCY SETS

The Red Cross has a long tradition of providing medical assistance to victims of natural disasters and of conflict situations. The League of Red Cross and Red Crescent Societies has espoused the WHO Kit as its main response to health needs following natural disasters. The International Committee of the Red Cross (ICRC) deals primarily with conflictual disasters and wars (*see* Chapter 8) and has devised standard units or sets to respond to these particular medical and surgical needs. Of the eleven different kinds of sets, only the following are detailed here: ICRC Dressing Material Set (*Table* 10.5), Dressing Material Set For Burn Wounds (*Table* 10.6), and Minor Surgery Set (*Table* 10.7).

STANDARDIZATION

In a book on medicine for disasters the need for international co-ordination and for adhering to standard medicines and equipment—both by providers and by recipients—cannot be overstated. Items unacceptable to relief agencies should not be sent (*Table* 10.8). The advantages of standardization are set out in *Table* 10.9. The opposite could mean a supply disaster on top of the real disaster.

Table 10.5. ICRC Dressing Material Set

1 parcel containing:

1 × 10	rolls gauze bandage 6 cm × 10 m
2 × 10	rolls gauze bandage 8 cm × 10 m
2 × 12	elastic bandage 8 cm
1 × 12	elastic bandage 10 cm
2 × 100	sterilized gauze compresses 10 × 10 cm
1 × 100	sterilized gauze compresses 10 × 20 cm
50 × 2	sterile gauze compresses 7·5 × 10 cm
1 kg	absorbent cotton wool
5	triangular bandages
1	adhesive bandage 5 m × 6 cm
1	adhesive bandage 5 m × 8 cm
1 × 12	rolls adhesive tape 2·5 cm × 10 m
1 × 6	rolls adhesive tape 5 cm × 10 m
1 l	skin disinfectant
1 pair	scissors + 1 forceps

Table 10.6. ICRC Dressing Material Set for Burn Wounds

1 parcel containing:

8	Sterile burns dressing 30 × 40 cm
5	Sterile burns dressing 60 × 80 cm
1	Box impregnated gauze pads 20 × 20 cm
2	Boxes impregnated gauze pads 90 × 12 cm
1	Bottle antiburns solution 250 ml
2	Tubes antiburns ointment
2 × 10	Metallized gauze pads 8 × 10 cm
2 × 10	Metallized gauze pads 10 × 12 cm
2 × 10	Gauze bandages 8 cm × 10 m
2 × 200	Gauze compresses 9 × 10 cm
2	Balloon catheters CH 12
2	Balloon catheters CH 16
2	Balloon catheters CH 20
1	Lubricating jelly
20	Urine bags

Table 10.7.   ICRC Minor Surgery Set

1 parcel containing:

One metal box consisting of:

—	1	Probe
—	1	Dissecting forceps
—	1	Tissue forceps
—	1	Splinter forceps
—	1	Scissors
—	25	Suture clips
—	3	Scalpel blades
—	1	Scalpel handle No 3
—	1	Clip applying forceps
—	1	Kocher forceps
—	1	Needle holder

1	Crile forceps, curved
2	Mosquito forceps
20	Safety pins
1	Box scalpel blades No 20
3 dz	Silk cutting needle 2-0
3 dz	Silk cutting needle 1
1 × 12	Chromic catgut 0 without needle
1 dz	Chromic catgut 1 atraumatic needles
2 m	Penrose drain 10 mm
2 m	Penrose drain 20 mm
1 m	Round drain 7 × 10 mm
1 × 50	Pairs surgical gloves 7·5
10	Operative drape 50 cm × 80 cm
5	Steri-strips 3
5	Vials Lidocaïne 1% 50 ml
30	Syringes 10 ml, Luer
20	Needles large size 0·9 × 55, Luer
20	Needles medium size 0·8 × 38, Luer
100	Suture clips
1	Tray for instruments
2 l	Skin disinfectant

Table 10.8. Unacceptable items. The need and acceptability of donations vary according to circumstances and to relief agencies

The items listed below are considered unacceptable to UNHCR's refugee programmes

1 **Certain types of food**

    a. some tinned fish (shrimp, crab, lobster, oyster, snail, squid, etc.) and meat (pork derivatives)
    b. tinned/fresh fruits and vegetables
    c. canned baby foods
    d. breast-milk substitutes, including any milk powder, condensed milk or baby formulas that can be put into bottles
    e. fruit or vegetable juice
    f. frozen or refrigerated foods

2 **Used clothing**

3 **Baby bottles**

4 **Mattresses**

5 **Water purification tablets**

6 **Multiple vitamins**

Table 10.9. Advantages of internationally standard supplies

WHO emergency health kit

Advantages

Reliable, standardized, inexpensive, appropriate, quickly available, essential drugs, standard simple equipment, weight known, price known, volume known, contents known, consumer/need known, easily adopted by others, encourages donors, no waste

Additionally

Stockpile for preparedness, essential baseline for primary health care

FURTHER READING

Gunn S. W. A. (1985) Anti-infective drugs in the WHO emergency health kit. *J. Hosp. Infection* **6**, 209–13.

Gunn S. W. A. (1986) Interventi dell'OMS in caso di catastrofe. In: Brenna A. and Tavazza F. *Protezione Civile e Servizi Sanitari*. Milano, Angeli.

International Committee of the Red Cross (1983) *The Red Cross in Emergency Medical Actions*. Geneva, ICRC.

Simmonds S., Vaughan P. and Gunn S. W. A. (1983) *Refugee Community Health Care*. Oxford, Oxford University Press.

World Health Organization (1983) *The Use of Essential Drugs. Technical Report Series No. 685*, Geneva, WHO.

World Health Organization (1984) *WHO Emergency Health Kit. Standard Drugs and Clinic Equipment for 10 000 Persons for 3 Months*. Geneva, WHO.

R. M. Weller

11

Patient Evacuation and Dispersal

DISPERSAL

After any disastrous accident, the sick and injured need treatment. This may be initiated at the scene of the incident and must be continued for as long as necessary in any available or appropriate hospital. Immediate care for small or large numbers is considered elsewhere (Chapter 2). Planning in both developed and developing countries is discussed in detail in Chapters 5 and 6 respectively.

In developed countries, where hospital facilities may be provided in quantity (which is not to say that they will not be overwhelmed by a major catastrophe), plans should be made to prevent overloading of one hospital, by dispersing patients to as many as possible. Specialist care may be needed; for instance, plastic surgeons skilled in the treatment of burns. This may only be available on a regional basis. Few hospitals, except the largest, can provide a fully comprehensive range of medical services. So for specialist care to be provided and, if it is available, it is only reasonable to assume that it should, either the specialist must be brought to the patient or the patient brought to the specialist. Examples of both exist in the last few years. In either case, an absolute requirement is that facilities must exist for the specialist to work as a specialist. The value of a specialist would be reduced or would disappear altogether if the tools of his specialty were unavailable.

After the Bradford City football stadium fire in 1985, in which 53 people died, 250 people were injured, 83 of whom required hospital admission. Fifty-five were treated by primary excision of their burns and skin grafting. They were fortunate that the regional burns unit was nearby. Nevertheless, surgical colleagues from London, Newcastle and Manchester came to help so that the extra operating time made available could be used.

Patients were brought for specialist care, fully sterile nursing care and bone marrow transplantation after the Chernobyl power station radiation disaster in April 1986. About 300 were flown to Number 6 Hospital, Moscow. Since transportation was readily available, it was considered preferable to bring the patients to the specialists and their immobile facilities, rather than vice versa.

The dispersal of casualties in the third (developing) world provides a different set of problems. Hospitals may be far away, poorly staffed or inadequately equipped. Specialist care may be completely absent or only available if brought from abroad. Even then, the lack of equipment and facilities to back up the work of specialists may reduce their value enormously.

Again, pre-disaster planning (Chapter 6) is needed. Local circumstances must prevail. There is no point in producing plans unless the means of implementing them exist. Inasmuch as the means of transport are likely to be minimal (or damaged) a much better case exists for bringing the medical care that can be offered into or close to the area of the disaster. Most patients will need to be treated locally. Only a few may be evacuated for sophisticated medical care in an established hospital. The rest, indeed the bulk, will be best treated in field hospitals, of no great degree of sophistication, but of great practical value and efficiency. They may be tented or may be created in existing buildings using portable equipment that can be brought by land, sea or air to the neighbourhood of the disaster.

TRANSPORT

No patients should be left, if possible, in a place where danger still threatens them. Having got them to a safe place, medical care must be provided. A decision can then be made, after the patients' condition has been stabilized, as to where treatment will be continued. This will involve transport of the patients. Before moving them anywhere, if at all possible, they should be in as stable a state as is reasonable. A balance may need to be struck between treating them where they are—almost certainly in an adverse situation—and the risk in transporting them to the better facilities of a hospital. The distance, journey time and means of transport will all need to be taken into the calculations. Patients may:

—walk or be carried
—be taken on horseback, or ox/mule/horse-drawn transport
—be taken by motorized transport. This would include car, lorry, or bus, as well as designated ambulance.
—be taken by rail
—be taken by sea
—be taken by air, be it helicopter or fixed wing aircraft. The distances could be very short, but could stretch to intercontinental dimensions.

No medical advice can really be given in the first two categories. The patient must be made as comfortable as possible before any journey commences. The seriously ill or injured will be unlikely to survive—infections, haemorrhage, dehydration, malnutrition and exposure will take their inevitable toll.

By Road

Provided resuscitation is started in advance, road transport over relatively short distances provides few problems to the injured. The driver must drive as gently as possible, avoiding steep cambers on the road, sudden acceleration and sudden braking. On poor roads or cross country much care will need to be taken. Patients should be accompanied by trained personnel. A critically ill patient will need a team of two to look after him. This really means that a 2-man ambulance team is inadequate, 3 being a better, but perhaps unrealistic, number to aim for.

Proper equipment in an ambulance is essential. This includes oxygen, a source of intermittent positive pressure ventilation, preferably with humidification, suction, monitoring and all the usual basic equipment. On good roads, long distances can then be travelled quite safely. A patient whose condition merits a real rush, a 'let's get to hospital quickly' call, will often do badly. Resuscitation and stabilization will probably have been inadequate, and a sprint across country or city is more likely to prove more dangerous to the lives of the rescuers than beneficial to the life of the rescued.

It goes without saying that a patient must be properly secured in any vehicle, as must any medical equipment, such as intravenous infusions, that may be attached to him.

By Rail

Hospital trains became a feature of military medicine from the early days of the railroad. They were used in the Boer War, during both World Wars in Europe, and are a vital part of the evacuation chain for casualties in Northern Europe at the present.

While plans exist to convert ordinary rolling stock, some designated purpose-built trains are available immediately. With three tiers of stretchers, it is only practical to offer much nursing care to patients on the middle level. They can carry up to 600 patients.

It is unlikely that trains will be of use in a civilian disaster, except in special circumstances, such as a rail accident in a tunnel (cf. Severn Bridge, Bristol, UK).

By Sea

Again, in the military context, hospital ships, protected by the Geneva Convention and clearly marked as non-combatant with the Red Cross, have been in use for many years. Most recently both British and Argentine forces employed them in the South Atlantic. Nevertheless, this does not confer immunity from radar-directed modern missiles.

Any ship with a doctor, nurses and medical assistants, and with a properly equipped sick bay, can offer help at a disaster near the coast. This may involve rescuing non-combatants from a war zone, as HMS Britannia did off Aden in 1986, and treating those needing care. Naval ships, better equipped with operating facilities, are often soon to be found at the scene of a disaster near the coast.

By Air

A number of factors need to be considered when moving patients by air. The principal two, the overall effect of reduced atmospheric pressure, and the specific effect of reduced oxygen tension are physical factors due to the effect of altitude. These will clearly be modified when a plane is pressurized, when the effect of altitude will be limited to between 5000 and 8000 feet depending on the aircraft used.

Transport of the sick and injured by air involves many aspects of their care. When a patient is moved by air in an emergency, risks may well need to be taken. At the same time, with foresight, the risk can be reduced. In a non-urgent situation, no risk should be taken, the patient being conveyed at the optimal time and in optimal circumstances.

Experience in air evacuation stretches back to the Great War, 1914–18. The rapid extraction of battle casualties from the battle scene reached its zenith in Vietnam, where helicopters were numerous and readily available. In parallel with the military, civilian air evacuation has increased in frequency as holidays are taken by larger and larger numbers of people in more and more exotic places.

Pressure Change

As the altitude of the plane increases, and the ambient pressure falls, so gas within a patient will expand. If that gas is within a closed cavity, it will almost certainly have a disadvantageous effect. The atmospheric pressure falls from about 760 mmHg at sea level to 380 mmHg at 28 000 ft (5 000 m). So gas will, if it can, double in volume. It can affect the following systems:

Gastrointestinal Tract

Gas in the bowel will expand. If the bowel wall has been weakened by ulceration or diverticulitis, or been interfered with by recent surgery, a risk of perforation exists. The distension caused by intestinal obstruction will be made worse. Flying is not advisable within 10 days to 2 weeks of abdominal surgery.

Pneumothorax

A risk exists of an increase in size of a pneumothorax. This may cause both respiratory difficulties and, by tearing adhesions, further bleeding. It is also possible that a tension pneumothorax might develop.

Spinal Cord and Joints

Patients suffering from dysbarism after a diving accident should not be transported by air for fear of aggravating 'the bends' or enlarging the air bubbles in the central nervous system.

Radiology

Air encephalography is an absolute contraindication to flight for a week. Any air introduced should by then have had time to absorb.

Fractures

Air within skull fractures may also expand. Limbs encased in plaster may swell, especially if there is any air in the tissues. This may embarrass the circulation. Plaster casts should thus be split before flying.

Equipment

Air within equipment will also expand on ascent, and contract on descent. Thus, it is worth reducing the volume in the cuff of an endotracheal or tracheostomy tube as the atmospheric pressure decreases, and reinflating as it increases during descent.

Similar care must be taken with inflatable orthopaedic splints and any method of pressurizing glass bottles containing intravenous fluids. Collapsible plastic bags are to be preferred.

Oxygen Partial Pressure

At 6000 ft a patient breathing air, whose normal PO_2 is 98 mmHg, will have dropped his PO_2 to 64 mmHg. At 8000 ft it will be 55 mmHg. Because of the shape of the oxygen dissociation curve, assuming a normal haemoglobin concentration of approximately 15 g/100 ml blood, the blood will still have a saturation of around 90 per cent.

This fall, of no importance to a fit patient seated in a normal commercial plane, may diminish the cardiopulmonary reserve of patients who have started from well below normal levels of either haemoglobin or oxygen saturation. Thus, patients should not be flown if their haemoglobin is below 8·0 g/100 ml blood, after a recent haemorrhage or within 3 to 6 weeks of a myocardial infarct.

Other Conditions

Wired Jaws

Wire cutters need to accompany patients with wired jaws, and somebody who knows which are the vital ones to cut in an emergency.

Pregnant Women

Flying after 32 weeks' gestation should be discouraged. After 36 weeks, any patient needs to be accompanied by a midwife or doctor prepared and equipped to deliver the baby, should labour start.

Infection

Patients with infectious diseases may be a danger to their accompanying attendants, to other passengers and crew, and to the toilet facilities on a plane. They are best not mixed with ordinary passengers. In severe cases, an air-portable isolation chamber may be needed. This is highly specialized equipment, and is only likely to be available to Air Forces.

Psychiatric Patients

For the safety of all, psychiatric patients should not fly unless they are calm, and even then should be escorted by a nurse and/or doctor. On a long flight, two escorts will be needed, so that one can rest at a time.

Practical Matters

Immobilization

Just as passengers have to fasten seat belts, so must patients be properly secured. Stretchers need to be properly mounted, and proper strapping is needed to prevent the patient moving about at take-off, on landing or during turbulence in flight.

For good immobilization, especially when any movement may be dangerous, a vacuum mattress is best. This is particularly useful in cases with a fractured spine or neck.

Equipment

Most is similar to that found in hospitals or ambulances. However, because of varying voltages and difficulties with electrical supply, battery power is usually necessary, with a fall-back to manual operation if needed. This includes suckers and ventilators particularly.

It should be noted that humidification is vital. Air in planes is dry. Endotracheal tubes and tracheostomies need either a blower humidifier or, more easily, one of the several expired air humidifiers that are available.

i.v. Infusion Rates

If it is essential that these remain constant, they can be controlled by a battery powered syringe pump or drip counter. Plastic bags are to be preferred to glass bottles. This also overcomes the problem, found especially in small planes, of the lack of headroom and consequently small head of pressure that exists between the fluid and the patient's arm.

Airborne Care

After a disaster, patients requiring transport are most likely to have suffered trauma. It is worth considering special aspects of these patients.

Head Injury

Changes in the level of consciousness of a patient must be recorded. The Glasgow Coma Scale is recommended, having achieved international recognition. Care of the airway is vital, especially as nausea and vomiting are both common with head injuries. Unconscious patients may be better paralysed, intubated and ventilated artificially, if the means are available.

Spinal Injury

A vacuum stretcher provides the best means of moving patients with fractures of the thoracic and lumbar spine. Cervical fracture creates a more difficult problem, especially if the patient is in some form of skull traction. This can be maintained by attachments on the stretcher. Alternatively, the head and neck can be supported by sandbags or rolled towels, and further secured with adhesive tape across the forehead.

A Stryker frame is too big for small aircraft, but can be used when large military aircraft are used.

Thoracic Injury

A chest drain is mandatory if a patient has multiple fractured ribs and a pneumo-thorax. Since underwater seal drains are large and easily knocked over, a Heimlich valve arrangement is to be preferred—a standard urine drainage bag will serve the purpose, for it has a built-in flap valve.

Abdominal Injury

Venting of expanding gas will be assisted with an open nasogastric tube. A colostomy bag should be changed before any flight, so the patient starts with a clean one in place. Spares are advisable.

Burns

A patient suffering serious burns may need moving to a specialist unit as a matter of urgency, while small burns should be able to be treated locally. These patients are ill and may indeed need more than a team of two to look after them. A larger than usual plane is useful because the patient may need not only fluid replacement but also respiratory care and thorough monitoring. Hypothermia should be avoided. If the distance is not too great, a helicopter has the advantage that movements of the patient may be reduced. The extent of the burns must be known before transport is arranged, so that adequate and appropriate intravenous fluids are available.

Haemorrhage and Anaemia

The effect of reduced partial pressure of oxygen is exaggerated by these conditions. This can be overcome by giving oxygen, even at sea level. It becomes essential as altitude increases.

SUMMARY

Dispersal

Basic medical care can often be brought to patients who have suffered in a disaster. For sophisticated and advanced care, it is more likely that the patient will have to be moved to the place where it is available. The treatment of burns is, perhaps, the exception to this rule, in that much specialist care can be provided without sophisticated equipment.

In any case, the dispersal of patients should be considered as a vital part of the planning for any disaster.

Transport

Patients whose condition has been stabilized can usually be transported safely. The support needed during a 5- or 6-day train journey is clearly quite different from that on a 2- or 3-hour flight. Advance planning and awareness of the possible problems should make both possible.

FURTHER READING

McNeil E. L. *Airborne Care of the Ill and Injured* (1983) Heidelberg and New York, Springer-Verlag. *Report of the Board of Science and Education Working Party on Air Transportation of the Sick and Injured* (1985) BMA.

P. Savage

12

Public Relations and the Media

All disasters are public relations exercises, and criticism may well follow the failure of a hospital to pay due attention to this often neglected part of disaster planning. With the natural concern to provide the best possible care for the injured, it is easy to overlook the needs of relatives and friends, to ignore the offers made by volunteers who come to the hospital and to antagonize the press corps by failing to provide accurate information about the disaster and its consequences.

CASUALTY IDENTIFICATION, LOCATION AND STATUS

On admission to hospital all casualties are tagged immediately with a disaster label bearing a unique number. The disaster label may also incorporate the initial emergency department triage category and space for recording the first clinical assessment and treatment. The number identifies not only the casualty but also his or her property, valuables and other documentation, X-rays and blood samples. In the early stages of hospital disaster management, this number is all that is required to identify the casualty. If disaster numbers are issued sequentially, it is an easy matter to find out the total number of casualties admitted.

Documentation teams are sent to the various treatment areas to record the disaster numbers of casualties and to document the name, age, address and next of kin of all casualties capable of giving these details. The clinical status of each casualty is sought from medical or nursing staff and recorded as 'critical', 'serious' or 'satisfactory'. These details are passed to the hospital information centre and displayed on a board which links each casualty's name, disaster number, location within the hospital and clinical status (*Fig.* 12.1). Once the system is working, the senior officers in the control room can see at a glance the total number of casualties admitted and their location, together with a rough idea of how many are in a critical, serious or satisfactory condition. It is also possible to respond to queries about an individual named casualty, indicating whether such a person has been admitted, their location in the hospital and their latest clinical status.

Written details of each casualty, once recorded on the display board, are transcribed on to individual cards which can be easily sorted into alphabetical order. Every 15 minutes or so while casualties are being admitted, these cards

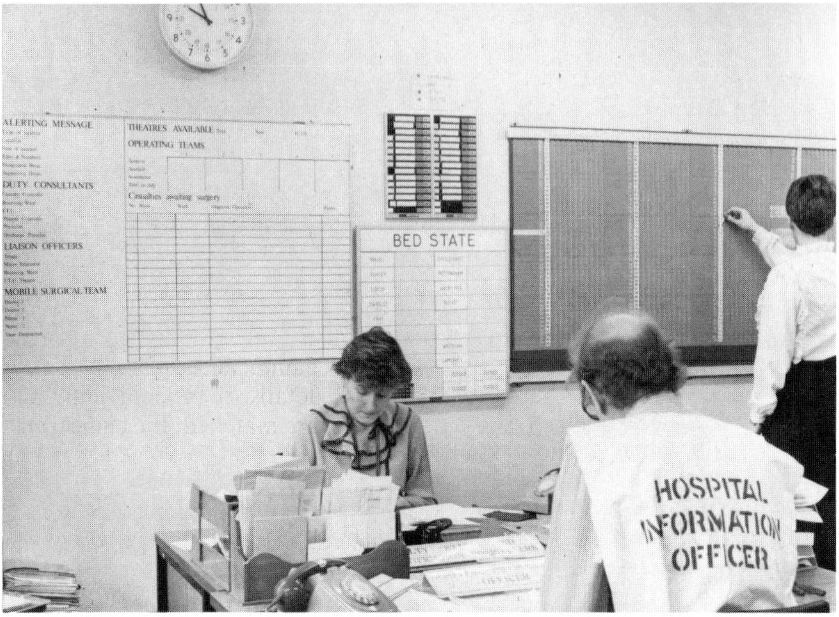

Fig. 12.1. The casualty identification, location and status board.

are used as the basis for making up casualty lists. The casualty list records the surname, first name, age and sex of identified casualties. An updated master copy is kept in the information centre and copies made available to the police documentation teams, the relatives' reception officer and the press officers.

In any large disaster, police documentation teams usually come to the hospital to assist with the production of casualty lists and to help with the identification of dead or unconscious casualties. Very often the police will open their own casualty bureau with a telephone number which is released by the media, thus relieving the receiving hospitals of the responsibility of responding to enquiries from anxious or distraught relatives and friends.

RELATIVES' RECEPTION

In many disasters, a large number of people arrive at the hospital looking for friends or relations who may have been injured. This particularly occurs in a local community disaster. In many disasters there will also be the uninjured victims who may not only have lost their means of transport or belongings, but have family members who are among the injured. This group of people must not be allowed to crowd into the treatment areas, but should be courteously but firmly directed to a relatives' reception area.

The relatives' reception area is best sited in a suite of rooms near to, but not actually in, the emergency department. The most important facility required is a source of accurate information about the casualties. Requests may be made concerning local hotels, car hire firms and local transport arrangements. Some individuals may have lost all their belongings and money. Visitors from abroad unable to speak the language will welcome the help of interpreters. Private rooms will be necessary for imparting bad news and for the sharing of grief. Nearly everyone will want to use a telephone at some time or other. A supply of light refreshments should be made available.

To the officers in charge of the relatives' reception area falls the responsibility of dealing with distraught men and women desperately seeking information. Every attempt must be made to ensure that the information given to individuals is correct. Copies of the casualty list received from the information centre may be displayed on a board, but clinical details or status should not be included.

Details about individual enquiries are noted on a card of a different colour to the one used for recording casualty data. The name, address and telephone number of the enquirer is noted together with details of the individual being sought and their relationship. Once the two cards are matched, the clinical status of the casualty can be sought and the relative or friend informed. Arrangements can then be made for the enquirer to be escorted to see the casualty.

A number of casualties with minor injuries will be able to leave the hospital once they have received treatment. They should also be directed to the relatives' reception area either to meet up with friends or relatives, or to be assisted with their accommodation or travel arrangements.

The painful business of identifying unconscious or dead casualties is carried out with the assistance of the police.

The relatives' reception area is staffed by members of the hospital social work department, assisted by the hospital chaplains. In addition to organizing the information service, they are able to use their skills as counsellors.

VOLUNTEER RECEPTION

During a disaster many people may come to a receiving hospital offering their services in a number of roles. Turning them away will cause offence and possibly adverse publicity. Able-bodied men are useful in augmenting the hospital portering staff in the movement of casualties, while first aiders may be deployed to assist the nursing staff. These individual volunteers will need to be paired with a member of the hospital's staff if their skills are to be of most use. A more satisfactory arrangement is to have had prior discussions with organized community groups. When an emergency occurs and the services of a particular group are required, a telephone call to a designated link-person mobilizes individuals who are not only used to working together, but are familiar with the hospital.

All volunteers coming to a hospital should be received by the volunteer reception officer who registers, identifies and deploys them. Registration is important as it not only allows the volunteer's service to be acknowledged subsequently, but enables any purported qualifications (particularly medical and nursing) to be checked. Groups who are not easily recognized by their own uniform (e.g. Scouts or Guides) are issued with coloured sashes to wear. These have the advantage of being visible from all directions and are cheap to produce in bulk. Different colours can be used to indicate different skill groups.

The problem of what to do with blood donors during a disaster often strains hospital resources. There is no doubt that it is better and safer to rely on blood supplied by an official blood transfusion service which has the facilities of screening donors and whose professional standards are monitored constantly. Trying to deal with a large number of unscreened potential blood donors while trying to manage a disaster is usually unsatisfactory and can be dangerous. It is better to send these volunteer donors to an official blood transfusion reception centre.

THE 'VERY IMPORTANT PERSON'

All disasters produce VIPs who are likely to visit the disaster site or receiving hospitals for a variety of motives. Local dignitaries, politicians, government and state officers, heads of state and royalty may wish to meet survivors, emergency services and hospital staff. Usually these visits are arranged with due consideration for work in progress and, depending on the status of the visitor, an appropriate escort should be provided.

MANAGING THE MEDIA

In the western world, where man-made disasters predominate, modern communications allow representatives of the media to become rapidly aware of any incident involving injury or loss of life, and very often newspaper, radio and television reporters arrive at the disaster site and receiving hospitals almost as soon as the emergency services. Modern telecommunication networks allow radio and television programmes to be interrupted for news flashes about any significant incident, and television pictures are often seen nationwide within a few hours.

In the third world, where there is a greater incidence of natural disasters, local media representatives are often able to give vivid descriptions of the disaster and, when the event is of sufficient size or significance to attract the attention of the world press and television, the disaster site and local health facilities are often invaded by journalists and camera crews from many countries.

The dividing line between individual privacy and public interest has never been clearly defined. The attempted assassination of a pope or president is a more newsworthy event than the injury of a commuter in a train accident. Should each individual be afforded the same degree of privacy? The severe injury or death of a pope or president would have international repercussions; the death of Jane Smith or John Doe, although equally distressing to family, friends and associates, would not.

UK National Health Service Advice

In 1956, the Ministry of Health in the United Kingdom produced a Health Management circular entitled 'Information to the press about conditions of patients'.[1] The recommendations in this circular had been agreed at a conference of representatives of the medical profession and the press.

It has been agreed that, following an accident, press representatives may be given the name, address and condition of an individual casualty, but not necessarily the diagnosis. The patient's relatives should be informed if possible before any press statement is made, but if this is not possible, the press should be so informed. Further information about the nature and extent of injuries should only be given with either the patient's consent or, if he or she is too ill, or is a minor, the consent of the nearest competent relative should be obtained. In accidents involving a number of people, the publication of casualty lists should not be unduly delayed, as such publication is important in allaying the anxieties of relatives and friends of other victims of the accident.

All hospitals are exhorted to ensure that a sufficiently experienced and responsible officer is at all times available to answer press enquiries. Media representatives should be requested to produce professional identity cards, and it may be necessary to check the authenticity of telephone enquirers.

The Ministry of Health note ended with this statement. 'Satisfactory co-operation between hospitals and the press will depend on the observance of conduct that will promote mutual confidence and good personal relations'.

Experience of Media Management

The problem caused by the arrival of a large number of media representatives at a disaster site or receiving hospital has been recognized for many years,[2] but two recent incidents have provided graphic descriptions of a number of problems and how they were tackled.

The Reagan Assassination Attempt

One of the most useful and analytical reports on modern media management has been made by O'Leary[3] who, as Dean of Clinical Studies at the George Washington University Medical Center, was responsible for providing information after President Reagan was shot on 30 March 1981.

Following the President's admission to the emergency room of the George Washington Medical Center, it was not long before 300 reporters, together with a large number of TV trucks, had turned the hospital grounds into what looked like an armed camp! As many hospitals in the past had been overwhelmed by the number of media representatives, all were excluded from the hospital, as it would have been impossible to care for the casualties and to look after the media at the same time.

Although the George Washington Medical Center had its own public relations department, it was decided at an early stage that a doctor would have more credibility on meeting the media, and would be better able to answer the inevitable clinical questions. Watching TV news bulletins before the first press conference allowed Dr O'Leary to see the media approach and to anticipate likely questions. He was also able to arrange for regular reports to be given to him from within the operating suite while the President was undergoing surgery.

Arrangements were made for the first press conference to be held in an adjacent building, and it was decided that, rather than read a written statement, Dr O'Leary would answer questions. An experienced press officer gave this important piece of advice: 'Now remember, just because someone asks you a question doesn't mean you have to answer it.' With a lack of hard facts, it was possible to fill the news vacuum with detail. Although there were risks that some errors would be made, these could be corrected at a later press briefing.

At the first press conference, the hospital press officer has a number of advantages. The media representatives will be 'newspeople' and therefore medically unsophisticated so that their questions are likely to be basic ones concerning facts rather than opinion. The press officer also has all the information, while the media has none. In the circumstances of President Reagan's injuries, there was also the advantage of having good news; it would have been much more difficult had he been more seriously injured, or there had been the possibility of permanent disability.

The second press conference was more difficult in that the media now had as much information as the press officer, and by now experienced science reporters and medical commentators were on the scene with more searching and detailed questions. Subsequent press conferences included doctors and nurses who were able to give more clinical details and to correct 'misinformation' that had been broadcast or published.

In all his dealings with the media, O'Leary emphasizes how important it is to remember that there are three major and different kinds of media—print, radio and television—and that each must receive due attention to keep the peace.

The Brighton Bomb Disaster

The bomb explosion at the Grand Hotel, Brighton, on Friday, 12 October was one of the biggest news stories of 1984.[4] Many leading members of the Conservative Party, including the Prime Minister and her cabinet colleagues, were staying at the hotel for the Conservative Party's Annual Conference when the building was split in two by a large explosion.

The greatest single problem was caused by the large number of reporters involved. For most of Friday, 12 October, over 70 reporters and photographers based themselves at the Royal Sussex County Hospital. They were controlled by setting up a press room and press waiting area close to the accident and emergency department and to the administrative control point. This made it easy for the hospital to control the release of information and, because the press were on the spot, eased the internal security problems that would have arisen had the press room been located anywhere else on the site.

The main difficulty arose when journalists sought interviews with some of the bomb victims. They found it impossible to agree amongst themselves to let a few of their number carry out interviews which would then be shared with other colleagues, and so casualties had to be interviewed by groups of up to 15 reporters at a time. This put such a strain on the victims that the interview arrangements were cancelled after the first half hour and no more interview facilities were granted until the following morning. The press officers were unable to convince the media representatives that 'pooling' would have been to their advantage.

A major problem in all disasters is the controlled release of information. It was tempting to make the press officer responsible for all announcements, but the scale of the Brighton bombing and the resulting media interest made this impracticable. In the event, statements about the condition of inpatients were drafted from information received from the administrative control room, cleared with the duty administrator, senior police officer on duty and, where appropriate, with Conservative Party officers who were present at the hospital, and with medical and nursing staff. Copies of the agreed statements were then given to the press officers and duty administrator who released this information as required. Initially, the information was given out at press briefings for all media representatives, but between one press briefing and the next statements were given out over the telephone or to individual enquirers.

As it was not possible to install a blackboard or wallchart in the press room, details given at press conferences were summarized in writing and copies handed to the journalists. This information was typed whenever possible, but at times of intense pressure, notes made in clear handwriting were photocopied for distribution.

The Brighton experience confirmed the need for a flexible approach to media management based on an understanding of their needs. The decision to site the press room near the accident and emergency department was in fact a departure from the official plan. Press conferences were held at fairly frequent intervals and were dictated not by any pre-set timetable but by the demands of the situation within the hospital and the changing needs of the media. The press officers, while nominally in charge of media management, never fronted a formal press briefing which was always conducted by the senior hospital administrator on duty at the time. An inflexible approach would have resulted in friction between the hospital and the media which in turn could have destroyed the atmosphere of mutual trust and confidence, which in retrospect was one of the hallmarks of the 3 days during which the press room remained open.

PLANNING FOR MEDIA MANAGEMENT

As in all aspects of disaster planning, dealing with an emergency situation is likely to be more successful if plans have been made and tested beforehand. Each hospital will have a recognized senior member of the administrative staff who liaises regularly with the media in his or her everyday work. Large institutions may have a public relations department and, in the United Kingdom, regional health authorities have experienced press officers available to assist in media management. When a large number of casualties are involved, or where figures of national or international importance or notoriety are injured, it would also be wise to designate a senior member of the medical staff as a medical press officer.

Phase One (The First Hour)

During the first hour or so following a disaster, the administrative press officer liaises with the hospital control centre, the senior police officer at the hospital and media representatives. At the same time the medical press officer obtains details about the casualty load and numbers and types of casualties.

On arriving at the hospital, it is useful if the press officer puts on an identifying tabard so that everyone knows who he is. A brief visit to the emergency department and a longer visit to the control and information centre will give him an overview of the size and severity of the disaster, and allow him to estimate the likely degree of media interest. While in the control centre he should confer with the administrator, head nurse and disaster co-ordinator and discuss with them the general principles of handling the media.

The press officer's next task is to identify the members of the media. This is not difficult as they will tend to congregate near the hospital's emergency entrance. After introducing himself, the press officer needs to find out and record the newscast deadlines for various radio and television stations, and similar deadlines for newspapers. Arrangements for opening the press room, the facilities available and the accessibility of telephones need to be outlined, together with the time of the first press conference. An initial press briefing may be made giving simple details of the disaster and how it is affecting the hospital (*Table* 12.1).

While this is going on, the medical press officer makes his own appreciation of the clinical workload, particularly the numbers and types of injuries, and the problems of informing next-of-kin. A visit to the control centre allows him to consult with the disaster co-ordinator, and to estimate the possible duration of the emergency. He should then meet up with the other press officer to exchange notes and to plan the next phase.

Phase Two (2–4 Hours)

The opening of the press room marks the second phase. The press room should be large enough to hold all the media representatives and be equipped with blackboard or flip chart on which can be recorded all the relevant information available for publication, together with the time of the next press conference. The provision of paper, typewriters, telephones and some light refreshments is always appreciated. Depending on the size of the disaster, the degree of media interest and the space available at the hospital, the press room can be in some large hall or lecture theatre, the hospital committee room, or near to the emergency room. The sooner the media representatives can be provided with a base and a source of reliable information, the less likely they are to start wandering around the hospital looking for a story.

The medical press officer meanwhile has been obtaining casualty details from the information centre and relatives' reception area, linking this with each casualty's clinical status, details of next-of-kin, and whether consent to release personal details has been obtained. From this detailed knowledge he is able to advise the press officer on what clinical information can be released to the media.

The press officer should have discussed with the senior police officer at the hospital any particular aspects of the disaster that should be emphasized or omitted, depending on the nature of the disaster. The likelihood of criminal proceedings or the involvement of important persons may be factors in deciding on the nature of press releases.

Taking into account the various media deadlines, the first major press conference opens with a review of the known circumstances of the disaster and details of numbers of dead and injured admitted to hospital. Where possible, details of the names, ages and addresses of casualties should be given together with the clinical status of dead, critically or seriously injured or those in a satisfactory condition. The number of casualties undergoing surgery, being

Table 12.1. First press release

. . . . .Hospital
. . . .(date)   . . . .(time)
. . . . .casualties have been received at the hospital of whom . . . . .have been admitted.
. . . . .casualties are seriously ill and undergoing emergency surgery. . . . . .casualties are being treated for minor injuries, most of whom are likely to be discharged.
The emergency work of the hospital is being co-ordinated by . . . .
A further press statement will be made at . . . . am/pm.
. . . .(signed) Press Officer.

cared for in the intensive therapy unit or who have been sent home should be stated. Where consent has been obtained from a casualty or his relative, clinical details of the extent of injuries may be given. Specific answers to previous queries that may have been made individually by reporters, or those that have been made in response to telephone enquiries should be repeated. Any erroneous statements should be corrected. Specific queries to which there are no immediate answers are carefully noted to be answered at the next press conference. The conference ends with details of the next briefing.

Phase Three (1–4 Days)
Phase Three lasts from when the flood of requests for information starts to die down until the incident loses its news value. The appearance of specialist reporters with specific lines of enquiry indicates the need for the medical press officer to handle their queries and to consider enlisting the support of nursing and medical colleagues at a special press conference. Reporters are also looking for human interest stories and would wish to interview survivors to hear first-hand of their experiences. A number of casualties will want to be interviewed, and moving these casualties into one ward or area makes the organization of a 'press hour' easier.

Due notice should be given to the media, including national and international press associations and radio and television networks as well as to major newspapers. At the appointed hour, the media representatives are allowed to interview casualties as follows: first, the newspaper photographers take their pictures, followed by the newspaper and radio reporters, and last come the television crews and reporters with their lights and equipment.

After some disasters, individual casualties although anxious to tell their stories may not be well enough to face this onslaught of media interest. In these circumstances, the media may agree to 'pool'—to share the copy, tape or film obtained by a small number of reporters with all the media representatives.

No reporter should be given an exclusive interview as this action would guarantee the loss of confidence of the media representatives with the hospital press officer. Senior medical staff in particular should be warned about this. However, during the later stages of a disaster as media interest wanes, facilities for interviews may be given to reporters from specialist journals and magazines, or to reporters from the casualties' locality who are writing up a particular aspect of the disaster.

REFERENCES

1. Ministry of Health (1956) *Information to the Press about the Condition of Patients.* (HM **56**:58) London, HMSO.
2. Department of Health & Social Security (1977) *Health Service Arrangements for Dealing with Major Accidents.* (HC **77**:1) London, HMSO.
3. O'Leary D. S. (1982) Managing a hospital under crisis. In: Cowley R. A. (ed.) *Mass Casualties.* Washington, US Dept. of Transportation.
4. Lelliott P. and Partington A. (1984) How Brighton stayed unrocked. *Health Soc. Serv. J.* **94**, 1286–7.
5. Partington A. J. and Savage P. E. A. (1985) Disaster planning: managing the media. *Br. Med. J.* **291**, 590–2.
6. Silver R. (ed.) (1985) *Health Service Public Relations—A Guide to Good Practice.* London, King Edward's Hospital Fund for London.
7. Savage P. E. A. (1984) Planning without panic. *Health Soc. Serv. J.* **94**, 170–2.

M. Tarry and P. J. F. Baskett

13

Communications

Good communications are essential to the management of any disaster. Many bodies and authorities are involved with disasters, and communications involve both inter-personal skills and relationships and the ability to use modern technology. The groups involved include:

The police force
The fire brigade
The ambulance service
The immediate care doctor scheme
The hospital
The local authorities
The military services
The specialist services (e.g. gas; electricity; airlines; shipping owners; tele-communications; recovery services, catering etc.)
The voluntary services
The media

INTER-PERSONAL RELATIONSHIPS

Each group will wish to meet amongst themselves to plan their major disaster response and to arrange methods of communicating with each other. It is then necessary for representatives of each group to meet together to discuss how they can communicate with each other and to ensure that their own group plans do not conflict with others. The best way of dealing with this is to establish a Joint Services Liaison Committee with appropriate representatives from all services. The Committee can draft plans and from time to time meet to agree changes and modifications, as required, by experience and developments. It is at this stage that inter-personal skills are essential and each group must be prepared to be flexible and compromise to ensure that integrated arrangements are possible. It is helpful if representatives from each group can give instructive talks to members of other groups through exchange visits, etc.

A typical chart of the communication requirements between the principal emergency services, the medical incident officer and his team and the hospital is shown in *Fig.* 13.1 (reproduced from Chapter 5 (Savage)).

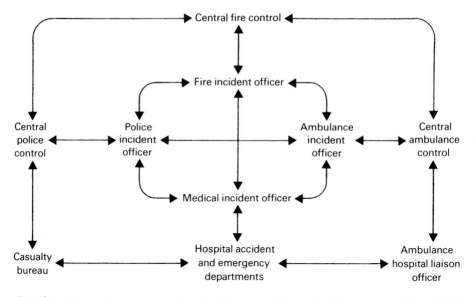

Fig. 13.1. Interservice communications at a disaster site. (Reproduced by courtesy of Hines, 1985, and *see* Chapter 5.)

TECHNICAL COMMUNICATIONS

Telecommunications and computer technology have made enormous strides forward in the last decade and can be harnessed effectively to enhance disaster management. Communications over relatively short distances are established by telephone, teleprinter, telex or radiotelephone. Over longer distances the international telephone, teleprinter or telex systems provide links using international cable networks and radiotelephones linked by satellite relays and computer systems. Two-way radio speech is now being supplemented by five-tone sequential signalling or Fast Shift Key (FSK) digital signalling. The system permits extremely rapid transmission—a complete message can often be sent in less than half a second. In this signalling arrangement data replaces the spoken word and a number represents the complete message. The number is interpreted by a computer and converted back to a written message which can then be displayed on a visual display unit (VDU) and recorded on paper by a printer. Naturally the message can be stored within the computer and transferred to another terminal, as required. Clearly the system requires trained operators.

COMMUNICATION ARRANGEMENTS AT A MAJOR INCIDENT

At a major incident both telephones and radiotelephones will be required to prevent one or other system becoming overloaded. Strict discipline in the use of both systems must be observed so that vital messages are given clearly and succinctly. All groups, particularly hospital emergency department staff, who may not be familiar with radio procedure, must be trained in radio phraseology, call signs and the radio alphabet.

Fig. 13.2 shows the outline of a typical major incident communications network based on ambulance control. Similar networks will be afforded to the police and fire brigade.

In this network the ambulance control will be the focal point of the communications network and all messages should pass through this structure. Some messages will be purely for information, e.g. monitoring the activity in the receiving hospital.

The ambulance control has direct contact with other emergency services, e.g. fire, police and the receiving and support hospitals. This contact is through both ordinary and dedicated land telephone lines. Ambulance control has also very high frequency (VHF) two-way radio contact with mobile radiotelephones fitted in the mobile control centre, ambulances and in the vehicles of immediate care doctors, senior officers and other key personnel working at the scene. The

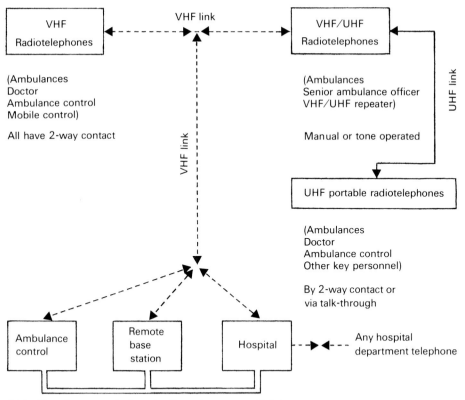

Fig. 13.2. A major incident communication system (simplified for ease of display).

VHF radio link may be direct to the mobile radiotelephones or indirectly via a remote base station. An ultra high frequency (UHF) hand-portable set is used as a forward radio link to the scene; this is linked to the VHF network by a VHF/UHF repeater, which may be either 5-tone sequential, continuous tone controlled squelch system (CTCSS) or manually operated. This forward link allows staff mobility when working away from their vehicles; it provides direct contact with other UHF hand-portable sets, the mobile control centre, senior officers and ambulances and through a VHF/UHF repeater system to the ambulance control, or via any department's normal telephone, to the receiving hospital.

The UHF hand-portable set may be single frequency working. This will allow direct contact with other similar UHF hand-portables within range. Alternatively, the UHF hand-portable set may be double frequency working which relies on a talk-through facility at the VHF/UHF repeater to contact other UHF hand-portables within range, but on a different frequency.

The receiving hospital uses two base station radios, one on remote base station frequencies, the other on mobile radiotelephone frequencies. They can both be connected to the hospital switchboard and communicate with any department's normal telephone. In the event of the remote base station failing, the hospital has direct contact with mobile radiotelephones at the base station. The base station is vital if the hospital switchboard is overloaded by calls seeking casualty information. The system also permits a consultant at the receiving hospital to speak to a doctor or ambulance officer at the scene through his car radio-telephone or a UHF hand-portable set by using the facility at the ambulance control and the VHF/UHF repeater system.

Finally, if the ambulance control, the remote base station and the receiving hospital base station all fail, it is still possible to use mobile radiotelephones working on base frequencies.

COMMUNICATIONS AT THE RECEIVING HOSPITAL

Notification of a major incident alert will be received by the hospital switchboard who will proceed to call key personnel according to the pre-arranged plan. Resident staff may be alerted by a hospital siren, public address system or bleep network and will attend their allotted place of duty.

Non-resident staff are best alerted through a cascade system to avoid over-loading the hospital telephone switchboard. Thus one surgeon is called by the hospital and he calls a colleague, who calls a colleague, etc. Similar arrangements are made for anaesthetists, physicians, radiologists, administrators, etc. (*See* Chapter 5.)

Experience has shown that hospitals also need mobile radiotelephones for key personnel who may move location during the course of their duty. It is essential that the Incident Control Room is kept informed of the bed state and all patient admissions, discharges and movements within the hospital.

Communications with enquiring relatives are vital and a person is required to be delegated specifically to fulfil this role. Communications with the media are discussed in Chapter 12.

ACKNOWLEDGEMENTS TO:

Mr. Alan Pinnell,
Staff Officer (Headquarters Support),
Northamptonshire Ambulance Service
for the technical information provided.

M. Midda

14

Identification of the Dead

In the course of the violent deaths of today from aircraft crashes, industrial accidents, fires etc., the human body is often mutilated beyond recognition. Obviously removal and subsequent treatment of the living is the prime consideration, but many disaster plans contain little or no provision for dealing with the dead in large numbers. There is considerable international variation in the legal obligations for such matters as settling the estates of persons who are victims of civil disaster or war. These require correct handling of evidence and procedures often differ from country to country. The accurate identification of the remains of victims of disasters of all kinds is a public duty and the following personnel are involved:

1. *The Coroner,* or his national equivalent, who requires to know who is dead. Where and when and by what means the deceased met their deaths must be determined to enable him to arrive at a verdict. His agents at the disaster site are the investigating police officers.
2. *The Pathologist,* who is responsible to the Coroner, with his findings of the cause of death and his satisfaction of identification.
3. *The Inspector of Accidents* of the relevant agency. For air crashes this person would be a member of the Civil Aviation Authority, and there would be his equivalent at a rail disaster. Where public buildings are involved, a representative of the appropriate government ministry would be in charge of accident investigation.
4. *The relatives of the deceased* usually wish to ensure accurate identification and occasionally request medical evidence to determine the order in which two or three relatives had died for the purposes of probate etc. Positive identification is absolutely essential for such reasons as insurance claims, estate settlements, inheritance, remarriage and prosecution of individuals in the case of criminal acts.

Other than the purely sociological needs of identification in the event of air, rail or boat accidents, a Board of Inquiry will wish to determine whether or not safety devices were used and if they were adequate and effective. They will also want to know if there should have been survivors, whether a medical condition contributed to the accident such as incapacitation of the operating crew, and if the medical evidence helps in the reconstruction of the accident or points to a non-medical cause. Only if the operating crew are identified is there any chance of demonstrating physical incapacity as a cause of the accident; if that is achieved, the cause of the accident may be identified and prevented on a future occasion.

A pilot may become incapacitated as a result of some environmental factor such as intoxication with carbon monoxide contaminating the cockpit, or hypoxia from the failure of his oxygen supply. Stevens[1] has reported a case where, after a very prolonged investigation in a particularly mutilating accident, he was able to identify the flight deck crew. Investigating these bodies for the presence of carbon monoxide, he found raised levels of carboxyhaemoglobin and he was able to point to the cockpit heater as the likely cause of pilot incapacitation. Carbon monoxide estimation on specimens of blood taken at post-mortem is not difficult to perform, but when blood cannot be obtained from a traumatized or burnt body, it should be taken from other tissues such as skeletal muscle. Techniques exist for the estimation of carbon monoxide on such tissue using gas or liquid chromatography. The problem of detecting ante-mortem hypoxia is difficult and currently there is little help from laboratory tests. Estimation of post-mortem lactic acid levels in nervous tissue is open to misinterpretation since raised levels may not only be due to a terminal hyperglycaemia resulting from hypoxia but also due to other causes of adrenal stimulation.

Only by personal identification can the casualties be related to their position at the time of the incident. Having achieved this, demonstration of specific injuries may lead to a reconstruction of the accident, the appraisal of safety factors and prevention of fatal accidents. In the investigation of the Comet disaster over the Mediterranean, 28 of the fatalities in the aircraft were placed with some certainty, and the pattern of their injuries indicated quite conclusively that the accident could not have been one involving a straightforward crash into the water. The pattern of blast and fragments indicated the presence of a bomb on board as the correct solution.

PRINCIPLES OF IDENTIFICATION

There is much to commend the Scandinavian system of a panel responsible for the identification of victims. Here a police officer is the chairman, aided by the pathologist who submits medical evidence. The panel meets to correlate all the information gathered from the disaster site, together with reports from the investigating officers who have been collecting data from the victim's relations, home and medical and dental practitioners. The central and fundamental part of the organization for the identification of mass casualties is the 'Secretariat'.[2] (See Fig. 14.1.) In an air disaster the panel has the advantage of rapid access to a list of crew and passengers which is presumed to be accurate. In a rail or bus disaster it takes time for the information as to who was travelling, or expected to travel, to become available. Following such a disaster there are often bodies to which there is no hope of putting any name. In these cases the help of those used to dealing with missing persons must be sought. A series of observations related to body numbers is made at the site and fed into the Secretariat which is simultaneously supplied with information from the investigating officers. The Secretariat is therefore in possession of two dossiers which are gradually being added to. Eventually certain facts begin to coincide. For example, information may have been received that Mrs. Smith was wearing a blue suit, whilst observation has shown that body number 6 was dressed in the remnants of a blue skirt. One can then form an 'engagement' of these two folders. If confirmatory

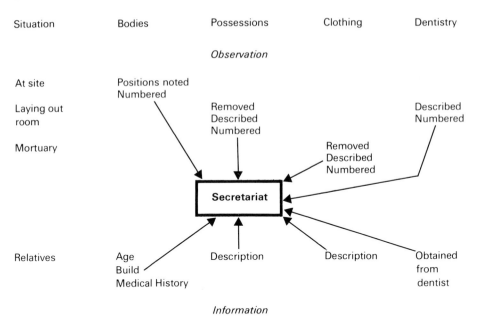

| Situation | Bodies | Possessions | Clothing | Dentistry |

Observation

At site — Positions noted / Numbered

Laying out room — Removed Described Numbered — Described Numbered

Mortuary — Removed Described Numbered

Secretariat

Relatives — Age Build Medical History — Description — Description — Obtained from dentist

Information

Fig. 14.1. Organization of the Secretariat for the identification of mass casualties.

evidence from another source is received, the engagement becomes a marriage; if the further evidence is contradictory, the marriage does not take place. The pattern of identification procedures is not identical in every case. If there is extensive fragmentation, inevitably there are a large number of unidentified remains. If the disaster is on water with rapid recovery of the bodies, visual identification will assume a greater importance. If, however, the bodies have been immersed for a long time, there is a greater dependence upon medical and dental information. Severe burning will also alter the pattern, and limit the value of documentary evidence.

In the absence of fire, men are easier to identify than women because they retain their documents on their person whereas women's handbags are inevitably separated from them. Where there is fire, women's jewellery is particularly helpful and assumes a particular significance in continental Europeans who wear more rings and tend to annotate them far more than in the British Isles. Children tend to be more easily identifiable by clothing as there is generally a member of the family who remembers the child's dress well.

Allowing for these many variations, the histogram (*Fig.* 14.2) has been prepared from 605 fatal cases in 13 fatal public transport accidents and gives some idea of the relative importance of the identification procedures.[2] The histogram has been constructed by charting every occasion on which each technique contributed to identification and tries to avoid built-in bias by recording every occasion on which means contributed to identification. Even this may not give a true picture of the most important methods of identification as it depends on the time available for study in depth, the motivation of the observers and the availability of a forensic odontologist or a radiographer. To get round this difficulty the terms primary and secondary identification are used. Primary

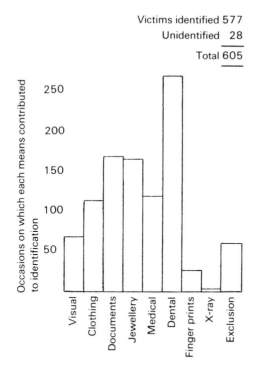

Victims identified 577
Unidentified   28
Total 605

Fig. 14.2. Means of identification in 13 fatal public transport accidents.

identification clearly indicates the probability of identification, whilst secondary identification is in effect the confirmatory method. This has the advantage of stressing the value of the simpler methods which are available to the initial investigators who are probably not specialists. As an example of the system, information is received that Michael Charles Anderson wears a signet ring on his left little finger. If a ring is found with the mark 'MCA' on the left little finger of a male body, this can be accepted as primary identification, provided there are no other persons involved in the incident with the same initials. The dentist may later come up with a perfect match, but the specialist identification will be of a secondary nature.

THE FIELD TEAM

It has been found that the smallest efficient working unit capable of dealing satisfactorily with an operation of this type is a team of 5. Where the total number of fatal casualties exceeds 50, an additional 2 operators are required in the early stage. One member must be a qualified embalmer and one a dentist with experience of forensic odontology. The duties of the field team are very flexible and members are expected to carry out any practical work according to the availability of labour at the accident site.

The team should be in possession of all necessary documentation. The recommended forms are:

1. Autopsy forms—male and female.
2. Clothing specimen forms.
3. External and dental examination charts—male and female.
4. Dental classification charts.
5. Fingerprint forms.
6. Property receipt forms.
7. Registration folders.

Procedure

The operation is usually divided into four main procedures:
1. Recovery of the remains and preservation of the evidence.
2. Identification and preservation of the evidence.
3. Arrangements for removal to the place of disposal by burial or cremation.
4. Recovery, renovation, cleaning and indentification of personal and other effects.

1. Recovery of the Remains

a. Before the bodies are removed from the wreckage or the disaster area, accurate charts, showing the location of the bodies, should be made and photographs taken. Numbered pegs are placed in the ground at the site of the body and this number is then used to refer to that body. The number will be tagged onto a part of the cadaver that is not easily disturbed and once placed in a coffin, it will be repeated on the box.

b. Recovery will normally be carried out by the local police and ambulance services who remove the remains to a mortuary or some convenient building. Every effort should be made to prevent personal effects and clothing being removed from the body prior to the arrival of the investigation team. These should only be removed and recorded in the presence of the pathologist and police officers. Permission must be obtained from the local coroner or police authorities before any examination can proceed.

c. Burial may have been carried out before the arrival of the field team where local regulations require disposal within 24 hours. However, every effort and diplomatic pressure should be applied to allow examination to fulfil the vital medico-legal and sociological obligations.

2. Identification of the Remains

a. Visual Identification

There are always a certain number of victims who are identifiable visually and in some countries this may be regarded as irrefutable evidence of identity. This is clearly a highly satisfactory means if the body can be reasonably viewed by a relative or acquaintance of the deceased. However, the investigators should be wary of this method. Relatives at the scene of a mass disaster are under intense emotional stress. Moreover, they have an overpowering desire to regain the body of a close relative and their powers of discrimination become distorted. In the case of aircraft accidents few bodies are suitable for viewing as most of the victims are smashed or burnt beyond any means of visual identification. Even a comparatively untraumatized body may be so altered in appearance from the living state that the emotional stress involved for a relative asked to identify the corpse is such that neither a negative nor positive answer can be accepted without other confirmatory evidence. It should also be remembered that most international aircraft carry many different nationalities and requesting relatives to attend the scene could cause considerable delay. The limitation of visual identification has been emphasized by Frykholm[3] and he notes how frequently even minor injuries and post-mortem exposure in sea or snow on a mountainside can distort appearances. Practice, therefore is to seek secondary confirmation of visually identified bodies, unless the absence of trauma is such that confirmation is clearly unnecessary. Even professional observers are not wholly immune to stress. On one occasion, three pathologists were given 3 hours to open and examine the contents of 114 coffins. Although they agreed on every case at the graveside, they ultimately found that they had misdiagnosed the sex in 3 cases.

b. Personal Effects

Identification by clothing is hardly more satisfactory. The days of laundry marks have gone and there is a widespread use of chainstore garments. However, it is surprising how often a really accurate description of a child's clothing can be obtained and, occasionally, there may be primary evidence such as a stewardess's uniform or a captain's rank badge, but even then it must be stressed that there may well be more than one person with apparently distinctive uniform. Military personnel should be carrying identification tags. In the author's experience, primary identification by clothing generally involves showing soiled clothing to distressed relatives and one wants to avoid such confrontations if at all possible. The contents of clothing are far more significant as evidence of identification. This is probably the most common and easiest method of identification in men in the absence of fire. Nearly everyone carries some form of identification with them and in the context of travel, this may be highly specific. At the same time, it should be stated that a number of people will be carrying documents which are misleading as to identification and the observer must be certain that he is reading the right thing. For example, he must make sure that he is reading the casualty's signature on a document and not that of the issuing officer. Of all the non-specialized items, jewellery is probably the most useful means of identification. It is uniquely described and commonly unique amongst a group of passengers; it is relatively resistant to fire and it is often distinctly marked. Rings and brooches are generally of sufficient specificity to allow primary identification and they have the enormous advantage of usually being presentable to relatives. Watches are in a different category as they are nowadays so standardized that even a close relative may make an incorrect identification.

c. Radiographic Evidence

Primary identification by radiographs, that is, by comparing a film or part of the cadaver with a radiograph taken in life, is, in the author's experience, extremely rarely of value in a mass disaster. It is only likely to be of use when there are only two or three bodies left which are otherwise quite indistinguishable. On the other hand, routine radiography of the bodies may reveal possessions which have been occluded within a burnt area and it is certainly useful in establishing the presence of foreign bodies which are significant in other contexts, i.e. bomb fragments. The main value of radiographs is in revealing the presence of orthopaedic devices etc., which are an intimate part of medical identification.

d. Medical Evidence

In this context, medical means of identification can be regarded as primary from the outset. Beyond this, care is needed and, in general, medical evidence should be of a secondary nature until there is a reduction to the 2 or 3 body stage. Assessment for stature in an incinerated body is difficult because of variable heat contraction and possible lengthening by opening up knee and hip joints. In addition, the accuracy of information supplied concerning a victim's height must not be accepted without question. Relations tend to give only relative estimates of a missing person's height.

Assessment by the pathologist can be made as to likely stature and age, the colour of skin, eyes and hair, and external identifying marks such as scars, moles and tattoos. Physical abnormalities have been found to be of help in some instances. In one, the finding of a marked deformity of the sternum corresponded with a description of 'pigeon chest' given by the relatives. In the other, a badly mutilated body had lobeless ears, a feature described by relatives and confirmed in a passport found in the wreckage. Internal examination may reveal the existence of post-surgical states or disease which may have been diagnosed in life. On one occasion, examination revealed the remains of a cheque book deeply embedded in the lacerated and charred muscle of the buttocks in a headless and limbless torso. The general run of operations such as appendicectomy or hysterectomy can be of value only in distinguishing between a very few bodies and, as such, are associated with identification by exclusion.

e. Identification by Exclusion

This method is almost unique to aircraft disasters for it is only in this type of accident that there is a passenger list. Thus, so long as the general physical descriptions tally, the investigator is justified in using exclusion as a basis for identification when reduced to one man and one woman. If there is some completely different feature such as a full denture or a hysterectomy, the principle can be extended to two bodies of the same sex. It is clear that the more bodies there are involved, the less precise must be evidence by exclusion.

An example of using this method is illustrated in *Fig.* 14.3. In this case 5 adult bodies remained unidentified, 3 bodies being females numbered 404, 451 and 482. Five passengers had not been identified of whom 3 were females named Jones, Smith and Green. A dental chart was available on passenger Jones but body 404 was partially decapitated and no teeth remained. However teeth remained in bodies 451 and 482 and showed that neither of them could possibly be Jones. It was therefore reasonable to exclude bodies 451 and 482 as being Jones and conclude tentatively that number 404 was Jones. In considering further information available it was known that Jones and Smith had very dark hair but Green was a true blond. Body 404 had dark hair, body 451 was blond and body 482, the scalp of which was missing, had dark body hair. On this evidence it could be again tentatively concluded that 451 was Green and by exclusion 482 was Smith. For this to be really acceptable all other clues must be found to fit and nothing must be found to contradict. In this instance, facts known concerning

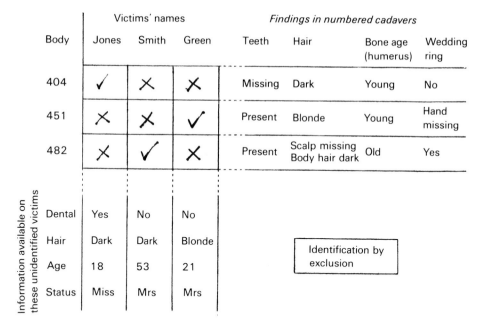

	Victims' names			Findings in numbered cadavers			
Body	Jones	Smith	Green	Teeth	Hair	Bone age (humerus)	Wedding ring
404	✓	✗	✗	Missing	Dark	Young	No
451	✗	✗	✓	Present	Blonde	Young	Hand missing
482	✗	✓	✗	Present	Scalp missing Body hair dark	Old	Yes

Information available on these unidentified victims

	Jones	Smith	Green
Dental	Yes	No	No
Hair	Dark	Dark	Blonde
Age	18	53	21
Status	Miss	Mrs	Mrs

Identification by exclusion

Fig. 14.3. Chart of identification by exclusion.

possession of wedding rings fitted and an estimate of age on the basis of the humerus which was sectioned from each of the bodies, corresponded with the ages of the passengers quite well. For non-criminal purposes, evidence as good as this can be regarded as entirely sufficient and acceptable.

f. Fingerprints

Identification by this means is of limited value as most passengers in licensed transport are law-abiding citizens and few countries routinely record the finger-prints of those without police records. A comparison of prints, therefore, involves a search of the casualty's home. This is a traumatic experience for the relatives, and should be avoided if possible. In the end, however, it is the availability of records which causes the gross discrepancy that exists between the importance given to fingerprints in the United Kingdom and, say, the USA. The field team should be trained in taking fingerprints but where there is decom-position of the body, expert advice should be sought from the police.

g. Dental Evidence

The importance of dental evidence in identification has been stressed in recent years, but to be of value there must be available both accurate information concerning the dental state of the supposed casualty and the cadaver.

Nevertheless, in forensic dentistry, one has something approximating the accuracy of a fingerprint, as the teeth, jaws and restorations show a vast number of individual details. It has been estimated that there are over 2.5 billion combinations in charting the human mouth and consequently in all probability no two mouths will be identical.

The task of dental examination of the victims is not one that the general dental practitioner should be called upon to perform, since with the best will in the world he cannot help but be sickened by the sights, nor can he be relied upon to give an accurate charting of the remains. This should be done by a dental expert who knows where to look for these parts. At one disaster, 9 dentists gave 9 different sets of chartings. The subject of forensic dentistry is not taught at undergraduate level and few countries give instruction at the postgraduate level. The dental surgeon works in close liaison with the pathologist and under his direction. He may be required to work only in the presence of the pathologist and to perform the dental examination at the same time as the post-mortem examination. The dentist must ensure that he has the permission of the pathologist to record the dentition on bodies and to remove any parts of the mouth he may feel would assist him in identification.

Charting of the bodies is undertaken as quickly and accurately as possible and here the first problems arise. Post-mortem changes make it difficult to open the jaws and so mutilating incisions may have to be made to expose the teeth. Obviously this should not be undertaken when a possible visual identification could be made. It is always better to remove the jaws to examine the teeth carefully. Severe mutilation of the facial skeleton in the high speed impact of crash may mean looking for fragments of jaws, as the maxilla readily disintegrates and teeth act as secondary missiles and become embedded in tissues distant from their normal position.

As bodies lie in coffins, imperfect lighting or soiling by blood and debris may mask the well-placed, tooth-coloured restoration and even a porcelain crown can go unnoticed. Fillings in teeth can be located by using a disclosing solution made up of 5 per cent methylene blue in methanol and chloroform.[4]

Dental Equipment
The following items are considered as the essentials of a forensic dentistry kit:
   Post-mortem apron or similar.
   Post-mortem or household rubber gloves.
   Scalpel handle with blades, size 22.
   Mouth mirrors, probes and excavators.
   Toothbrushes.
   Large scissors.
   Hunt's syringe.
   Saw or large osteotome.
   A means of illumination: a head lamp is invaluable as it leaves both hands free.
   Disclosing solution.

The kit may be supplemented with a tape recorder with spare batteries, as clerking may not be available, a 35mm single lens reflex camera with a ring flash or similar and plenty of film, and facilities for radiographic examination if possible. Fractured teeth may give no clue to the restorations they may have held and severe burning can cause shattering of the enamel leaving the teeth looking like multiple crown preparations. Dentures and prostheses should be a valuable aid but full upper and lower dentures frequently disintegrate in high speed impacts and are often removed as part of the safety drill in an impending aircraft crash. About half of all denture wearers have the appliance in their

Table 14.1.   Telex code based on Zsigmondy's classification

```
UP LT    R  S  T  V  W  X  Y  Z
UP RT    R  S  T  V  W  X  Y  Z
LR LT    R  S  T  V  W  X  Y  Z
LR LT    R  S  T  V  W  X  Y  Z
```

R = central incisor   Z = third molar

Abbreviations
MIS	– Missing
UE	– Unerupted
DEC	– Deciduous
AMAL	– Amalgam
CEM	– Any tooth-coloured filling
GOLD	– Gold

All filled anterior teeth are CEM unless otherwise stated.

CR	– Crown followed by material, i.e. GOLD or CEM
F	– Replaced by denture or bridge
BRIDGE	– To state which teeth involved

All 32 teeth *must* be transmitted except if edentulous.

Table 14.2.   Typical signals

Dental information for Mr John Albert Doe aged 63 years

UP LT ZMIS Y DO AMAL X OP O AMAL W MIS F V MIS F T B CEM S D CEM
  R MIS F
UP RT Z MIS Y MOD AMAL X DO AMAL W B AMAL V MIS F T S R M CEM
LR RT Z MIS F Y MIS F X MIS F W MOD B AMAL V DO AMAL T S R
LR LT Z MIS F Y MIS F X MIS F W MIS F V MOD AMAL T S R

End of John Albert Doe

This transferred to a chart:

	B														
–	MOD DO	B	–	.	.	M	–	D	B	–	–	OP MOD	–		
8	7	6	5	4	3	2	1	1	2	3	4	5	6	7	8
8	7	6	5	4	3	2	1	1	2	3	4	5	6	7	8
–	–	–	MOD DO							MOD	–	–	–	–	
	B														

Patient wears partial dentures replacing

```
        41    45
        ----------
        876   5678
```

mouths at examination, but these are usually partial plates. Having recorded this information the details of the victim's dental records are awaited.

This can present a major problem as there are 12 major and minor variations in dental recording systems used throughout the world. In order to overcome this problem a system was devised by the British Dental Association Working Party on Forensic Odontology[5] which is easily transmittable by telex without the possibility of error (*Tables* 14.1 and 14.2). The quadrants are described by using the symbols UP, LR, RT and LT followed by letters only. An all letter code enables speedier transmission as the operator does not have to change the keyboard in order to type numerals on a typewriter. 'R S T V W X Y Z' are the symbols used, R being the central incisor and X the first molar, U is omitted as it would be confused with upper. None of these symbols are used in the shorthand description of any dentistry performed on the patient.

This information is transcribed on to cards similar to the body chartings and the process of matching begins.

The presence of the unusual, e.g. temporary crowns, is very helpful and the use of gold or porcelain makes for a speedy match. If, however, the restoration is not of gold, comparison of ante- and post-mortem radiographs can be of the greatest importance and may give conclusive proof of identity. The knowledge that a gold inlay is present in the lower right second premolar becomes useless if the mandible is missing, and more often than not it is only portions of the jaw with two or three teeth that remain. In an ideal world removable prostheses should be marked in some way. These marks should be easily distinguishable and unambiguous, and of such manufacture as to be preserved under extreme physical or chemical assault. The patient's name typed on tissue paper and inserted into the acrylic during the construction of the denture would be invaluable. In the Royal Air Force, laboratory numbers are placed in each appliance, thus leading to a rapid and accurate identification. On metal appliances the name can be neatly engraved on a fitting surface.

Radiographs can be used to show the presence of root fillings and also to determine age by the presence of unerupted teeth and the stages of tooth development. Dental ageing is fairly accurate up to the age of 23 to 25 years, but after that it becomes more difficult. For further details of the value of dental evidence the reader is referred to the suggested reading list.

3. Disposal of Remains and Personal Effects

The disposal of the remains and personal effects will vary from country to country, but specialized firms of funeral directors exist with the expert personnel who are under contract to various state airlines etc. The majority of victims, when identified, are usually repatriated to their place of residence, but there may be requests for local burial.

For repatriation, purpose-made zinc coffins must be used to ensure against leakage of gases and arrangements must be made for them to be brought to the site as soon as possible. Before repatriation of the remains either at home or abroad, certificates of death showing the cause of death must be signed by the local coroner or his equivalent and endorsed by the Consul of the country of the victim. In the United Kingdom, unidentified remains may be cremated using

Cremation Regulations 1965, 1146, Para. 7b. Final death certificates are applied for by the next of kin.

The personal effects removed from the bodies and salvaged from the wreckage require permission from the police to be handed over to the relatives. A detailed list of unidentified property should be prepared for circulation to all relatives as well as survivors. In the interests of public health, badly damaged articles of little value and stained and torn clothing are extracted, thoroughly searched, and destroyed by burning. Jewellery, especially if removed from charred bodies, must be cleaned before any attempt is made to return it to relatives. Discretion must be exercised when dealing with very personal documents such as private letters, diaries and confidential business papers to ensure that they are delivered into the appropriate hands. Receipts are obtained for all articles handed over and passports are returned to the passport office of the relevant country.

REFERENCES

1. Stevens P. J. (1970) *Fatal Aircraft Accidents: their Medical and Pathological Investigations.* Bristol, Wright.
2. Midda M. (1974) The role of dental identification in mass disasters *J. Irish Dent. Assoc.* **20**, 51–62.
3. Frykholm K. O. (1956) Identification in the 'Ormen Friske' disaster. *Acta Odontol. Scand.* **14**, 11–22.
4. Midda M. (1969) A disclosing solution for synthetic filling. *Br. Dent. J.* **127**(11), 519–20.
5. British Dental Association (1969) Forensic odontology: report of working party. *Br. Dent. J.* **127**, 521–5.

FURTHER READING

Cameron J. M. and Sims B. G. (1973) *Forensic Dentistry.* London, Churchill Livingstone.
Luntz L. and Luntz P. (1973) *Handbook for Dental Identification: Techniques in Forensic Dentistry.* Philadelphia, Lippincott.

Roberta E. Steadman

15

Nursing Aspects of Disaster Management

The occurrence of disasters is an undeniable fact of life upon planet Earth. A 'disaster' is commonly defined as a sudden, catastrophic event, producing great material damage and loss to persons and/or property, overwhelming the natural order. Morbidity and mortality figures, the extent of environmental damage, the destruction of personal property and industry comprise the statistical information gathered following disasters and attempt to illustrate the degree of impact the event has had upon the course of human history. The frequency of mass casualty incidents has escalated over the past decade. Disasters attributable to human error increase with the escalating complexity of technology. Those disasters due to nature's whims are still predominantly not controllable by humanity; at best, we can sometimes predict natural disasters and can therefore improve our ability to plan and take defensive action. This too, is dependent upon the technology at our disposal and varies from situation to situation, nation to nation. At the annual convention of the American Geophysical Union in May of 1986, Dr Joseph V. Smith of the University of Chicago urged that the 1990s be dedicated to the study of natural disasters. This suggestion was echoed by Dr Frank Smith, President of the National Academy of Sciences, who emphasized the lack of information, funding for research, and public attention directed toward natural disasters.

The role of the nurse prior to, during and following a disaster depends upon educational preparation for disaster nursing, location of practice (community or hospital), individual experience, and where the nurse happens to be at the time of impact, or occurrence of the disaster. It is not possible to report what all nurses have to offer at the time of a disaster; individual nurses are not necessarily interchangeable. As a profession, nursing has become increasingly specialized and the skills each nurse brings to disaster planning and implementation differ markedly. This chapter will explore each of these variables, to emphasize the unique role of the nurse in disaster management.

EDUCATIONAL PREPARATION FOR DISASTER NURSING

Emergency care in disasters is not a succinct topic and would be difficult to add to an already overcrowded nursing school curriculum. Continuing education courses, articles and books are rare indeed. This is unfortunate since the result is not only less efficiency at the time of the disaster, but less creative input in planning and, ultimately, less quality in health care delivery. Nurses must seek learning opportunities and expand their knowledge bases in order to add their special services to the disaster management team.

The individual nurse can find some help in courses provided for the Red Cross such as 'Providing Red Cross Disaster Health Services' and 'Disaster Health Services in Radiation Accidents'. If the nurse is employed within a hospital or community health care agency, the educational services department can be approached with a request to offer classes in disaster management. Specialty nursing organizations can be encouraged to design courses geared specifically to the needs of nurses in given specialties, such as the emergency department. Continuing education programmes focusing on general first aid techniques and crisis intervention skills are also very helpful. Naturally, it is expected that nurses will maintain their proficiency in cardiopulmonary resuscitation, and advanced life support (including drug therapy, defibrillation and cardioversion, and oxygen therapy). Courses for physicians, but open to nurses, can add breadth to a nurse's preparation for disaster, but the depth should be in general disaster theory and the role of the nurse.

Articles and books are available in medical and nursing libraries associated with schools of medicine and nursing, and in health care agencies. A reference list of materials can be prepared and kept with the agency disaster plan. Seeking out this information will take some time and effort. The reference and further reading lists presented at the end of this chapter will provide a starting point.

LOCATION OF PRACTICE

Whether the nurse's practice location is the hospital or the community will have an impact upon the specific roles assumed during all phases of a disaster. Skills of nurses in differing settings are very diverse and each must bring their own expertise to bear upon the disaster. It should be remembered that it is not only how well nurses do their own jobs, but their ability to support others in doing their jobs which will result in the best possible outcome in a disaster.

Hospital-based nurses are involved in hospital disaster planning and the dissemination of the plan, stockpiling of supplies, arranging for inter- and intra-hospital patient transfers, arranging for staffing and the needs of staff for food and rest, designing methods of record keeping, identifying communication methods and conducting practice drills. The extent of involvement in each of these facets will vary depending upon the individual nurse's position within the hospital organizational structure: staff or managerial/supervisory nurse. These roles will be examined in more detail later in this chapter.

Nurses whose location of practice is outside hospital may be found in such diverse settings as industrial or occupational health, family practice, public health agencies, or working in a variety of their local or national health services. The major common skills they have to offer are their resourcefulness and flexibility. Community nurses can contribute to the designing of a community disaster plan and its articulation with the hospital disaster plan. This primary intervention for the community includes the delivery of health care and the meeting of basic needs in the circumstances imposed by disaster.[1] Inherent within the disaster plans are arrangements for field triage, transportation and distribution of casualties, stockpiling essential supplies, maintaining communication between agencies, organizing rescue teams, establishing shelters, designing methods of record keeping, teaching first aid and cardiopulmonary resuscitation, and conducting practice drills. These responsibilities are based upon the community nurse's thorough assessment of the health needs of the community.

INDIVIDUAL EXPERIENCE

Few nurses have any experience in the area of disaster management or planning. However, certain types of nursing experience will assist in preparing the individual nurse for a role in disaster nursing. The nurse should go through a personal assessment, seeking to identify previous experience which might prove to be most helpful.

There are many professional and personal experiences which could be of value in disaster nursing. Management or supervisory expertise can be helpful both in the planning phase and during the disaster itself; the experienced leader is always a valued member of the health care team. Skills in emergency nursing or the emergency aspects of a specialty such as obstetrics or psychiatry are particularly useful. However, health care during a disaster period consists not only of the management of acute trauma, but also of the continuing care of diseases such as diabetes and chronic pulmonary and heart disease. Thorough knowledge of community or national resources means the nurse is aware of the emergency services that can be called upon in time of disaster. The nurse often knows the options available to meet the health care needs of the community, the type of equipment and personnel each has at its disposal, and the extent and variety of supplies. A thorough, current assessment of the cultural diversity, general state of health and socio-economic status of the community can be very helpful. Political awareness and contacts which might improve the allocation of resources or legislation regarding disaster intervention are always of value. In some communities, nurses are part of task forces, gathering information and data to aid political decision-making and providing an impetus to overcome the inertia which often precedes disaster planning.

Every nurse has something to offer; some skill, some energy, which can assist the community to pass through the destruction and grief which accompany a disaster.

LOCATION AT THE TIME OF THE DISASTER

It is most desirable for the entire community as well as the individual health care delivery agencies to have well designed plans for the sequential courses of action to be initiated at the time of a disaster. In this plan, the individual nurse will have a clearly identified role, assigned tasks and position, to be assumed at the time of the disaster. This is based upon the nurse being either on duty at his or her place of work or able to be called in at the time the disaster plan is activated. Things may be different, however, if the nurse is close to the scene of the disaster. In this case, the nurse might prove to be of more value in immediately assisting the rescue or triage teams, moving people to shelters, or providing services in some other capacity, regardless of his or her order planned role. However, sometimes the nurse's planned role within the agency is imperative, in which case that role should take precedence. This decision needs to be made on an individual basis.

ROLES OF THE NURSE IN DISASTER MANAGEMENT

Primarily, the role of the nurse in disaster management depends upon location. Occasionally, nurses are involved in disaster management both within the hospital and within the community, but it is more likely that their role will be in one or the other.

The Nurse in the Hospital

Every hospital (acute or intermediate care agency), should have a Disaster Planning Committee with representatives from the various key groups most likely to be involved at the time of a disaster. Areas which will require representation include: security, medical services, ancillary personnel, maintenance, pharmacy, nursing service, emergency department and operating room. Nurses may represent the emergency department and operating room, as well as the nursing service in general. There is certainly no such thing as a 'good' disaster, but there can be disasters in which planning can be the crucial factor in minimizing problems for all those involved.

Certain basic assumptions serve to guide the Hospital Disaster Planning Committee in their preparations to receive large numbers of casualties with maximum efficiency.[2] These assumptions are illustrated in *Table* 15.1.

Table 15.1. Basic assumptions regarding disaster situations

1. Disasters that cause mass casualties occur with little or no warning.
2. As the density of the population increases, the danger of a disaster producing mass casualties increases.
3. Disruptions may occur in communication and all community services, including transport and utilities.
4. Normal hospital operation will be disrupted by a disaster.
5. Control of traffic flow, information and security will be necessitated.
6. Planning and drilling for mass casualty situations helps to prepare the hospital for maximum efficiency.

Planning

As a member of the Hospital Disaster Planning Committee, the nurse may be involved in considering modifications of the existing structure which might be necessary to produce more efficient management of disaster casualties. Certain essential facilities need to be provided for in the hospital (*see* Chapter 5). First, there must be an area for patient triage on their arrival. This area should be located near the casualty delivery point, have separate entrances and exits, and plenty of open space. Generally, the emergency department best fulfils these criteria. Areas for preoperative, operative, postoperative and non-operative patient care must be designated. It is important to identify a place for family and friends to congregate where they can be kept out of the way of the health care team. Advance identification should be made of those persons who will work in this area, to deal with the families' anxiety and to keep them informed of the patients' progress. Nurses may be used here, or this may be a good position for the well trained volunteer and/or mental health worker. The early designation of an area for the press to be located and a responsible person to interact with them will reduce the likelihood of problems developing which are due to incomplete, inaccurate information. The final essential area is a morgue. Existing facilities in the hospital may well be overwhelmed and require more space. The morgue serves both as a store and as an area where the deceased may be identified and thought should be given to this dual function. Here again, nurses can provide support to the families as they search for their loved ones.[3]

The Planning Committee should also establish the communication centre or Centre for Disaster Operations (CDO) to direct the action within the hospital during the disaster, liaise with other health care agencies and, as much as possible, communicate with those at the scene of the disaster. Nurses working in the CDO provide continuous, current information regarding the number of available patient beds, nursing staff numbers and locations, and types and quantities of supplies available. Methods for gathering this information must be established early since important nursing and medical decisions will be based upon the results.

Before casualties arrive at the hospital, the patients already there may need to be moved within the hospital, or discharged, to make space for the disaster victims. Nurses on duty in the patient care units should assess the state of patients for potential discharge or transfer as soon as notification of the disaster reaches the hospital. Depending upon the particular hospital's disaster plan, this assessment and evaluation may be done by nurses only, or by teams of nurses and doctors. Guidelines need to be established for those who must make these decisions, to accelerate the operation and eliminate potential sources of dissent. Nurses should assist with the discharge and transfer of patients and their belongings, complete minimal paperwork and arrange transport to their destination. Some disaster plans are designed to allow for the movement of hospitalized patients between departments and even hospitals, in order to make more acute care beds available. In these situations, transfers can be activated by nurses between acute care hospitals and nursing homes, convalescent centres, or rehabilitation agencies.

The disaster plan should also include arrangements for extra staffing of nursing units during the time of the emergency, such as holding over staff and calling in additional personnel as necessary. In most cases, 12 hour shifts work well during a disaster. A telephone cascade system should be activated by the nurse manager of each unit so that personnel can be reached and activated as needed. Each nurse will call two nurses who in turn each call two further nurses and so on, until the entire staff of the unit has been notified of the disaster and given instructions.

In addition to calling in nursing personnel, consideration should be given to the probable need to provide internal housing and catering for staff. Transport difficulties, combined with the long shifts, often require these actions to maintain staff in the best possible physical and mental condition to perform their functions under hardship circumstances. This presents an entirely new set of problems to the nursing management. Most hospitals have few or no facilities for housing or backup staffing but, ideally, both should be considered.[4]

Accurate inventories of supplies and equipment should always be maintained by the hospital. These should be reviewed by the Planning Committee and modified to include the possibility of mass disaster. During the disaster, these inventories must be kept current and will most certainly have to be rationed. Guidelines as to the use of supplies will help, but each nurse should attempt to be as frugal as possible.

Nursing Care

Nursing care itself must be limited to the essential. Priorities in direct patient care must be made and indirect patient care eliminated as much as possible. Direct patient care activities which can be reduced include bathing, daily bed linen changes, frequent dressing changes, and four hourly observation and recording of vital signs. Indirect patient care which may be reduced or eliminated during a disaster includes patient teaching, frequent changes of intravenous equipment, patient care conferences and referrals. *Table* 15.2 presents a summation of guidelines for nursing staff on duty at the time the disaster occurs.[5]

Nurses should strive to make record keeping during a disaster as simple as possible. Usually, abbreviated forms and/or checklists work best. Over-reliance upon computers, which may 'go down' during power failures, power surges or structural damage, is to be discouraged. Nurses assigned to a task force by the

Table 15.2. Guidelines for hospital nursing personnel

All nursing personnel should take the following action:
1. Remain calm.
2. Inform patients and family of disaster situation and request co-operation.
3. Notify on-duty staff and call in off-duty staff as needed, sending extra personnel to the personnel pool.
4. Obtain an initial count of available beds.
5. Evaluate patients to determine who can be discharged or transferred, should the need arise.
6. Determine minimum care required and revise bed availability as patients are discharged.
7. Reallocate resources to the treatment areas (e.g. wheelchairs, stretchers, i.v. poles).
8. Conserve supplies and resources left on the unit.
9. Avoid use of telephones and lifts except for disaster activities.
10. Assign someone to make an inventory, i.v. poles, wheelchairs, stretchers, etc.; to submit requisitions; and to keep a running count of supplies.
11. Arrange for patients, staff and visitors entering or leaving the unit to sign in or out so that an accurate head count can be maintained.
12. If the need to evacuate patients arises, rehearse the preparations for evacuation (i.e. chart preparation, transportation, dress of patients, essential items to be sent with patients) and make staff assignments for assisting with the evacuation.

Planning Committee can be responsible for designing a form or forms to be used in the disaster situation. Staff nurses are in the best position to help with the design of such records because of their experience in history taking and documentation. The record should attempt to combine thoroughness and precision with brevity.

Telephone and computer services are subject to damage with resultant disruption of communication throughout the hospital. Nurses should avoid using the telephones in the unit, unless their function in the disaster plan is essential. Two-way radios or human 'runners' are often used to pass information within the hospital during a disaster. All efforts should be directed to reducing communication gaps.

Failure to disseminate the plan adequately and incomplete evaluation can spell disaster for the plan itself. The nursing service must assume the responsibility of ensuring that nursing personnel who currently work in the institution are appraised of the disaster plan and that it is included in the orientation for all new employees. After the introduction of the plan, there must be periodic drills to test the plan and the people involved, and assess weak areas in the finished product. It is in the conduct of the drills that many disaster plans fall by the wayside. Often the problem is not in the quality of the components of the plan itself, but the infrequency of drills and the pervasive attitude of levity with which employees sometimes approach the drill. This poses a serious management problem, similar in many ways to the sense of community and/or national inertia which may retard the design of a disaster plan on the larger scale. Nursing management and hospital management must draw upon all of their resources to prepare a realistic drill which thoroughly tests the plan in all its aspects and provides sufficient motivation to guarantee the committed involvement of all personnel.

The Role of the Community Nurse

Nurses are not only working in the hospital setting when disaster strikes. Many nurses have roles within the community during the immediate disaster response and following the event, in the days, months and years it may require the community to reach its new equilibrium.

Prior to the disaster, community health nurses bring in-depth information to the committee whose task it is to prepare a blueprint for a community disaster response. As the Community Disaster Committee gathers data upon which to base their plan, they will include a thorough assessment of the services and resources available to them, locally, nationally and internationally. Specifically, community health nurses provide information regarding the pre-disaster status of the community, its current health needs, available services, susceptibility to disaster and possible response methods to deal with disaster.[1] Designing a community disaster plan requires such knowledge in detail and meticulous attention to the strengths and weaknesses the community possesses.

The Community Disaster Committee must work closely with the Hospital Disaster Committees in order to facilitate the best possible response to the disaster. Nurses are often in a position to bridge the gap between these two bodies, enhancing the transfer of information and clarifying any unclear areas of responsibility. The well-informed, motivated community health nurse is a valuable participant in such pre-disaster planning.

Nurses in the community may be called upon to take part in casualty priority allocation at the scene (field triage) in preparation for transport to the hospitals. The literature abounds with methods for classifying the injured. The method selected is not as important as the consistency with which it is applied to the situation. In the field, leadership is mandatory. The nurse may be the triage officer initially, relinquishing this role as soon as others arrive who are more qualified. During a disaster, it is not only how well one does one's job, but how well one permits others to carry out theirs. Once the injured are classified, skilful nursing care at the scene is imperative to stabilize the patient and prevent any deterioration prior to transport. This is a very important role. Experienced nurses are by far the most valuable and should be divided between the stations to direct the work of less knowledgeable and skilled volunteers. Nurses who are the most effective in providing care directly at the scene of the disaster are usually those with a strong background in trauma. However, nurses with general skills will find they are able to function quite well with direction from other, more specialized personnel.

Transport

Specific arrangements need to be made for the movement of casualties from the scene of the disaster to the hospitals. Usually, teams are dispatched from the hospitals. Some communities have ambulance services staffed by trained paramedical personnel. There may even be more sophisticated Emergency Medical Services Systems which are designed on a national level and then activated locally. Any vehicles which are near the site of the disaster will be pressed into service for the transport of the injured. Care needs to be taken, however, since more damage may be produced during the transport of casualties than occurred at the scene of the disaster. It would be ideal if only disaster/trauma-trained individuals actually transported the injured, but there are rarely enough to go around. There must also be arrangements for the distribution of casualties among the various health care agencies within the community to avoid overwhelming the resources of one hospital and under-utilizing others. Nursing homes and other extended care facilities may be used to house casualties, transfers from hospitals, or as shelters for the homeless. A single hospital or health care agency should be designated as the communication centre for the co-ordination of transport. As soon as possible, communication lines should be established between the scene of the disaster and the Centre for Disaster Operations (CDO) located in the co-ordinating hospital.

The practice of stockpiling supplies, food and even water varies considerably from community to community. It is most commonly done in those communities which are in particularly disaster-prone areas. If such stockpiling is instituted, public health nurses are often involved in the selection of materials and locations, based upon their knowledge of the community needs. With the loss of personal shelter, the destruction of the home often means that individual personal effects such as food, water, clothing and medicines for the treatment of chronic diseases are inaccessible. The services normally provided to the community are profoundly affected by disaster: water, power, sanitation and so forth. These breaks in community continuity may be mollified through stockpiling of canned and dehydrated food stuffs, drinking water, chemicals for rendering water safe for drinking, chemical toilets, blankets, candles and alternative lighting sources and basic first aid supplies. The expiry dates of such supplies should be carefully listed, and thorough plans made in advance for their distribution.

Communication

Nurses in the community may find themselves involved in the search for alternative communication systems to provide information between the scene of the disaster and the health care agencies, between the various health care agencies and the shelters. If the telephone services are interrupted, inaccessible or overwhelmed, there must be predetermined methods by which communications can be continued. Two-way radios have been the major alternative, used by the military and carried over into the civilian system. However, in the past five to ten years an even more accessible system has developed in the citizen's band (CB) radio. Disaster teams have found the CB radio to be extremely beneficial in reaching and directing the disaster response.

Methods for organizing rescue teams need to be considered in the community disaster plan and forethought will be rapaid by less confusion and wasted effort at the time. This is an excellent area for participation by nurses since poorly prepared workers can result in prolonged rescue manoeuvres, and increased morbidity and mortality. A thorough assessment of resources available may identify agencies or services, usually on a national level, especially prepared for search and rescue and general support.

Shelter

With the destruction of personal property, disasters usually displace large numbers of people. Meeting their basic needs for shelter, food, water, clothing and health care is a major part of disaster relief. Selecting, equipping and staffing emergency shelters is a role nurses in the community are frequently called upon to assume.

In the ideal scenario, specially trained personnel will be available to manage the shelters. Nurses may be these managers or work under their direction. Sites most chosen for shelters are schools, churches, auditoriums and other public meeting places. These locations have the essential components of large open space, cooking facilities, water and sanitary services.

The responsibilities of the nurse in the shelter will vary. The manager deals with the administrative functions of allocating and arranging the space, scheduling staff to operate the shelter and providing the necessary services. The manager will establish and maintain records, distribute supplies and provide such regulations and enforcement as the situation requires. Skills in the field of mental health and counselling are especially valuable to the nurse working as a member of the shelter staff. Individuals who have lost homes and loved ones are in various stages of the grieving process and have a need for emotional support as great as their need for food and rest. The threat of communicable disease in the shelters is ever-present; it can be brought into the shelter or develop there later. Nurses must be attentive to hygiene, food preparation and the storage of food and water. Established protocols for the monitoring of these facilities should be prepared in advance. Immunization programmes may be initiated. Illnesses in the shelter setting are many and varied. During the process of triage at the scene of the disaster, individuals are often identified whose injuries place them at the lowest priority for health care. These individuals, who may have sprains, contusions and abrasions, even minimal burns, are often sent to the shelter to have their injuries attended to. In addition to their first aid needs, they may also have chronic illnesses which require various levels of intervention. Nurses working in shelters therefore need skills ranging from basic first aid to sophisticated physical assessment and clinical judgement.

Documentation

Record keeping is a significant problem during a community disaster. Some method needs to be identified to assist in tracking people; frequently, the process of ascertaining whether individuals are among the living or the dead is directly dependent upon the records kept. A simple method should be chosen, sometimes using modified checklists. If possible, of course, casualties should be identified by name. If that is not possible, vital statistics and the location where the individual was found are recorded; this is often a primary method of identification. Nurses are actively involved in the record keeping in acute care agencies, at the scene of the disaster during rescue operations and in triage, and at shelters and/or first aid stations. Since they are routinely involved in the data gathering, nurses are of great help during the planning phase, when forms are being selected and/or devised for disaster use. Prepared forms which have been used and refined and are the most broadly applicable are to be preferred.

Teaching basic first aid and cardiopulmonary resuscitation is an important pre-disaster community service nurses are in an excellent position to provide. The more individuals in the public sector with these skills, the greater the pool of volunteers to draw upon in time of need. Nurses should have on-going programmes in their communities to provide this necessary education, and also the records to locate these individuals. Their use during the actual disaster can be built into the plan.

Drills should be community-wide and repetitive since no disaster plan is ever truly complete; it needs to be continually evaluated and modified. As the community population, services and geography change, the plan must grow. The community drill should be interactive and shared with the health care agencies. Nurses must evaluate their individual function during drills, and also their function within the total operation. Any suggestions they can make to improve the role of nursing or the efficiency of the entire plan should be brought forward. Nursing brings a unique perspective to disaster planning and care and should not hesitate to share it.

SUMMARY

Disasters are not totally avoidable in the world today. Survival of individuals and communities is directly related to the knowledge and preparedness they possess. Research is desperately needed to expand the understanding of the short- and long-term impact of disasters and improve methods of implementing and evaluating care. To provide the best possible conclusion to disaster preparedness and intervention, all members of the health care team must develop new skills and knowledge and apply previous expertise in new ways. Nurses, by virtue of their eclectic experience, education and locations of practice are in a position to play a very substantial role in health care during the demanding period preceding and following a disaster.

REFERENCES

1. Switzer K. H. (1986) Functioning in a community health setting. In: Garcia L. M. (ed.) *Disaster Nursing: Planning, Assessment and Intervention* (pp. 229–77). Rockville, Aspen Systems Corp.
2. Lansky G. Y. (1982) Disaster! Planning for the worst. *Health Services Manager* 1–3.
3. Ballinger W. F., Rutherford R. B. and Zuidema G. D. (eds.) (1973) *The Management of Trauma.* Philadelphia, Saunders.
4. Hargreaves A.,Krell G. I., Blakeney B. et al. (1979) Blizzard '78: Dealing with disaster. *Am. J. Nursing,* **79**, 268–71.
5. Wieland M. P. and Hattan D. K. (1986) Disaster decision making in the acute care facility. In: Garcia L. M. (ed.) *Disaster Nursing: Planning, Assessment and Intervention* (pp. 71–100). Rockville, Aspen Systems Corp.

FURTHER READING

Berren M. R., Beigel A. and Ghertner S. (1980) A typology for the classification of disasters. *Mental Health J.,* **16** (2), 103–11.
Butman A. M. (1982) *Responding to the Mass Casualty Incident: A Guide for EMS Personnel.* Westport, Educational Direction Inc.
Cohen R. E. and Ahearn F. L. Jr. (1980) *Handbook for Mental Health Care of Disaster Victims.* Baltimore and London, John Hopkins University Press.
Demi A. S. and Miles M. S. (1984) An examination of nursing leadership following a disaster. *Top. Clin. Nurs.,* **6** (1), 63–78.
Demi A. S. and Miles M. S. (1983) Understanding psychologic reactions to disaster. *J. Emerg. Nurs.,* **9** (1), 11–16.
Disaster Services Regulations and Procedures: Administrative Regulations. (1984) (ARC 3003) Washington DC, American Red Cross.
Disaster Services Regulations and Procedures: Disaster Health Services. (1982) (ARC 3050) Washington DC, American Red Cross.
Disaster Services Regulations and Procedures: Disaster Health Services in Radiation Accidents. (1985) (ARC 3076-R) Washington DC, American Red Cross.
Disaster Services Regulations and Procedures: Providing Red Cross Disaster Health Services. (1983) (ARC 3076) Washington DC, American Red Cross.
Disaster Services Regulations and Procedures: Shelter Management: A Guide for Trainers. (1985) (ARC 3078) Washington DC, American Red Cross.
Ellison D. (1967) Education for nursing care in disaster. *Nurs. Clin. North Am.,* **2**, 299–307.
Emergency Health Management After Natural Disasters. (1981) Pan American Health Organization Scientific Publication No. 407. Washington DC, World Health Organization.
Garcia L. M. (ed.) (1986) *Disaster Nursing: Planning, Assessment and Intervention.* Rockville, Aspen Systems Corp.
Hargreaves A. G. (1982) Coping with disaster. *Am. J. Nurs.,* **80**, 683.
Lindemann E. (1944) Symptomatology and management of acute grief. *Am. J. Psychiat.,* **101** (10), 141–8.
Maxwell C. (1982) Hospital organizational response to the nuclear accident at Three Mile Island: implications for future-oriented disaster planning. *Am. J. Public Health,* **72** (3), 275–9.

Richter L. L., Berk H. W., Teates C. D. et al. (1980) A systems approach to the management of radiation accidents. *Ann. Emerg. Med.*, **9** (6), 303–9.
Skeet M. (1977) *Manual for Disaster Relief Work.* Edinburgh, Churchill Livingstone.
Steadman R. E. (1986) Disaster: knowledge is critical. *Focus on Crit. Care*, **13** (1), 20–8.

Ellen G. McDaniel

16

Psychological Response to Disasters

OVERVIEW OF THE IMPACT OF STRESS

Stress can be defined as the subjective experience of increased tension in reaction to a perceived view of environmental, interpersonal or somatic events. It is an inherent part of psychological development, moving the growing child forward toward increasingly more adaptive and mature ways of thought and behaviour. Episodes of frustration and disappointment limit the rewards of remaining infantile and encourage the child to seek alternative pathways in the search for survival and satisfaction. This is not to minimize the enormous role parents have in providing security, comfort, protection and narcissistic gratification (important in the building of self-esteem) for their developing progeny. An infant needs to be enveloped in an emotionally supportive sanctuary which gradually opens its doors to the challenges of the external environment at a rate compatible with the growing youngster's cognitive and psychological abilities. If the doors are not opened at a timely pace, fixation at an infantile stage of development is encouraged. Overprotection can be as crippling to emotional growth as neglect and abuse. In this sense, experience of stress is a vital part of maturation.

What happens when the youngster is deprived of an age-appropriate sanctuary—when the doors of the refuge open too fast at certain developmental stages? The child's psyche becomes overwhelmed, for he does not have the cognitive, psychological or physical ability to tackle properly the stress to which he is exposed. He has only a few limited options, none of them being particularly beneficial. He might regress to an earlier mode of functioning in an effort to cope, which will be manifested by immature behaviour. He might withdraw increasingly into himself to avoid the overwhelming stress, which can result in a loss of contact with reality. Or he might continue on as best he can, but with an increasingly fixed distortion in character development. This distortion may be necessary in order to survive the trauma psychologically, particularly when the stress is too intense and too repetitive. However, the adaptation necessary to preserve self-esteem and survival may well result in a pathological response when viewed by a wider society. For example, youngsters growing up in abusive families and poverty-stricken communities may fail to develop appropriate levels of tolerance to frustration, may form idiosyncratic ethical systems, and may learn to relate to others in the aggressive and combative style necessary for survival in their own neighbourhoods. These character adaptations are seen as distorted and pathological when viewed by the outside community with whom these youngsters eventually interact. Stress in these instances has crippled development.

Finally, stress can occur in a sudden, overwhelming, massive assault, in response to the natural and man-made disasters that have been part of our civilization for centuries. Although not commonly recognized, these severe stresses ultimately may result in a better overall adaptation for some individuals relative to their pre-trauma function. However, for most of the survivors, families, communities and rescue workers, these events are formidable psychological ordeals which may provoke regressive and maladaptive behaviour, either for a limited period or forever, permanently clouding their adjustment to life. The normal, predictable world, at least momentarily, is changed in a disaster and the mind is unprepared. Symptomatic behaviour is common but in contrast to the child, adults have more options available for coping. The majority of adults will recover their previous equilibrium.

TYPICAL PSYCHOLOGICAL RESPONSES TO A DISASTER

Although every disaster is distinct and each individual brings his own unique personal history to the situation, some generalizations can be made about the typical responses of people to catastrophies. These responses usually are categorized by the stages of the disaster in which they occur.[1-6] The stages typically are divided into the period of forewarning, the event, the period of recovery, and the resumption of a stable routine of living. The following describes the stages of a time-limited, acute disaster. One must realize that chronic trauma, such as participating in prolonged war or living in a refugee camp, exact a toll on the involved populations in a more insidious, often more malignant and permanent manner.

Forewarning

A reasonable prediction might be that if people are warned about an impending disaster, they will take the necessary steps to avoid it. Yet people do not commonly act in this manner. The use of cigarettes and the disregard of seat belts while driving are two very ordinary examples of the limitations of hazard warnings. State and local governments sometimes use legal restrictions to prevent people from ignoring, self-destructively, certain hazard warnings. Interestingly, these restrictions are often met with protest by those same people, who would rather accept the hazard than have their freedom to choose restricted.

Research has been conducted into the human response to predictions of hazards and disasters. One study concluded that 'the evidence supporting the casual link between hazard awareness and protective responses is minimal and, correspondingly, the evidence documenting the failure of such educational efforts is considerable'.[7] Suggestions made to enhance the value of warnings for a population at risk include: (1) the warning must be clear, (2) it must convey the appropriate response, (3) it must be perceived as coming from a credible source, (4) it must be reinforced socially and at the local level, (5) the medium used to disseminate the warning is important and has to be chosen with consideration for the community involved and the situation, and (6) the type of appeal (i.e. supportive or through the use of fear) made by the warning must be carefully assessed.[7]

Why do some people ignore the prediction of catastrophe? The answers are varied. People who have chosen to live in an area that has an above average likelihood of sustaining some type of disaster, whether man-made (e.g. surrounding a toxic chemical plant) or natural (e.g. resting in a flood plain) do so for economic, cultural and/or social reasons. They adjust to the constant threat by diminishing the significance of the predicted threat (a defence mechanism known as denial), and underestimating the possibility of an occurrence that may happen as infrequently as once in several generations. They may respond to warnings of an impending disaster with a casualness that comes from having heard repeated previous threats of such calamities that never came to fruition. In contrast, the individual may become desensitized to the presence of disaster in an environment where such danger is omnipresent, such as in a high crime area. A sense of resignation to what is believed to be inevitable, or a psychologically protective grandiose belief that one is immune to these tragedies, also prevents proper attention being given to forewarnings.

The above is not to disparage the dissemination of disaster information in the period before the impact. Other studies[8,9] describe the value of communicating a warning. Contrary to the myth that if someone yells 'Fire!' in a theatre, everyone will panic, confrontation with the possibility of disaster not uncommonly brings out appropriate and constructive organizational behaviour in families, neighbourhoods and communities. People become concerned and goal-directed in preserving the lives and properties of those important to them.[10,11] This fact, nevertheless, raises a difficult question. In the pre-impact phase, when preparation for evacuation, protection of life and property and planning for the aftermath might be possible, should emotionally neutral outsiders be brought into the area to direct and assist, or should any organized efforts use mainly the resident population? The argument against the latter is that people naturally think first of preservation of family and self and preparatory efforts for the community might be thwarted by the universal tendency to take care of one's own kin first. Usually, the need to respond immediately to an impending disaster makes this question a rhetorical one.

The Event

Consideration needs to be given to the duration of a disaster when considering the psychological aspects of this stage. In some situations, the trauma occurs so rapidly that there is virtually no warning and no time for reaction during the impact, e.g. a plane explosion in mid-air in an otherwise smooth flight. A shipwreck resulting in a lifeboat full of survivors adrift at sea for days represents a prolonged trauma in which the acute episode cannot be considered over until the survivors have been rescued. Finally, one might consider the case of a community which is located beside a toxic waste depot. The event theoretically can be considered as long as successive generations wait to see if medical problems will arise in themselves or their offspring. Each situation presents different types of psychological difficulties.

Initially, the most common responses by those directly involved in a disaster situation will be bewilderment, disbelief, emotional numbness and reflexive behaviour (*Fig.* 16.1, p. 233). The majority of the population will be able to respond in a restricted manner to the demands of the situation and will follow

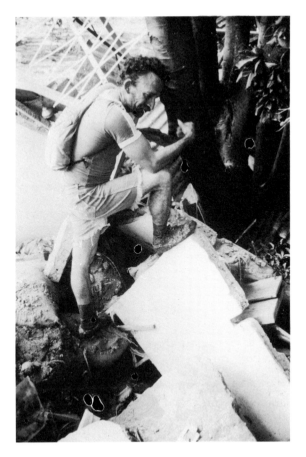

clear directions from a readily identifiable leader. But they may not be able to appraise the situation beyond their narrowed focus of attention, or make decisions based on a projection of the situation into the future. Two of the most significant forces pushing a potential victim to keep trying to preserve life until rescue comes are a strong attachment to someone else and hope that the efforts to survive will be successful. Many a survivor has stated that he had to keep trying in order to see his children (wife, husband, parents) again. It can also be predicted that when confronted by disaster, a small number of people will rise above the majority and be capable of providing remarkable leadership for the masses. In an account of the World War II atomic bombing of Hiroshima, Shinzo Hamai, chief of the Municipal Distribution Section, became a major organizer and support to the population. There was nothing obvious that would have identified this individual as being a leader with such remarkable courage as well as organizational abilities.[12] After a shipwreck, 10 men drifted for 9 days in a raft. The survivors were not discovered on a beach until the thirteenth day. All of the men spontaneously identified one individual as the recognized leader of the group within a few hours after the sinking. His leadership qualities included the ability to make decisions, to understand the technicalities involved, to discipline the men who endangered the group and to provide compassion and hope.[13]

Along with the remarkable individuals who emerge as strong leaders in a disaster-stricken population, there will be another group of people who, for a wide variety of reasons, will be psychologically incapacitated, as demonstrated by uncontrollable emotional outbursts that prevent appropriate action being taken, and by cognitive impairment such as confusion, disorganization of thought processes, inability to attend to the immediate tasks at hand, and overwhelming and paralysing anxiety. In a tiny percentage, a sequel of physiological reactions to the psychological shock of the disaster may even result in death.[14–16]

Recovery

In addition to the rebuilding of lives and communities, recovery must include the psychological integration of the disaster and its consequences into the victim's perception of himself or herself and the world. This includes the necessary period of grieving for the losses sustained, which are not restricted to the dead

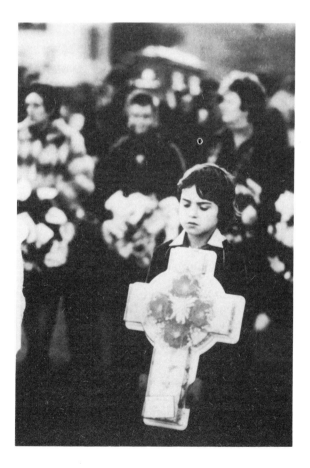

but include a changed body, home, or society. Most survivors eventually become desensitized to the memories of the disaster, accept the personal and environmental changes that have resulted, and focus attention increasingly on the present and future. Although the character structure and outlook on life may be permanently altered to some degree, life returns (nearly) to normal.

On the journey to this successful outcome, many difficult and distressing psychological events are experienced. Intrusive and recurring images of specific aspects of the catastrophe will invade the consciousness despite a desire to have these memories recede or disappear. The images are accompanied by very distressing affects and may occur very frequently in the days or weeks after the impact, but lessen with the passage of time. They may occur particularly during moments when the attention is not specifically focused, such as on a long car ride or before falling asleep. And they may be evoked when some environmental stimulus rekindles the memories through an associative link. As with any emotionally highly traumatic event, however ordinary and predictable, these painful memories rarely (if ever) totally disappear. But they eventually recede so that the ability to function and to enjoy the present is not handicapped.

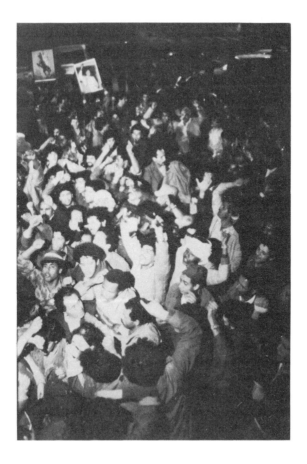

The sadness over the losses is pernicious and pervasive (*Fig.* 16.2, p. 234); but other troubling emotions follow. For example, anger is very commonly experienced . In a disaster considered entirely natural, such as that caused by a tornado or cyclone, some survivors work toward acceptance of the consequences by a spiritual interpretation of their changed lives, such as believing the events were 'Acts of God', and thus preordained or of spiritual importance, even if the meaning is obscure. A problem arises when these people do not find a focus for their painful, uncomfortable, anxiety-provoking feelings of rage. The survivor feels a need to conceal this 'illogical' affect, which then becomes a hidden source of both somatic and psychic distress. In a man-made disaster, the victim may be tormented by obsessional ruminations (e.g. if only the dam/reactor/building had been built differently), with attendant feelings of being deceived, misused and disregarded by whomever is perceived as the responsible party. Often, the target of the anger is logical and justifiable but, not infrequently, the target is irrational and reflective of misunderstanding and previously existing stereotyping and prejudices. Institutions, corporations and governments, as well as individuals (including rescue workers and relief organizations), may become scapegoats. One extremely dangerous consequence of the need to target anger outside of oneself is the development of a mob reaction, in which many more losses are sustained in a pathologically diverted attempt to achieve psychological repair (*Fig.* 16.3, p. 235).

Guilt is another commonly experienced emotion. The reasons for this are numerous and include the well-known 'survivor's guilt'[18] which arises out of the realization that one has survived while others have perished. 'Survivor's guilt' may also stem from the actions which had to be taken in order to survive and/or help others to survive, such as an excruciating decision to save the life of one child at the expense of another. Guilt may also arise from those events which occurred moments to years before the catastrophe but which have become psychologically linked to the disaster. Imagine the added pain of a couple who had a bitter argument in the moments before the disaster which killed one of them. The surviving member may blame himself for the demise of the spouse, irrationally linking the feeling of wishing the spouse would disappear during the heat of the argument with the actual loss of the person. The survivor is left with the pain of never being able to make amends.

Other symptoms of anxiety are common in the recovery phase of the disaster. The perception of the immediate environment may be significantly altered, as evidenced by an exaggerated startle response and an excessive vigilance for danger, or by a sense of helplessness and humiliation that one could do so little in the face of such devastation. Insomnia, nightmares, avoidance behaviour (even to the extreme of phobias or isolation), decreased interest in work and recreational activities, somatic complaints and emotional lability are all commonly experienced.

What is the time limit within which one may consider these psychological consequences normal? The grieving period after a major loss usually lasts at least 6 months and commonly 1–2 years. However, psychological interventions should not be delayed until the first anniversary of the disaster has passed. On the contrary, early intervention may prevent an unnecessary prolongation of common but distressing symptoms.

Survivors of a disaster are not the only people affected in the above manner.

Consider how many other people may be involved: family, bystanders, neighbourhoods and communities, rescue workers, clean-up crews, morgue attendants, medical personnel, those involved in the administration or technology of a structure involved in a man-made disaster (such as the scientists and administrators in the space shuttle explosion). All of these groups are subject to the same recovery phase distress, and about 10–20 per cent will proceed to a stage of chronicity, or will have a delayed and pathological response at some time later in their lives. For a small number, psychological recovery, in the sense of resuming a reasonably satisfying and psychologically stable life, will never take place.

Table 16.1. Factors that prolong psychological recovery

1. Helplessness
2. Confrontation with death
3. Mutilation and decay of bodies
4. Identification with the victims
5. Death of children
6. Psychological immaturity of survivors and rescue workers
7. Loss of community
8. Uncertainty of future effects of the disaster
9. Specific personal losses
10. Pathological reaction of family members
11. Continued economic dependency on source of disaster
12. Delayed or absent treatment
13. Secondary gain
14. Malingering
15. Impending litigation

Psychological Recovery

What are the factors that prolong psychological recovery? *Table* 16.1 shows a list of some of them. A sense of helplessness is one of the most distressing experiences reported. To be unable to contribute constructively to the care of family, neighbours, and other victims provokes feelings of inadequacy, guilt, anger and restlessness, regardless of the cause. Confrontation with death is always a distressing event, especially for those not used to dealing fairly regularly with dying; and the distress is increased when the toll has been massive, the bodies have started decaying or have otherwise been mutilated, and identification of the victim is difficult (*Fig.* 16.4, p. 238). Rescue workers and survivors develop disturbing olfactory and visual memories of this assault on the senses. If rescue workers closely identify with the victims, either through community ties or by association with the age, race or other obvious aspects of the victims, the distress is again intensified. The mutilation and death of infants and children is particularly difficult to witness (*Fig.* 16.5, p. 239), and, of course, the relative degree of immaturity and the presence of certain predisposing personality factors also contribute to the ability (or inability) to maintain a healthy psychological equilibrium.[19]

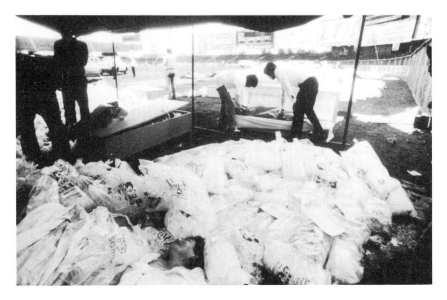

Predisposing Personality Factors

The significance of the pre-existing personality structure on the development of a post-traumatic stress disorder has been debated for decades.[21-23] In general, the presence of basic trust, a positive orientation to life, and the ability to attach to others in a reasonably mature manner will diminish the prolongation of mental suffering (as well as assist the survivor to get through the disaster itself). If the disaster has a particular symbolic meaning for the individual involved, the emotional response may be exaggerated because what is being expressed may reflect an accumulation of conflicts over past events, e.g. an individual who comes from an abusive family environment which severely damaged his self-esteem might personalize his involvement in a recent disaster as reflecting his general unworthiness and incompetence. Certain well-established defence mechanisms, used to ward off anxiety, may impair the ability to grieve and move on with life after the disaster. For example, the use of denial and of withdrawal into fantasy may interfere with dealing with the demands of the recovery phase realistically. The use of projection (e.g. the person who blames others for his own shortcomings and failures) might result in a grossly exaggerated expression of rage.

Loss of Community

Some disasters are described as centrifugal, i.e. an event destroys a specific space or vehicle, in which the affected population comes from many different communities. An example of this would be an aeroplane crash. In another type of disaster, a centripetal one, the event destroys a wide area which encompasses

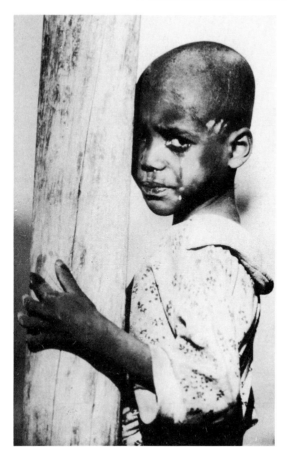

intact communities and neighbourhoods. Floods and hurricanes would belong in this category.[24] The distress over the loss of the lives of family and friends and of the home is clearly understood. Not always considered is the damage done when a community is destroyed, particularly if that community has a long-standing cultural and economic history.[25] The extensive network of relationships, often going back for generations, may be lost in the recovery phase, particularly if a large segment of the population has been lost or if a geographical move to another area is required. Also lost may be the source of economic support, which often cannot be replaced. Consider the consequences of the rural coal mining community which was wiped out by a flood in the Buffalo Creek disaster in 1972. The community was permanently destroyed; families had to move from homes to trailer camps scattered over a wide area; and the very interdependent, rural nature of that society was lost forever. Consider the cultures of African nations whose populations have died or have been evacuated to refugee camps far from their homes (*Fig.* 16.6, p. 240).

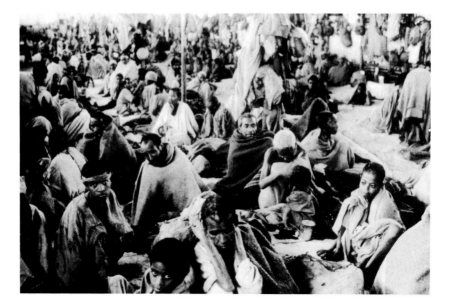

TREATMENT

Treatment can be provided at three critical points in the life history of a disaster: at the moment of impact, during the recovery phase, and at some point after life has returned to a routine. The goals of treatment at each point are quite different, and the methods used to reach the affected populations and achieve the therapeutic goals vary enormously, according to the type of disaster and the stage of intervention.

Early Treatment

At the time of the catastrophe (assuming for the moment that the disaster is sudden and of short duration), three groups of people need attention to reduce the psychological impact of the disaster. These are the survivors, their families and the personnel involved in the rescue, evacuation, handling of the dead and clean-up. The treatment goals are to provide emotional support, minimize the assault to the psyche and offer cognitive assistance.

Commonsense dictates many of the ways of achieving these goals. Because each disaster presents with a unique set of problems, the immediate response often has to be highly individualized, creative and quickly operational. One approach is to reduce the sense of helplessness in the population involved. Another aims at minimizing the exposure to the full visual, auditory and olfactory assault of the calamity. A sense of some degree of helplessness is inherent in most confronted with a massive disaster and, conversely, the desire to help by those not numbed by the ordeal can become a problem in itself. Following a

Mexico City earthquake, a bulletin from a branch of the Health Department noted that 'the necessity to express our generosity and genuine desire to help can have negative effects: contribute to the disorder, obstruct technical workers, and cause even more pain . . .'.[26] A sense of helplessness can be reduced to the minimal levels possible (which can still be considerable) by the emergence of an identifiable leader(s) who co-ordinates the tasks required for survival, by keeping waiting families occupied and in communication with accurate sources of information, and by organized community efforts in the immediate recovery phase which acknowledge the benefit of having the surviving population active and useful. A sense of helplessness also can be lessened by minimizing the exposure of individuals to the disaster. Rescue operations should be structured (when possible) to prevent rescue workers from unremitting exposure to the death and destruction involved. Families of the dead can be cordoned off from the vision of mutilated bodies and the morgue and, when possible, placed in a protective setting (both physically and emotionally) where they can be cared for appropriately.

Emotional support is essential for all concerned. Those involved in the handling of the injured and dead often welcome an opportunity to ventilate their feelings in a debriefing session after their shift has ended and/or the rescue/evacuation/clean-up phases have concluded. These sessions might include a recognized representative of the community, corporation or country involved who acknowledges the efforts of the task forces and gives the workers positive reinforcement while they continue their onerous tasks and/or after their work has been completed. For families of potential victims, creative interventions have been described which vary enormously, depending on resources available and the type of disaster. For example, following the crash of a commercial aeroplane on 2 August, 1985 at a Texas airport, a nearby hotel housed the victims' families and the uninjured survivors for up to 6 days, during which time mental health workers, clergymen and representatives of the airline provided organized and informal counselling to groups and individuals. This idea was described as a 'libidinal cocoon' concept,[27] not unlike the metaphor of the psychological sanctuary so necessary for healthy development in children. In another situation, two aerial walkways spanning a crowded lobby of a Kansas City hotel suddenly collapsed on a Friday night in July, 1981. Using the media to communicate information, support group activities were immediately set up by the community mental health centre in every part of the metropolitan area and training in crisis intervention was offered for professionals, such as clergymen, who would be natural sources of support for the community.[28]

Many times, the opportunity to provide emotional support has to be postponed until after the rescue and clean-up phase has ended. In crisis intervention, the main goal is to restore the individual's previous level of psychological function, to attain symptom relief and to provide cognitive assistance in sorting out what has happened and what to do in the aftermath (with such matters as relocation, financing, employment) and to prevent prolonged or delayed psychiatric problems. At this stage, treatment can still be considered preventative and supportive to a population undergoing a normal reaction to an overwhelming assault on its psyche. The goal of crisis intervention is not to facilitate changes in previously existing psychological difficulties.

Later Treatment

Treatment should be offered within 3 months after the disaster, preferably in a setting that does not suggest that the individuals being counselled are psychiatrically impaired. Traditional community centres for a variety of activities may be preferable places for counselling, because psychiatric hospitals and physicians' offices support the belief that someone undergoing a grief reaction or experiencing symptoms of anxiety is ill, rather than suffering a normal response to a tragedy. Examples of these centres might be schools, churches and government buildings. Treatment, most practically, is offered in small groups with trained group leaders, who may be psychiatrists and other mental health workers but certainly could also be empathic and qualified teachers, clergy or community leaders. Individual counselling of some participants is typically necessary. The media and community organization can be used to reach the appropriate populations involved.

Treatment is active, short-term, lasting from one session to up to ten, the number being arbitrary. But it should not be prolonged and thereby encourage a sick role or unnecessary dependency, or increase the possibility of delving into pre-existing psychopathology. A supportive and non-judgemental atmosphere of acceptance and empathy is essential. Methods used to help re-establish the participants' psychic equilibrium include allowing individuals the opportunity to identify verbally and express painful feelings in this supportive setting, sustaining and even encouraging healthy responses and appropriate coping behaviour to deal with the painful memories of the disaster (e.g. supporting the use of reasonable amounts of denial and intellectualization, encouraging an active, future-oriented perspective) and providing concrete advice on practical matters that have to be addressed in the months ahead.

How does this type of intervention work? First, the participants are able to relive verbally and emotionally their experiences until such time that they have more or less fully identified the issues, have had the opportunity to voice them in a setting that offers empathy and validation, and have had the time to desensitize themselves to the memories. The group works toward the acceptance and integration of the experience into their lives. Second, the group, along with the group leader, offers encouragement of healthy coping behaviours rather than supporting regressive maladaptive responses. Third, the sharing of the personal experience with others in a structured way offers participants a helping as well as a recipient role, and it reduces the feeling of helplessness as well as making obvious the normality and universality of the symptomatic behaviour.

The Trauma Membrane

Survivors of disasters, despite their distress, sometimes shun outside intervention. The concept of the trauma membrane originated from this observation.[29] The trauma membrane is a protective shield formed around the survivors by spouses, family members and friends to protect the individual from what is viewed as potentially disturbing intrusions into the life of someone who is already experiencing intrusive imagery and symptoms of depression and anxiety. Compassionate effort is required to penetrate this membrane, to help a community or family see the agencies and professionals as helpers instead of intruders. For example, when a mental health worker assists the family in that highly charged moment when the identification of a victim is made, a bond is often established that can be used in helping the family members in the aftermath. Nevertheless, professionals must respect the anxiety contained within the trauma membrane, being very careful not to push for the expression of affect if they are not spontaneously forthcoming from the participants. Survivors, rescue workers, and families are not homogeneous in their values, goals, beliefs and socio-economic resources, and emotional maturity (particularly when the disaster has affected people from various communities) and psychological progress will have to be achieved at different rates for those involved.

Not everyone, of course, benefits from crisis intervention. Many participants in a disaster have the ability to work through the necessary therapeutic steps on their own, or with the help of families and friends. And others, whether or not they have had the benefit of timely outside intervention, will develop either a prolonged and pathological response to being overwhelmed psychologically by the disaster, or will show a delayed reaction at some time in the future (even years later).

Other Help

Finally, various support services are needed to ensure as rapid a return to normality as possible. This could include housing, relocation assistance, financial aid, prolonged medical care, insurance information, legal advice, etc. The bureaucratic entanglements can be confusing at best and, not atypically, another source of significant stress. Assistance in guiding survivors through this quagmire can be invaluable.

PROLONGED PROBLEMS

In a certain number of individuals, the symptomatic behaviour that initially was considered predictable and normal, continues on in an unremitting manner for longer than normal. The external environment returns to some semblance of normality but the individual is impaired from functioning at his previous level by symptoms of depression, anxiety, or what is known as a post-traumatic stress disorder (*Table* 16.2). Earlier in this chapter, the factors that increase the possibility of this complication (and others) were discussed.

In another type of situation, the difficulty may not be seen until years after the disaster. After the usual symptomatic period, the individual appears to have regained his psychological equilibrium. However, months or years later, symptomatic behaviour returns, perhaps precipitated by an event that the individual symbolically associates with the original disaster. Not uncommonly, one notes that in retrospect, some character changes have occurred after the original trauma, rendering the individual more vulnerable, more restricted, less attached and thus less able to compensate when faced with another difficult situation. For example, a woman in her late 30s lost her entire family (husband, children and parents) in a motor vehicle accident. Her way of coping, which reflected previously existing character traits, was to re-establish her life in a manner that isolated her from others, outside her work. In other words, she insulated herself from making new emotional attachments. When incapacitated for a few months

Table 16.2. DSM-III diagnostic criteria for post-traumatic stress disorder

---

1. Existence of a recognizable stress or that which would evoke significant symptoms of distress in almost everyone.
2. Re-experiencing of the trauma as evidenced by at least one of the following:
    a. Recurrent and intrusive recollections of the event
    b. Recurrent dreams of the event
    c. Sudden acting or feeling as if the traumatic event were recurring because of an association with an environmental stimulus or association of ideas
3. Numbing of responsiveness to or reduced involvement with the external world, beginning some time after the trauma, as shown by at least one of the following:
    a. Markedly diminished interest in one or more significant activities
    b. Feeling of detachment or estrangement from others
    c. Constricted affect.
4. At least two of the following symptoms that were not present before the trauma:
    a. Hyper-alertness or exaggerated startle response
    b. Sleep disturbance
    c. Guilt about surviving when others have not, or about behaviour required for survival
    d. Memory impairment or trouble concentrating
    e. Avoidance of activities that arouse recollection of the traumatic event
    f. Intensification of symptoms by exposure to events that symbolize or resemble the traumatic event.

(Adapted with permission from (1980) *Diagnostic and Statistical Manual of Mental Disorders,* 3rd edition. Washington, DC, American Psychiatric Association.)

due to cancer surgery (itself a psychologically traumatic event), intrusive imagery of the accident and renewed grieving over her significant losses were experienced.

In approaching the treatment of these prolonged or delayed reactions, a combination of both insight-oriented and supportive psychotherapy is indicated, by trained professionals. The use of other forms of treatment should be considered, e.g. medication, behaviour modification, hospitalization.

SUMMARY

The psychological ramifications of a disaster are numerous. No group of involved people is spared. Survivors, families, rescue workers, clean-up crews and entire communities may display symptoms of a normal, predictable response to being confronted with an extremely emotional and overwhelming event. These symptoms are intrusive imagery, sleep disturbances, sadness, anger, guilt, a sense of helplessness and anxiety. Depending on the degree of environmental and human destruction experienced, the symbolic meaning of the disaster, the maturity of the survivor, predisposing personality factors and other determinents, these normal symptoms should resolve within a few weeks to a year after the trauma. In about 10–15 per cent of those involved, a prolonged or a delayed reaction will occur, necessitating additional treatment.

Crisis intervention is the treatment of choice within the first few hours to months after the disaster. The goal is to reduce symptomatic behaviour and return the individual to a previous level of function.

REFERENCES

1. Tyhurst J. S. (1951) Individual reactions to community disaster. The natural history of psychiatric phenomena. *Am. J. Psychiatry* **107**, 764–9.
2. Horowitz M. J. (1973) Phase oriented treatment of stress response syndrome. *Am. J. Psychotherapy* **27**, 506–15.
3. Horowitz M. J. (1976) *Stress Response Syndromes*. New York, Jason Aronson.
4. Dynes R. R. (1970) *Organized Behavior in Disaster*. Lexington, MA, Heath Lexington Books.
5. Friedman P. and Linn L. (1957) Some psychiatric notes on the Andrea Doria disaster. *Am. J. Psychiatry* **114**, 426–32.
6. Rangell L. (1976) Discussion of the Buffalo Creek disaster. The course of psychic trauma. *Am. J. Psychiatry* **133**, 313–16.
7. Sims J. H., Baumann D. D. (1983) Educational programs and human response to natural hazards. *Environment and Behaviour* **15**, 165–89.
8. Draber T. and Stephenson J. (1971) When disaster strikes. *J. Appl. Soc. Psychol.* **1**, 187–203.
9. Perry R. W., Lindell M. K., Greene M. R. (1982) Threat perception and public response to volcano hazard. *J. Social Psychology* **116**, 199–204.
10. Baker G. W., Chapman D. W. (eds.) (1962) *Man and Society in Disaster*. New York, Basic Books.
11. Edwards J. G. (1976) Psychiatric aspects of civilian disasters. *Br. Med. J.* **1**, 944–7.
12. Wyden P. (1984) *Day One Before Hiroshima and After*. New York, Simon and Schuster.
13. Henderson S. and Bostock T. (1977) Coping behaviour after shipwreck. *Br. J. Psychiatry* **131**, 15–20.
14. Scully R. E. (ed.) (1986) Case records of the Massachusetts General Hospital *N. Eng. J. Med.* **314**, 1240–7.
15. Engel G. L. (1971) Sudden and rapid death during psychological stress: folklore or folk wisdom? *Ann. Intern. Med.* **74**, 771–82.
16. Cebelin M. S. and Hirsch, C. S. (1980) Human stress cardiomyopathy: myocardial lesions in victims of homicidal assaults without internal injuries. *Hum. Pathol.* **11**, 123–32.
17. Drabek T. E. and Quarantelli E. L. (1967) Scapegoats, villians and disasters. *Trans-Action* **4**, 12–17.
18. Krystal H. (ed.) (1968) *Massive Psychic Trauma*. New York, International Universities Press.
19. Raphael B., Singh B., Bradbury L. et al. (1983–4) Who helps the helper? The effects of a disaster on the rescue workers. *OMEGA* **14**, 9–20.
20. Hershiser M. R. and Quarantelli E. L. (1976) The handling of the dead in a disaster. *OMEGA* **7**, 195–208.
21. Kardiner A. and Spiegal H. (1947) *War, Stress and Neurotic Illness*. New York, Hoeber.
22. Hendin H., Haas A. P., Singer P. et al. (1983) The influence of precombat personality disorder on post-traumatic stress disorder. *Compr. Psychiatry* **24**, 530–4.
23. Horowitz M. J. (1985) Disasters and psychological responses to stress. *Psychiat. Ann.* **15**, 161–7.
24. Lindy J. D., Grace M. C. and Green B. L. (1981) Survivors: outreach to a reluctant population. *Am. J. Orthopsychiat.* **51**, 468–78.
25. Lifton R. J. and Olson E. (1985) The human meaning of total disaster. *Psychiatry* **39**, 1–18.
26. *American Medical News* (11 October, 1985) p. 20.
27. *American Medical News* (18 October, 1985) p. 22.
28. Gist R. and Stolz S. B. (1982) Mental health promotion and the media. *Am. Psychol.* **37**, 1136–9.
29. Lindy J. D. (1985) The trauma membrane and other clinical concepts derived from psychotherapeutic work with survivors of natural disasters. *Psychiat. Ann.* **15**, 153–60.
30. *Diagnostic and Statistical Manual of Mental Disorders*, 3rd edition (1980) Washington D.C., American Psychiatric Association.

17

Environmental Problems in Disasters

INTRODUCTION

Disasters often occur in adverse environmental conditions. For example, blizzard conditions and the icy waters of the Potomac River were the setting for the Air Florida crash in Washington, DC. Environmental illness or injury can affect both victim and rescue worker, complicating traumatic injuries, hampering relief and rescue efforts as workers succumb to heat or cold exposure, and affecting homeless individuals when shelter is limited. Understanding heat and cold, and the recognition, treatment and prevention, of their related illnesses is the foundation for a disaster environmental assessment.

HEAT ILLNESS

Three clinical types of heat illness are recognized—*heat cramps, heat exhaustion* and *heat stroke*. Rather than being clearly distinct illnesses, these conditions represent a continuum of homeostatic imbalance of heat loss and gain.

Heat Cramps

Rescue workers are especially susceptible to heat cramps. The individual complains of brief, intermittent, severe cramps after muscular work in a hot environment. Cramps usually occur in the muscle groups most stressed by the labour, e.g. arms after digging or shovelling rubble. The core body temperature is normal and other signs and symptoms are absent.

Sodium depletion is the primary cause of heat cramps. A person tends to replace sweat salt and water losses with water alone. Treatment consists of resting the person in a cool area and providing fluid and electrolyte replacement. Those with heat cramps usually tolerate oral fluids such as lemonade, tomato juice, commercial drinks for athletes or other balanced salt oral rehydration solutions. A 0·1 per cent saline solution can be prepared by dissolving 2 (600 mg) salt tablets in one litre of water. This solution is made palatable by adding some lemon or other citrus flavour.

Providing an adequate supply of water and electrolyte solution and urging workers or victims to drink helps prevent heat cramps. Because of problems of potassium balance, salt tablets alone are no longer recommended.

Heat Exhaustion

Heat exhaustion is the next step along the continuum of heat illnesses. The individual exhibits a wide range of systemic signs and symptoms. Indications of volume depletion include hypotension, tachycardia, syncope and thirst, and are the hallmark of heat exhaustion. Central nervous system disturbances are also prominent and include headache, vertigo, irritability and faintness. Other signs and symptoms include anorexia, vomiting, weakness, malaise and muscle cramps. Body temperature is normal or slightly elevated.

Heat exhaustion is caused by either water or sodium depletion. Water depletion heat exhaustion occurs when the supply of drinking water is limited or when individual intake is curtailed in trapped victims and patients who are injured or unconscious. These individuals have a slightly elevated temperature and hypernatraemic dehydration and may rapidly progress to heat stroke. Sodium depletion heat exhaustion is similar to heat cramps—sweat salt and water losses being replaced by water alone.

Individuals with signs and symptoms of heat exhaustion should be rested in a cool shaded area and given replacement electrolyte solutions. Alert patients usually tolerate oral solutions as recommended for heat cramps. Others may require intravenous fluids, usually normal saline. A 3 per cent saline solution may be used in the hospital setting to correct hyponatraemia in salt depletion heat exhaustion. Measures to prevent heat exhaustion are the same as for heat cramps—an adequate supply of fluids and careful observation of victims and workers to ensure that they have a sufficient fluid intake and work-rest cycles.

Heat Stroke

Heat stroke is a true medical emergency with a mortality rate of up to 70 per cent in various reported series of patients. Any person who is unconscious after heat exposure should be presumed to have heat stroke until proven otherwise.

Two heat stroke syndromes are recognized. *Classical heat stroke* is usually seen at the extremes of age, and may occur in association with some injury or systemic disease. Sweating is absent and the skin is hot and dry. The rectal temperature is greater than 40·6°C. Central nervous system signs and symptoms are prominent. The patient may be markedly confused, comatose with dilated or poorly-reactive pupils, or exhibit grand mal seizures. Classical heat stroke may occur in injured or trapped disaster victims exposed to heat and sun for long periods of time.

The second type of heat stroke, *exertional heat stroke*, occurs in normal, healthy individuals while performing intense muscle work and is more likely among rescue workers. These individuals have hot, moist skin, a rectal temperature greater than 40·6°C and central nervous system symptoms similar to those in classical heat stroke. In addition, they may develop severe rhabdomyolysis resulting in acute renal tubular necrosis, disseminated intravascular coagulation and severe electrolyte and acid-base disturbances including lactic acidosis. Ventricular ectopy, tachyarrhythmias and conduction defects occur in both types of heat stroke.

Management of heat stroke must begin in the field with rapid cooling using whatever means is available. The patient should be moved to a cool, shaded area and dowsed with cool water which can be evaporated by fans. The airway should be cleared and adequate ventilation (with oxygen if available) ensured. In the first instance 1·0–1·2 litres of i.v. fluids (normal saline or lactated Ringers solution) should be given in the first 4 hours. Heat stroke victims require rapid transfer to a medical treatment facility.

Hospital care includes continued rapid cooling to a temperature of 38·9°C and then more gradual cooling to normal values, ventilatory support, fluid replacement, and careful monitoring of cardiac function and electrolyte and acid-base balance. Osmotic agents, such as 20 per cent mannitol or furosemide (frusemide) are given if acute tubular necrosis develops.

In a disaster situation, prevention of heat stroke depends on carefully observing very young or old victims and comatose casualties and having a shaded, cool victim-holding area with water available. Exertional heat stroke is far less predictable than the classical type.

Summary

To prevent or minimize heat illness in a disaster situation, it is essential to be aware of the environment and its potential for heat stress. Rescue personnel must avoid becoming victims themselves. They must drink fluids regularly, observe work-rest cycles, and avoid direct sun exposure by using head gear and sunscreen. Shelter for victims should be provided with ventilation, shade, oral and intravenous fluids and other appropriate measures. Patients with heat cramps or mild heat exhaustion can frequently be treated on site but those with heat stroke will require rapid evacuation to a medical treatment facility.

COLD INJURIES

Cold injuries fall into two categories—*local cold injury* and *generalized hypothermia*. The core temperature remains normal with local cold injuries but the peripheral areas (ear-lobes, cheeks, hands and feet) are affected. Hypothermia occurs when the core temperature decreases to less than 35°C. Several factors contribute to cold injury including the degree of cold, the duration of exposure, the wind velocity, whether the patient was subjected to water submersion, dependency and immobilization of the extremities, and skin contact with metal or fluids.

Local Cold Injuries

There are two types of local cold injuries. *Non-freezing injuries* are a result of vasoconstriction and thrombosis. *Freezing injuries* result from extracellular ice crystal formation and, in addition, vasoconstriction and thrombosis.

Non-Freezing Injuries

Chilblains, trenchfoot and immersion foot are the three types of non-freezing injuries. Chilblains are the mildest form of local cold injury resulting in painful, red, pruritic, swollen skin in exposed areas. The erythematous areas blanch with pressure. Occasionally vesicles, bullae or ulcers form. Chilblains are easily treated by warming and gently massaging the affected areas. Placing the affected areas in the axilla, groin or against the abdomen is a simple warming method. After treatment, the skin areas must be protected from further cold exposure.

Trench and immersion foot can be discussed as a single entity for the purpose of disaster medicine. These injuries occur in individuals who have been immobilized with dependent extremities for long periods in a cold, wet environment as may occur in some rescue situations. The person complains of cold, numb feet and leg cramps. The affected extremities are swollen and erythematous. Vesicles or gangrenous changes can occur. Pedal arterial pulses are absent. Initially, the patient should be placed at rest in a warm, dry area and any wet or constricting garments removed. The affected extremity should be elevated moderately. No amputation or surgical debridement should be performed because demarcation of non-viable areas may take up to one month or more.

Freezing Injuries

There are three types of freezing injuries, again representing a spectrum rather than separate and distinct processes. Frostnip is the mildest form of frostbite, often affecting fingertips, toes, nose, zygomatic arch area and ear-lobes. The patient reports a sensation of severe cold in the affected area, then numbness followed by pain. The skin is tender and red without vesicles or oedema. Frostnip is quickly and adequately treated by warming the affected parts against the warm body areas and then protecting them from further cold exposure. Superficial frostbite extends from the surface into the subcutaneous layers of skin. The skin is blanched, hard and waxlike. The patient describes a progression from coldness to numbness to a pleasant, warm sensation in the affected part. Oedema, vesicle or bulla formation occurs 24–36 hours after injury. Deep frostbite extends below the subcutaneous skin layer and exhibits the same signs and symptoms as superficial frostbite. A distinguishing feature is the formation of small, haemorrhagic blisters.

The treatment for both superficial and deep frostbite begins with removing any constricting and wet garments and wrapping the affected part in a dry blanket or clothing. Rewarming is the definitive treatment. This should be done only once and should not be initiated outside a medical facility if there is any risk of refreezing. A person can walk long distances on frozen feet without increasing injury but once the feet are thawed, he must be carried by stretcher. Tissue damage is significantly increased by repeated thaw-freeze cycles. Rewarming should be done carefully using a water bath at a controlled temperature of 40·6–43·3°C in a container large enough to permit immersion of the affected part without touching the sides or bottom. Immersion should be continued until the colour returns or the area has been immersed for about 40 minutes. If a carefully monitored water bath is not available, use the warm body areas (e.g. axilla, groin). Once the affected area has been thawed, the tissues must be handled in a delicate manner similar to a burn. The digits should be separated and padded, a loose dressing applied and the extremity elevated. Blisters are left intact unless they appear infected. No ointments should be applied to the areas. Surgical debridement or amputation should be delayed for one month or more, allowing for the complete demarcation of non-viable tissue. The affected area should not be rubbed with snow, exposed to vehicle exhaust, open flame or dry heat. The person may drink warm liquids but must avoid cigarettes and alcohol.

Hypothermia

Hypothermia is a true medical emergency with a mortality rate of 21–87 per cent depending on the severity. Mild hypothermia with a core temperature of 32·2–35°C has a lower morbidity and mortality than severe hypothermia with a core temperature less than 32·2°C. In a disaster, trauma victims with immobilizing injuries or unconsciousness are at high risk of developing hypothermia in adverse climatic conditions.

The clinical signs and symptoms of hypothermia include: cold, cyanotic skin and mucous membranes; markedly decreased heart and respiratory rates, and alterations in mental status ranging from apathy and poor concentration to coma. It is important to note that apnoea occurs at 24°C and asystole at 15°C. The myocardium is very irritable at or below 30°C and arrhythmias develop that are refractory to the usual management until the patient is rewarmed. The hypothermic patient may appear dead but should not be pronounced so unless resuscitation is unsuccessful after rewarming to above 30°C.

The on-site treatment of hypothermia begins with moving the person to shelter out of the wind as much as possible, removing wet clothing and replacing it with dry blankets or other warm garments. The victim can be warmed by placing him skin-to-skin with a rescuer in blankets or a sleeping bag. The patient may need cardiopulmonary resuscitation, oxygen, and i.v. fluids, which should be warmed if possible. Hospital management consists of careful monitoring, vigorous supportive measures and various techniques of passive and active core rewarming.

Just as with heat injuries, recognizing the potential for cold injuries in the disaster environment is essential to prevention. Rescue workers must have adequate cold weather equipment, dress in layers of non-constricting garments which should cover head, ears and hands and use a protective balm on the nose, lips and zygomatic arch area. When operating in a cold disaster environment it is necessary to have available a sheltered warm environment, blankets and other support supplies.

Further details of the problems and treatment of cold injuries and hypothermia appear in Chapter 25.

SUMMARY

Environmental injuries and illness can affect both the rescue worker and the disaster victim. It is thus very important to assess not only the number of casualties and their injuries, but also the environment where the event has occurred and to be concerned with possible heat or cold injury or illness.

DISCLAIMER: The opinions and assertions in this paper are not to be construed as official or reflecting the views of the United States Air Force, the Uniformed Services University or the United States Department of Defense.

FURTHER READING

Abramowicz M. (ed.) (1976) Treatment of frostbite. *Med. Lett. Drugs Ther.* **18** (25), 105–6.
Boswick J. A. (1976) Cold injuries. *Major Probl. Clin. Surg.* **19**, 96–106.

Clowes G. and O'Donnell T. (1974) Heat stroke. *N. Engl. J. Med.* **291** (11), 564–6.

DaVee T. and Reieberg E. (1980) Extreme hypothermia and ventricular fibrillation. *Ann. Emerg. Med.* **9** (2), 100–2.

Knochel J. (1974) Environmental heat illness: An electric review. *Arch. Intern. Med.* **133**, 841–64.

Maclean D. and Emslie-Smith D. (1977) *Accidental Hypothermia.* London, Blackwell Scientific Publications.

Miller J. et al. (1980) Urban accidental hypothermia: 135 cases. *Ann. Emerg. Med.* **9** (9), 456–60.

O'Donnell T. (1975) Acute heat stroke: Epidemiologic, biochemical, renal and coagulation studies. *JAMA* **234** (8), 824–8.

O'Donnell T. and Clowes G. (1972) The circulatory abnormalities of heat stroke. *N. Eng. J. Med.* **287** (15), 734–7.

Schrier R. et al. (1970) Renal, metabolic, and circulatory responses to heat and exercise. *Ann. Intern. Med.* **73**, 213–23.

Skitkata J. et al. (1964) Studies in experimental frostbite. *Arch. Surg.* **89**, 575–84.

Stine R. J. (1977) Accidental hypothermia. *J. Am. Coll. Emerg. Physicians* **6** (9), 413–16.

Stine R. J. (1977) Heat illness. *J. Am. Coll. Emerg. Physicians* **8**, 154–60.

Ward M. (1974) Frostbite. *Br. Med. J.* **1**, 67–70.

Welton D. E. et al. (1978) Treatment of profound hypothermia. *JAMA* **240**, 2291–2.

C. de Ville de Goyet and J. L. Zeballos

18

Communicable Diseases and Epidemiological Surveillance After Sudden Natural Disasters

During the last decade, disasters from all causes have stirred growing interest among the authorities and the public in the stricken countries and in scientific quarters. This rebirth of interest is unquestionably due as much to the brutality and spectacular nature of major disasters, which have triggered international concern, as to the increasing risk of disasters in most developing countries.[*] These hazards are associated with expanding population settlements in areas under threat from natural disasters such as floods, earthquakes and hurricanes. The rapid urbanization of many countries inevitably increases the number of victims and the potential amount of damage in future disasters.

The problems raised by these and other disasters are many and varied. Health problems are only one, and often not the most important, aspect of a complex situation. In disasters, confusion, if not actual chaos, and a lack of objective health information and unsubstantiated rumours, make up the general background from which vital and far-reaching decisions have to be determined.

Hearsay reports of imminent outbreaks of communicable diseases rapidly reach the epidemiological services of the government and, unfortunately, the mass media which is too often ready to amplify indiscriminately the concerns of the population traumatized by the natural disaster.

In this chapter the risk of increased incidence of diseases following disasters will be analyzed, the principle of epidemiological surveillance under emergency conditions will be outlined and appropriate control measures proposed. The analysis will be limited to natural disasters such as earthquakes, hurricanes, tornados, floods and volcanic eruptions.

The problems for countries afflicted by chronic famine or protracted conflicts, when acute clinical malnutrition and total disruption of the public services occurring as a consequence of a sudden disaster add a new dimension to the already dismal situation, will also be considered briefly.

---

[*] In 1985 alone, catastrophic earthquakes devastated Chile on 3 March, when 150 people were killed and 2000 injured, and Mexico City, where an estimated 10 000 persons died or were reported missing following the seisms of 18 and 19 September. Over 420 buildings totally collapsed and 5000 hospital beds were instantly destroyed. (Source: Epidemiologia, Boletin Mensual, Mexico, Vol. 1, 1 enero 1986, p. 5.)

In Colombia, the dormant volcano Nevado del Ruiz brutally erupted following several weeks of precursory seismic activity and mild emissions of ashes and gas. The moderate-sized eruption of 14 November 1985 caused the thawing of an estimated 5·7 per cent of the glacial ice cap. Forty-five minutes later, the mudflow obliterated the city of Armero, resulting in a death toll of 23 000.

RISK FACTORS FOR INCREASED INCIDENCE OF COMMUNICABLE DISEASES FOLLOWING DISASTERS

An epidemic is generally defined as the occurrence of cases in greater number than normally expected. In the special and emotional context of emergency situations when dead bodies are counted by thousands, we will reserve the use of the term 'epidemic' or 'outbreak' for a sudden and geographically-defined occurrence of a large number of cases—a definition more akin to that accepted by the general public, the press and the politicians. The term 'increased incidence' will be used otherwise.

Undeniably, disasters, in the absence of preventive and corrective measures, can favour the transmission of certain diseases. The major plagues of earlier centuries were often associated with natural disasters. There are three ways in which an increased incidence can be triggered by a disaster: by the increased transmission of local pathogens, by a change in the receptivity of the population and by the introduction of a new specific pathogen into the environment.

Enhancement of Transmission

Disasters may increase the transmission of communicable diseases by a wide variety of devices: (*a*) an increase of promiscuity, (*b*) a deterioration of environmental health and (*c*) a partial or total disruption of control programmes. To judge the extent to which these factors are affected by a disaster, it is necessary to know the situation prior to it. In developing countries, the scarcity of baseline data on environmental health services and the lack of effective immunization coverage associated with widespread disease may lead inexperienced relief medical personnel or researchers to blame a natural disaster for chronic problems in the health situation erroneously.

Promiscuity most often increases when temporary settlements quickly become overcrowded, resulting in 'outbreaks' of scabies and lice and flea infestations. The sanitation and administration problems that inevitably arise, and the tendency of such camps to become permanent, are some of the many reasons for the authorities to avoid encouraging their establishment (*Fig.* 18.1).

Deterioration of sanitary conditions in the environment is the most important factor and the one most responsive to energetic action. The potential impact of the disaster on health is determined by the level of sanitation prior to the disaster. If there is no sanitary infrastructure, no water supply network, no sewage system, and personal hygiene is poor, a natural disaster can hardly aggravate the existing situation. At the other extreme, an urban area where sanitation services are strained to the limit of their capacity by population growth is particularly vulnerable.

Water Supply

The most critical and best known environmental factor is the provision of water. A few commonsense observations are worth stating:

1. People will need and seek to obtain the basic amount of water regardless of its quality, cost, time or the legal considerations to acquire it.
2. A supply of bacteriologically safe water is a priority for relief personnel,

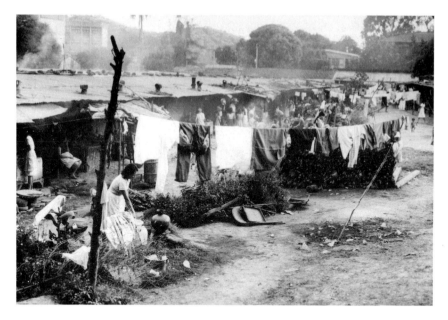

Fig. 18.1. Overcrowding and the lack of basic sanitation in temporary settlements is a major factor in the incidence of communicable diseases following disasters.

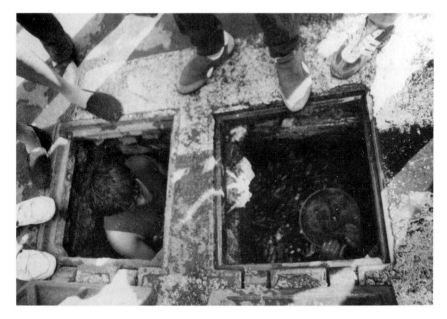

Fig. 18.2. Unsafe break-in into the main water pipe following the earthquake in Mexico, 1985.

health authorities and a small educated segment of the population in developing countries.

3. Short-term (days/weeks) emergency measures to provide drinking water to large populations are a logistical nightmare and extremely expensive. Each natural disaster may affect the amount of drinking water available in a distinctive manner.

4. Direct physical damage to water plants and distribution networks is common following earthquakes. Leak detection and emergency repair became a top health priority immediately after the initial treatment of mass casualties following the well-studied urban earthquakes in Nicaragua (1972), Guatemala (1976), Chile and Mexico City (1985) (*Fig.* 18.2). Similar shortages of drinking water were reported following floods (Jamaica, June 1986) and mud flows (volcanic explosion of Nevado del Ruiz, Colombia, 1985).

5. Indirect effects such as lack of electricity or failure of key staff to report for duty are both common following any large scale catastrophe, and have caused water shortages, usually of short duration.

6. A large population increase in the areas served by an existing (and intact) water supply system is the direct consequence of migration towards urban centres. The formal establishment of temporary settlements/refugee camps will not be considered in this chapter.

In relief operations or emergency situations, the quality of the water is not the issue. What matters is the potential *change* in water quality experienced by the population as a consequence of the natural disaster or subsequent population movements.

Earthquakes affecting areas with water and sewage systems increases the possibility of cross-contamination. However, daily bacteriological monitoring of water samples following the earthquakes in Latin America did not reveal any massive water contamination.

It is accepted that the flooding of wells or other water supply sources may lead to an increased incidence of water-borne disease. However, hard data and research results are scarce on the magnitude of the problem. The possibility of a beneficial dilution of pathogens following heavy flooding or tidal waves (e.g. Bangladesh 1970 and 1984) in densely populated rural areas cannot be discarded.

Outbreaks of leptospirosis caused by direct contact with water contaminated by infected animal urine has been reported following floods in Portugal (1967), Amazonia, Brazil (1973) and Jamaica (1979).

Food Hygiene

In the past, increased incidence of disease has been attributed more to poor hygiene of relief foods than to contaminated water supplies. Small outbreaks of mass food poisoning are commonly reported among victims and relief personnel in the aftermath of earthquakes or other natural disasters.

Vector and Rodent-Related Diseases

The importance of vector-related diseases following natural disasters is well summarized by the Pan American Health Organization.[1] Mosquito-borne diseases, especially malaria, dengue and arboviral encephalitis, eventually cause significant concern after disasters associated with heavy rain and flooding. The immediate effect is, however, the destruction of larval habitats and a reduction of the vector population with the secondary creation of new larval habitats. It is difficult to determine the probability that greater adult densities will be produced in these habitats and whether an increase in disease transmission will occur subsequently.

Vector-related diseases such as endemic typhus and certain rickettsial diseases, will be of concern when they are already endemic in or near a disaster area. In addition, fly, cockroach, bedbug, human louse and rodent infestations may pose problems. Immediately after a natural disaster, the fly and rodent densities may appear to be greater, either because they become more visible or have indeed really increased. This is partly due to disruption of sanitary services, such as garbage collection and disposal, and also because human overcrowding is accompanied by an increase in the numbers of rodents and other vermin seeking the same sources of food and accommodation.[1]

One of the best documented examples of a vector-born outbreak occurred in Haiti in 1963 when hurricane Flora struck shortly after households had been sprayed with DDT in the malaria eradication campaign. The availability of breeding sites, the destruction of homes protected by the insecticide and migration of the population helped to cause an explosive epidemic of malaria from Plasmodium falciparum (more than 75 000 cases were reported). A resurgence of malaria with high mortality has often been seen following the rains ending a prolonged period of drought.

Other examples include the dramatically increased incidence of malaria following major floods in Ecuador and Peru.

The extensive rains and consequential flooding which characterized the El Niño phenomenon during 1982–3 along South America's Pacific coastline created an ecological environment which favoured the spread of malarial diseases into susceptible geographical areas.

In Peru the northern provinces of Piura and Tumbes suffered the heaviest rains. In 1983 alone, 11 075 new cases of malaria were recorded there. The number of cases reached a peak in September and October registering a figure 7 times greater than the average between 1976 and 1982.[2]

The simultaneous flooding which occurred in Ecuador encouraged a similar situation. Not only were new breeding places for mosquitos created but many carriers and potentially susceptible people moved out of rural areas into areas where malaria was already endemic, creating suitable conditions for additional outbreaks, such as those which occurred in Guayaquil. The incidence of malaria in Ecuador's coastal area jumped from 4000 registered cases in 1982 to 28 000 cases in 1984.[3]

Corpses

Other factors may exist but often they are given exaggerated importance: the public and the administrative authorities seem under a misapprehension concerning the part played by corpses in the transmission of diseases. Examples abound in which the press and television have evoked the spectre of cholera, typhoid fever or plague epidemics, to which the population is supposedly

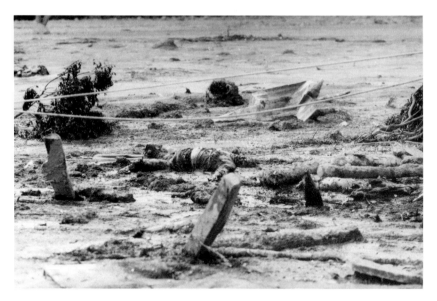

Fig. 18.3. Dead bodies are not a major public health problem following natural disasters (volcano eruption, Colombia, November 1985).

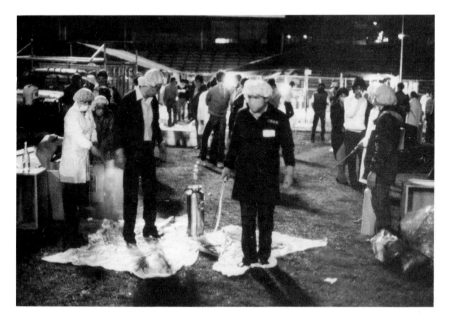

Fig. 18.4. Unsubstantiated fear of epidemics leads to the disinfection of relief personnel handling dead bodies following the 1985 earthquake in Mexico.

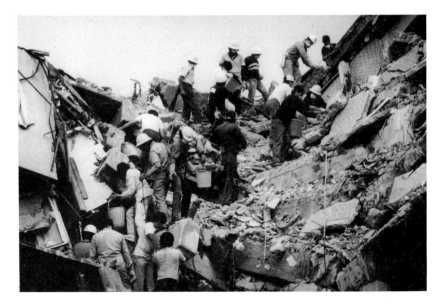

Fig. 18.5. Over 500 patients and health personnel were buried under the ruins of the Hospital Juarez in the Mexican earthquake of September 1985.

exposed by the presence of human corpses. These alarmist claims overlook the fundamental epidemiological fact that these diseases are transmitted by *Vibrio cholerae, Salmonella typhi* (or *paratyphi*) and *Yersinia pestis* respectively, and not by the bacteria of putrefaction. Therefore, there seems to be no public health reason for cremating corpses or mass burial without respect for traditions and legitimate demands from the families (*Figs.* 18.3 and 18.4).

During the Mexican earthquake in 1985, the health authorities used polyethylene bags and ice to slow down the process of organic decomposition in order to allow relatives to identify the victims. After 72 hours the unclaimed corpses were transferred to wooden coffins for final disposal in common graves (*Fig.* 18.5).

During this experience a seminar for the press on 'health aspects in disaster situations' and the dissemination of properly documented information calmed public fears and contained a wave of rumours about the possibilities of epidemic outbreaks such as the plague, typhoid fever, typhus and other diseases.[4]

Disease Control Programmes

The interruption of regular disease control programmes is probably one of the most often overlooked factors. The epidemic of malaria from *P. falciparum* triggered by hurricane Flora in Haiti may be indirectly blamed both on the suspension of normal spraying and on ecological change itself. Temporary interruption of the ambulatory tuberculosis treatment in Bangladesh has also been cited as the cause of many complications reported in the wake of the cyclone of 1970. Though few reliable statistics are available for assessing the importance of this factor, it is essential to resume normal primary health care and disease control activities as quickly as possible rather than to divert scarce material and human resources to highly visible improvized emergency programmes of dubious health benefit.

Receptivity of the Population

The importance of the host–pathogen relationship cannot be overestimated. No further proof is needed of the synergism between malnutrition and infections. In famines caused by serious and prolonged food shortage, infectious diseases are the major cause of death. Measles, gastroenteritis and respiratory ailments have a higher than normal fatality rate. In times of famine the mortality from diseases rises considerably (up to 50 per cent for measles), but evidence of increased incidence and transmission of disease during the same period remains controversal.

The role of weather and climate is still more difficult to gauge. It is generally accepted by the public that exposure to severe cold following an earthquake, for example, inevitably raises the incidence of respiratory infections. This association between exposure and the incidence of respiratory infections is not reflected in the morbidity statistics in tropical or warm climates.

Paradoxically, some disasters have left behind a surviving population that is temporarily more resistant, as a group, to communicable diseases. The hurricane that ravaged the coasts of Bangladesh in November 1970 took about 250 000 lives. Two consecutive surveys made on representative samples reported high mortality, attributable to the hurricane, in the groups that were also the most vulnerable to diseases; children under 5 years (29·2 per cent), persons over 70 (20·7 per cent), and those who were too weak or ill to escape from the force of the hurricane and its accompanying tidal wave. This natural selection of the inhabitants most resistant to the elements and to diseases resulted in a lower morbidity during the months following the disaster.

Introduction of a New Pathogen

When the causal agent of a disease is not present in the environment, it is not possible for that disease to be transmitted. *Vibrio cholerae*, for example, is, for all practical purposes, not prevalent in Latin America. Hence, no natural disaster (either flood, earthquake or hurricane) is likely to affect its incidence. Similarly, since the prevalence of *Salmonella typhi* is very low in most industrialized urban areas, the risk of an epidemic outbreak of typhoid fever during temporary stoppages of sanitary services is somewhat fanciful.

In special situations with widespread massive migration over long distances, pathogens or new strains might be brought into areas of low prevalence and immunity or, conversely, immunized populations might traverse an area of high prevalence (e.g. malaria). The significance of this mechanism is usually negligible compared to the magnitude of population flow and local travel during normal times.

In the first 6 months following the March 1983 earthquake in Popayan, Colombia, 49 cases of imported malaria (an increase of 245 per cent over the preceding year) were reported. The majority were residents from high endemic areas on the Pacific Coast seeking employment in the reconstruction of the city.

Independent of nationality and culture, populations and communities affected by sudden impact disasters tend to remain as close as possible to their land and major properties. Displacement is limited and generally accepted only for the most compelling reasons (rising water level, etc.). One tragic example was the failure of the population living on the slopes of volcano Nevado del Ruiz to follow official evacuation instructions prompted by alarming signs of a likely second catastrophic eruption in mid 1986.

Heightened surveillance at borders and a stricter enforcement of national and international regulations already in force will suffice to contain the problem without recourse to further restrictions (new requirements of immunization certificates, vaccination on arrival, quarantine, etc.).

OCCURRENCES OF INCREASED INCIDENCE OF COMMUNICABLE DISEASES (*see Table* 18.1)

In a few well-documented instances, satisfactory evidence points to a direct causal relationship. Nevertheless, in most cases, the comparison of reported cases before and after the disaster cannot be regarded as a valid estimation since post-disaster reporting and case finding generally improves with the influx of attention by health officials or the temporary increase of health services by volunteers and outside medical teams.

In Latin America, a region highly vulnerable to disaster, considerable epidemiological efforts have been made to detect and document an increased incidence of diseases after disasters with remarkably little success so far.

A recent study of the relationship between the incidence of disease and the impact of a sudden natural disaster concluded that, following natural disasters, such outbreaks have been the exception rather than the rule.[5]

Reports of lower levels of disease after the impact probably reflect the acutely increased awareness of the authorities and public for basic hygiene and water safety rather than the 'success' of improvized high profile medical measures.

In brief, review of past disasters indicates that severe oubreaks, a common occurrence following famine and mass starvation, are far from inevitable and even rare following natural disasters such as earthquakes, cyclones, hurricanes and floods. When a moderate increase of incidence is reported, it concerns local endemics with which the health authorities are already familiar, rather than exotic diseases unknown to the affected area.

Epidemiological Surveillance

For a traumatized population in need of protective measures, the most sensible decision is to set up close epidemiological surveillance that will enable the authorities to make the most of the resources available to keep the public informed and their fears allayed.

In countries where surveillance systems are already in operation, the following actions must be taken:

1. Identification, preferably prior to the disaster, of the diseases already

Table 18.1. Summary of a number of recorded occurrences of communicable diseases associated with national disasters (excluding prolonged drought)

Disease	Location	Disaster/date	Observations
Malaria	Haiti	Hurricane 1963	75 000 cases[1]
	Peru	Floods 1983	28 560 cases[2]
	Ecuador	Floods 1982–3	28 000 cases[3]
	Colombia	Popayan earthquake 1983	35 imported cases[4]
Leptospirosis	Brazil	Floods 1966, 1970, 1975	100+ cases[5]
	Jamaica	Floods 1978–9	40 cases[5]
	Portugal	Floods 1967	Under 10 cases[5]
Gastroenteritis	Dominican Republic	Hurricanes 1979	28 000 cases[6]
	Jamaica	Floods 1979	70 cases from fish poisoning[7]
Typhoid fever	Puerto Rico	Hurricane 1956	23 cases[5]
	Chile	Earthquake 1985	Significant decline in case numbers[8]
Diarrhoea	Colombia	Popayan earthquake 1983	15 000 cases[4]
Tetanus	Colombia	Floods from volcano eruption 1985	4 cases[9]
Gangrene	Colombia	Floods from volcano eruption 1985	30 cases, all died[9]
Hepatitis	Colombia	Popayan earthquake 1983	241 cases, 121% increase over previous year[4]

SOURCES
1. Mason J. and Cavalie P. (1965) Malaria epidemic in Haiti following a hurricane. *Am. J. Trop. Med. Hyg.* **14**(4), 1–10.
2. Poves P. R. (1985) *Epidemia de Malaria Post Fenómeno del Nino, 1983.* Lima, Peru, Ministerio de Salud, pp. 1–25.
3. Cedeno J. M. (1985) *Lluvias e Inundaciones en la Cuenca del Guayas y sus Efectos sobre la Incidencia Palúdica, 1982–1985.* Quito, Ecuador, pp. 1–15.
4. Gomez N. G. and de Sarmiento N. (1985) Comportamiento de algunas enfermedades transmisibles con posterioridad al desastre, Terremoto en Popayan, Colombia, 1983. *Crónicas de Desastres* No. 1. Organización Panamerican de la Salud, pp. 1–10.
5. Leus X. (1985) *Natural Disaster and Communicable Diseases.* Paper presented at the Symposim on Natural Disaster, Epidemiology and Environmental Health, 14–17 October, 1985, Havana, Cuba, pp. 1–12.
6. Bissell J. (1983) Delayed-impact infectious disease after a natural disaster. *J. Emerg. Med.* **1**, 59–65.
7. *Fish Poisoning, St Elizabeth, Jamaica.* (1979) CAREC Surveillance Report **5**(9), 1–6.
8. Ortiz M. R. (1985) *Las Infecciones Eutericas en el Terremoto de Marzo de 1985.* Santiago, Chile, Ministerio de Salud, pp. 1–10.
9. Oxtoby M. (1986) *Foreign Trip Report to Colombia following the Nevado del Ruiz Volcano Eruption.* US Department of Health & Human Services, pp. 1–8.

Table 18.2. Representative form for daily report of disease surveillance/post-disaster surveillance

Daily Report by_____   For_____
                 Name of Reporter

                                                Date _____

From   Evacuation Centre   Location Address   Phone No.

       Hospital OPD

       Health Centre

       Clinic

       Other

       Specify_____

Number of new cases with	Total
1. Fever (100°F+ 38°C+)	
2. Fever and cough	
3. Fever and diarrhoea	
4. Vomiting and/or diarrhoea	
5. Fever and rash	
6. Other new medical problems Specify_____	

Comments

Complete for evaluation centre only
No. of persons accommodated today

Report significant changes in Sanitation/Food Supply Situation

Note: Complete back portion of the form for first report only.

(Reproduced from: *Epidemiologic Surveillance after Natural Disaster.* (1982) Scientific Publication No. 420, Pan American Health Organization, pp. 31.)

under surveillance which will require enhanced monitoring: diseases whose transmission could be increased by the disaster, diseases whose epidemic potential is recognized in the country and diseases about which the public or the political authorities are especially concerned.

2. The selection of particularly sensitive indicators even before disaster strikes. It is preferable to trade off some specificity in exchange for sensitivity. Symptom or syndrome-based reporting is recommended. *Table* 18.2 presents a sample form used for gathering symptomatic data for daily reports during disease surveillance.

3. The routine frequency (weekly or monthly) and means (by mail or administrative report) of disease reports may not be suited to the needs of the emergency. Reports must be sent to the central level by the most rapid means (telecommunications networks of the armed forces, police and Red Cross) and with increased frequency (on a daily basis). Negative reports, that is, the absence of cases should be included but lack of information should not be assumed as lack of disease.

4. The investigation of rumours of epidemic outbreaks. When a natural disaster strikes, rumours frequently circulate about epidemic episodes that have purportedly followed in its wake. So long as they are not officially investigated by the health services, such rumours can only grow and nullify the benefits of surveillance, based exclusively on reports received at the central level. While it may not be possible to track down the source of each rumour, a maximum of resources (personnel and vehicles) must still be assigned to the task. There can be no doubt, however, that any unusual event detected by the surveillance system must be immediately investigated in order to determine its nature and magnitude and to take any specific measures of control that may be necessary.

5. The rapid circulation and use of results. In the situation created by major disasters, it is particularly desirable to circulate epidemiological information promptly and widely. The bureaucratic obstacles and resistance that are often encountered in disseminating sensitive information must be overcome. A summary of the main results and their interpretation in terms of operational decisions may be usefully circulated to, for example, the national emergency committee and to any other official bodies in charge of relief co-ordination (such as civil defence), the local representative of the United Nations Disaster Relief Office (UNDRO), the Red Cross, and the major voluntary agencies in the health field. A daily summary report should also be given to the press. If necessary, or if there is some particular problem, a periodic press conference will prevent the media from paying too much heed to alarmist rumours.

6. A gradual return to the regular surveillance system. Most emergencies are fairly short-lived, and special operations should give way to the normal programmes as soon as possible. The epidemiological characteristics of diseases placed under intensified surveillance in a disaster must determine the moment when such heightened attention is no longer needed. The incubation period and the time needed for an epidemic to break out are essential factors. For example, massive water pollution might give rise to gastroenteritis epidemics in the very first week. Since the risk can persist as long as pollution is a possibility, the surveillance must also be continued.

Conversely, an epidemic of type B viral hepatitis—a real possibility after mass immunization campaigns which in major disasters are all too often conducted in conditions of uncertain asepsis—is only likely to break out between 45 and 160 days after the campaign.

In some regions the surveillance system cannot provide the required infrastructure for intensified monitoring. It may then be necessary to organize a provisional surveillance system which, as happened in Guatemala in 1976 and in Italy in 1980, can provide the stimulus for a permanent programme.

Circumstances are unlikely to allow the recommended stages to be followed in strict sequence. Surveillance in times of disaster cannot be improvized without some compromise on the quality of the data and hence on the validity of conclusions and decisions based on them. Problems may occur with broken lines of communication and insufficient means of transportation can thwart effective surveillance. The principal difficulty, as illustrated by the surveillance set up following the earthquake in Italy in 1980, lies in translating the findings into decisions at the highest level. Too often, surveillance conclusions have been overshadowed by emotional or political considerations leading to counterproductive health measures.

Epidemiologists and public health experts should refrain from taking shelter behind rows of statistics and tests of significance and instead should actively seek the support of the relief co-ordinator, politicians and the public opinion to implement the most appropriate and cost-effective action based on technical evidence.

PREVENTION AND CONTROL MEASURES

The techniques and methods of national prevention and control of communicable disease programmes in normal times often remain the most effective and inexpensive under emergency conditions. A disaster is not necessarily a commanding reason for changing to more sophisticated methods whose effectiveness has not been demonstrated in the country.

Public health measures to prevent or control communicable diseases fall into two categories: environmental health and medical measures.

Environmental Health Measures

Emergency environmental health measures aim to restore the situation (and risk level) prior to the disaster. Emergency measures (expensive and temporary by essence) must give way as soon as possible to rehabilitation and reconstruction efforts directed towards permanent improvement. During the emergency phase, particular focus should be placed on public water supply, food hygiene, human waste disposal and vector control.

Water supply: Access to minimum quantity (at least 10 litres per person per day with up to 40 litres in urban areas) of reasonably safe water is the first concern in most instances.

Bacteriological quality control follows. In urban areas, heavy chlorination is recommended to counteract possible cross-contamination. However, risk of contamination has been demonstrated to be much more serious at temporary

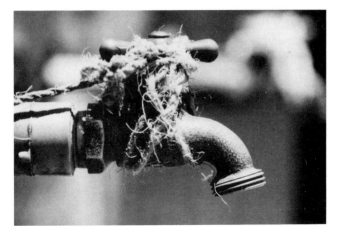

Fig. 18.6. The amount of available water is often more critical than its bacteriological quality in the immediate aftermath of a disaster.

storage sites (tanks, cisterns, home containers). Public education to boil water is more effective than mass distribution of water purification tablets, an item routinely requested from the international community. It is recommended to limit the use of water purification tablets to small groups of educated populations or relief workers able to read and understand the instructions for their use. The diversity of presentations (amount of water treated, duration, etc.), the lack of standardized containers for domestic use, and the risk of inaccurate quantities of disinfectant (too low or too high) make mass use counterproductive.

Hauling of drinking water (in bags, containers or tanks) is technically effective but difficult. It is only justified where availability of safe water has been interrupted by the disaster. Digging of wells or the extension of the existing water distribution network is preferable for temporary settlements likely to last over one month.

Food Hygiene

Community kitchens, donations of food and power failures make increased surveillance and control of food quality necessary. Although botulism has not been reported following disasters, measures should be taken to screen incoming food donations and to destroy suspicious or spoiled items.

Human Waste Disposal

Personal faecal habits are highly resistant to rapid change. Relief programmes focusing on the construction of latrines without investing considerable time educating those who are supposed to use them, enhance the after-action reports of the sponsoring agency rather than improve the actual public health situation. The sophistication (from trench latrines to chemical toilets) and privacy (communal or private facilities) will be determined by the prevailing cultural and social pattern.

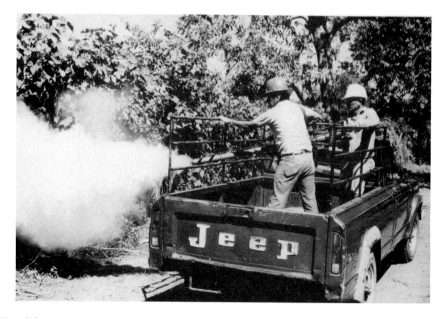

Fig. 18.7. Insecticide spraying following volcano eruption in Colombia, 1985.

Vector Control

Time-tested methods used in the country remain the best approach. Biological cycles, habits and vector characteristics of the local species are unaffected by natural hazards. The environment may become more favourable to the vector or the human being more vulnerable or accessible to infective contacts.

In any case, vector control should not be an immediate priority from a technical point of view, although it may become so from a political standpoint.

The decision to implement vector control measures is determined first by their impact on disease transmission and not by the nuisance of the vector itself. Filth, flies and rodents are best controlled by sanitation measures (waste disposal and proper food storage). Massive aerial spraying against flies has little health benefit and large scale use of rodenticide is unlikely to bring satisfactory results.

Mosquito control in malaria or dengue endemic areas should be a continuous integrated approach covering areas often larger than those affected by the natural disaster and continued after the immediate post-disaster period. Insecticides are hazardous in themselves, expensive and quickly become obsolete by vector resistance (*Fig.* 18.7). Labour-intensive control of breeding sites should be promoted with the active participation of the communities. Mosquito control where no transmissible disease exists is not a health concern.

Medical Measures

Medical measures range from chemoprophylaxis and vaccination to case treatment and the sanitary isolation of infected areas. Chemoprophylaxis has very limited application in disasters. Antibiotic prevention of gastroenteritis/diarrhoea

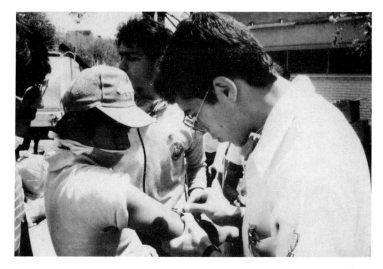

Fig. 18.8.   Unnecessary immunization against T-fever following earthquakes.

is strongly discouraged by the World Health Organization. Chemoprophylaxis of malaria can be considered under some circumstances for non-immune populations migrating towards high endemicity areas, an uncommon occurrence in natural disasters. The decision is best left to experts in this field. (Individual prophylaxis for expatriate relief workers is, of course, a must!)

The drive toward mass immunization generally has full public and political support (*Fig.* 18.8). It is usually not an appropriate disease control measure under the special circumstances of a natural disaster for the following reasons:

a. Lack of epidemiological justification.

b. Difficult logistics (transportation and a cold chain) in an emergency situation.

c. Failure to keep records of the people vaccinated. They may be accidently vaccinated again by different teams or organizations, and it is difficult to arrange for the requisite booster shots to be administered.

d. Secondary effects are particularly unwelcome during rehabilitation and reconstruction.

e. Vaccines against typhoid fever and cholera in particular, confer only partial and short-lived immunity and do little to impede transmission of the disease or prevent epidemics.

f. The fact that massive vaccination campaigns induce a false sense of security in the population and the authorities outside the health sector is often overlooked by relief workers, and consequently the aspects of sanitation and education are neglected.

When epidemics mistakenly regarded as inevitable fail to materialize, the illusion can be reinforced that the campaigns were effective and support the maintenance of a counterproductive strategy. While massive campaigns that mobilize enormous amounts of resources should not be encouraged, strengthening routine immunization programmes or their careful expansion to particularly vulnerable groups remains a tool of high value. The Guatemalan experience is an example. Following the 1976 earthquake, the public demanded increased protection from predicted outbreaks through vaccination. Typhoid fever was a major concern. In response to the public demand for official action, the Ministry of Health advanced the date of the annual vaccination campaign (DPT and measles). The participation of the public in this previously planned routine campaign of established effectiveness exceeded all expectations. This experience illustrates the approach of reinforcing the quality and extending the coverage of usual activities instead of adopting entirely different methods and strategies when a disaster strikes.

Immunization (or booster) against tetanus should be encouraged for relief personnel and, of course, for every person wounded.

In temporary settlements of a population otherwise scattered, major efforts should be undertaken to improve the expectedly low coverage of routine immunization. It is, however, taking advantage of the situation for developmental purposes rather than an emergency-related measure.

Sanitary isolation or quarantine is increasingly less used as its ineffectiveness is recognized. It is often too late (transmission has already taken place) and unenforceable (people will bypass the check points). The best approach remains to re-establish and improve the delivery of primary health care through the restoration of affected health services.

Basic health services should continue to be provided and to contribute to disease control after outside medical teams (national or expatriate) have left the affected areas.

It is perhaps the time to emphasize that relief medical teams should not undertake disease prevention or control measures on their own initiative without approval or instruction from the local health authorities. Too many resources are wasted, and sometimes too much harm is done by well intentioned relief workers or medical personnel unfamiliar with the local conditions, priorities and resources for follow-up.

CONCLUSIONS

Epidemiology is defined as the discipline that studies the dynamics of health phenomena with a view to proposing the most effective control measures. Its usefulness in periods of general disaster can range from the surveillance of communicable diseases to the study of the surge of medical emergencies, the occurrence of mental disturbances, etc. The enhanced part played by epidemiologists in recent disasters has permitted a start to be made on the development of techniques and methods that have helped to improve relief work and its integration into the long-term development programmes of disaster-stricken countries.

The solution to health problems created by disasters calls for a flow of accurate and viable information. Active participation of the health sector in national disaster preparedness planning will avoid costly improvization. Preparation for disasters, including public health activities such as the prevention of automotive and industrial accidents and the control of environmental pollution, must be a technical programme with its own funds and staff.

Only an on-going planning effort in conjunction with a research and personnel training programme will give the needed basis for the health services to promote a more effective and organized action in major national disasters.

REFERENCES

1. *Emergency Vector Control after Natural Disaster* 1982) Pan American Health Organization Scientific Publication No. 419.
2. Poves P. R. (1985) *Epidemia de Malaria Post Fenómeno del Niño, 1983.* Lima, Peru, Ministerio de Salud, pp. 11–13.
3. Cedeno J. M. (1985) *Lluvias e Inundaciones en la Cuenca del Guayas y sus Efectos sobre la Incidencia Palúdica, 1982–1985.* Quito, Eduador, Ministerio de Salud Pública, Anexo 6.
4. Zeballos J. L. (1986) *Health Aspects of the Mexico Earthquake, 19 September 1985.* Pan American Health Organization, pp. 4–5.
5. Leus X. (1985) *Natural Disaster and Communicable Diseases.* Paper presented at the Symposium on Natural Disaster, Epidemiology and Environmental Health, 14–17 October, 1985, Havana, Cuba, pp. 1–12.

SPECIFIC SECTION

Natural Disasters

T. Lusty

19

Famine

DEFINITION, CHARACTERISTICS AND CAUSES

Famine is not a scientific term and can be interpreted in different ways by different people. For the purposes of this chapter it is considered to be a situation of unusual food shortage resulting in abnormally high levels of starvation and death among reasonably large populations (say, over 20000 people).

Of course, many poor communities suffer from starvation every year in the pre-harvest period when the previous season's crop is insufficient to last the family for the whole year. The suffering and death that this causes, mainly among children, is probably considerably greater than in classic famines but, because it is part of the accepted (if not acceptable) pattern of life and does not attract the response from media or the international agencies, it is excluded here.

However, these poor communities that suffer such seasonal hardship are the same people who are most likely to suffer in famines. Marginalized onto a small acreage of poor land or even totally landless, they are most vulnerable to any change in climate as well as fluctuations in food prices. The more marginal a family economy, the smaller the deterioration needed to precipitate disaster.

Famine, therefore, is a problem of the poor. Except in very unusual situations, such as military sieges, rich people do not starve. Indeed, as Chen has pointed out, families often starve due to the victims' lack of purchasing power, rather than an overall food shortage in their vicinity. Crop failure, therefore, has a double effect on families: it reduces both their income and their food stocks.

By and large, urban areas do not suffer from famine, or only do so secondarily when large numbers of rural people migrate, as in the Brazil famine of 1984–5.

273

Usually, governments make sure that urban populations are fed, partly because these provide the industrial work force, as in the case of the Bengal famine of 1942–4 and partly because it is politically dangerous to have a starving population right on the government's doorstep. However, this does not mean that there is no starvation in cities; to some degree the problem of malnutrition among the urban poor is even more intractable than that in rural areas: families have little or no opportunity to grow significant amounts of their own food and are, therefore, totally dependent on income and the cash economy.

While it is certainly true that almost all recorded famines are linked to poor harvest and bad climatic conditions, such as rain failure, nevertheless it is not unusual for famine to exist in the presence of local food surpluses; there is evidence that during the 1973 famine in Wollo, Ethiopia, food was actually exported out of the area: it is also clear that food prices did not rise astronomically during that famine, which once again indicates that people starved because they could not afford food rather than because it was not available.

Characteristics of famine clearly vary from situation to situation, but it is commonly accompanied by unusual migrations: in the earlier stages it is the men who seek work, often some distance away from their homes and later the women and children also leave home to seek food. There is also a tendency for precious items such as the silver Ethiopian crosses and other family possessions to be sold in order to generate income. Perhaps one of the most depressing features is the sale of the means of livelihood itself, so that poor farmers sell or kill their draught animals, eat their seed and even dispose of what land rights they have.

One of the most telling differences between seasonal starvation and true famine is that during seasonal shortages, families and communities tighten their belts and manage to continue living their lives without any outside assistance, whereas during famine the means of livelihood of whole communities is destroyed and outside support is needed to reinstate them.

Patterns and Indicators of Famines

By their nature famines are slow in onset unlike, for example, earthquakes, cyclones and epidemics. An overt famine usually only occurs after a succession of poor rains and bad harvests which gradually weaken the economic position of poor communities. Due to this long lead time, it should be possible to predict periods of acute food shortage and to take the necessary actions to mitigate them: famines should not occur. India, in particular, has had some success in this field, notably in the Bihar famine of 1968 and more recently in Maharashtra in 1972. However, against these successes are the total failures in the Horn of Africa both in 1972–3 and again in 1984–5. In both these cases, the Ethiopian government and other agencies forecast the onset of a famine but in both cases the main international input of food came too late to prevent hundreds of thousands of deaths.

There is clearly a need for a series of long- and short-term indicators linked closely to relevant interventions: there is no point in forecasting famine if that forecast does not trigger the relief process. Various systems are in the process of being worked out and tested. These usually combine a mixture of harvest forecasting and food price monitoring. Where livestock husbandry is significant it is useful to watch fluctuations in the relative value of animals and grain; in the later stages, some measurement of household stocks of food and levels of malnutrition among children can be added. Unfortunately, the cost of close surveillance is very high and few countries have the resources to continue it for a long period of time over large areas. Therefore, what is needed is a simple system of monitoring data which is collected routinely for other purposes, such as market prices and rainfall. Where these give cause for alarm more detailed, specially planned surveys can then be mounted. At the same time, those concerned with food aid can be alerted that a crisis is developing. Planning this 'graded response' is probably one of the greatest challenges in famine relief for the 1980s and beyond.

While famines are largely caused by our inability to forecast food shortages accurately, they are also influenced by the long lead times in getting food supplies to an area once the problem has been recognized. Therefore, in addition to devising systems of graded response, strong emphasis should also be given to the stockpiling of buffer stocks of food in countries and regions where famines are likely to occur.

CRISIS MANAGEMENT IN FAMINE CONDITIONS

Analysis of the Situation

Once a serious food shortage situation is suspected, an analysis has to be made as to how severe it is and what internal and external resources will be needed to prevent catastrophes.

Early on in any situation some sort of a measurement of the level of malnutrition is essential in order to assess the severity of the problem and to decide in which particular areas food is most urgently needed. Apart from trying to obtain some figure on mortality (usually of children) the most common measurements taken are:

1. The middle upper arm circumference of children under the age of 5 years, or less than 115 cm tall where age is not known.
2. The ratio of weight (kg) to height (cm) compared with normal values.

Both of these measurements have international standards against which the findings can be compared. The exact relationship between arm circumference and weight to height is not clear but both are apparently useful; various studies are underway at the time of writing to try to establish which is best in any given situation. Basically the arm circumference is easy and quick, while the weight for height involves more mathematical dexterity and record-keeping as well as needing continual checking of scales. Currently the cut-off points for malnutrition and severe malnutrition are:

arm circumference—malnutrition less than 13·5 cm, severe malnutrition less than 12 cm.

weight for height—malnutrition less than 80 per cent of normal, severe malnutrition less than 70 per cent. Normally a situation is considered severe if more than 20 per cent of children are less than 80 per cent of weight for height or fall in the malnourished category.

In order to obtain an accurate impression of the situation, it is necessary either to measure all the children (which is usually impossible) or to select random samples of between 200 and 400 children (more in large camps). Detailed advice on how to organize surveys and analyse data can be found in the books recommended at the end of this chapter.

Clearly, anthropometry is limited; it measures what has happened in the past and gives some idea of the present situation. In order to decide what interventions should be taken, it is important also to make some forecast for the future. For this, one needs to know what sort of foodstuffs are presently available in the famine area for the people most needing them, how long it is until the next harvest is expected, how large that harvest will be, etc. One also needs to know to what degree the population has lost its earning capacity. For example, have the nomads lost so many of their cattle that they can no longer be self-sufficient or do agriculturalists have the necessary seeds and equipment to sow the next season's crop?

Having made these judgements, it is then necessary to assess what resources are available, both locally and overseas, and what more is needed and for how long. Wherever possible, food should be purchased locally provided it does not push up market prices excessively. Local purchase is both cheaper and encourages the development of a higher agricultural production, whereas large food imports can sometimes depress local production and may even compete for storage space.

Assistance usually takes one of the following forms: cash donations, provision of personnel, logistic facilities (transport and storage) and food itself. Often famine victims migrate into camps or nearby urban slums where in addition to starvation they suffer from the problems of overcrowding which include an increased incidence of infectious diseases, such as diarrhoea, measles and respiratory infections (*see* Chapter 18). Use of the various check lists in the appendix may be useful on these occasions.

There are various methods for calculating the nutritional needs of communities. For the sake of simplicity, one can presume that a normal population of men, women and children need around 2000 calories per head per day. The bulk of this energy requirement is usually supplied in the form of grain of one kind or another. Where total feeding is required, it is usually reckoned that around 500 g of grain plus other supplementary rations are needed daily for each person. This involves providing 15 kg per head per month (15 metric tons per 1000 people per month).

When the population is at risk, but not totally dependent, the amount of grain needed can be reduced, possibly to around a third of the quantity or 5 metric tons per 1000 head of population per month.

The longer an emergency continues the more important it is that the rations should be balanced, containing sufficient protein, minerals and vitamins. It is therefore important to involve nutritionists at an early stage of planning and to continue to deploy them for monitoring the situation. In particular, it is common to find deficiencies of vitamins A and C and these should be watched for. Most people now advocate the routine supplementation of milk powder with vitamin A.

It is important to realize that there are 3 general types of ration available in famine situations:

1. General ration, which supplies most of the calories and which is indispensable.

2. Supplementary ration, either added to the general ration to give it variety and flavour or specially aimed at vulnerable groups such as children under the age of 5 and lactating or pregnant women.
3. Therapeutic foods, specially designed with low bulk and high palatability for the severely malnourished who are on the point of death.

The priorities in any situation will vary according to its severity but it is vital to realize that supplementary and therapeutic rations on their own will not be able to improve the situation where the general ration is lacking.

In circumstances where food supplies are severely limited it is, of course, essential to target the food to those in most need. As well as looking to the particularly vulnerable groups mentioned above, it is usual to find that certain geographical areas and certain types of people are worse off than others: they need and should receive correspondingly more assistance. A form of nutritional triage, whereby only the fit are fed and the malnourished left to die has been advocated in the past. This is totally unacceptable to this author and most other relief workers.

There are, then, basically 3 types of relief food:
a. The staple or bulk ration, usually cereal.
b. Mixed rations often used to supplement the general ration (e.g. corn, soya, milk).
c. Other supplements such as oil and sugar, dried skimmed milk etc. which are used either to balance the general ration and ensure an adequate quantity of protein, vitamins and minerals, or separately as a supplementary or therapeutic ration for particular groups.

Where the bulk ration (*a*) is imported, this usually consists of one of the grain foods, commonly wheat, maize or rice. Ideally, this should be compatible with the normal food practices of the famine population, but sometimes this may not be possible. However, the problem of exotic staples not being acceptable has probably been exaggerated. In fact, the difficulty is usually that the population does not have the necessary knowledge or equipment to prepare the food (e.g. mills to grind wheat or fuel to cook with) and once these have been provided they adapt fairly quickly. This has been demonstrated particularly with special foods such as energy biscuits which appear to be acceptable and palatable wherever they have been given, even among people who had not previously seen a biscuit.

It is, therefore, essential that when deciding upon types and quantities of relief food the difficulties of food preparation are not forgotten. It is important to have a clear idea of how the population will use these foods.

In most situations a choice has to be made between giving the ration 'dry', to be prepared and cooked in the home, and 'on the spot' mass feeding, where food is cooked in a soup kitchen and people come to consume it there. Sometimes the 'general ration' is distributed 'dry' and the supplementary 'on the spot' but this may vary according to conditions, e.g. fuel may not be available for family cooking. In general, the more normal feeding habits can be, the better it is. Family feeding is an important part of social life and should be encouraged. It is important to realize that when children are given an extra 'on the spot' supplement, their mothers may reduce their share of the 'general ration' in the home so that the benefit of the supplement is reduced or lost.

Therapeutic or intensive feeding is always supervised and usually residential, as it entails at least 4 meals a day (usually 6) and the patient is almost always suffering from concomitant infectious disease.

Logistics and the Delivery of Food

Although it may complicate logistics, food should always be distributed as near as possible to the homes of the people who will eat it. This reduces migration and makes subsequent rehabilitation easier. Once people have left their homes it is hard to restore their independence.

There are several stages in the delivery of foodstuffs into the famine area, namely:

1. Purchase and loading in the donor country.
2. Transport from the donor to the recipient country and unloading and storage in the docks.
3. Transport from docks to regional stores.
4. Transport from regional stores to the periphery.

There may, in fact, be yet another level of distribution if the terrain is difficult, which may involve the use of livestock such as camels and donkeys, as in Ethiopia in 1985. It is seldom worthwhile to use aeroplanes or helicopters to deliver anything but very specialized foods or drugs. The only exception to this may be where groups of people are beleaguered by armed forces who will not let civilian supplies through by land routes.

Food for Work

In any food distribution programme, the risk of creating a dependent population exists. Where the famine is not too severe, some independence can be maintained by asking people to work for their food. There are many suitable activities for both men and women. These may include road building, cultivation and planting, terracing, etc. The amount of food given for a day's work varies, but usually it is more than the family needs so some will be exchanged or sold. In severe famines where the population is weak, food for work may be inappropriate as the most needy will not benefit.

Related Health Problems (Table 19.1)

In any famine the level of infectious disease tends to rise. This is partly because malnutrition lowers the individual's resistance to disease and partly because people migrate and crowd together close to points where food is distributed. Where such crowding occurs it is common to find high rates of diarrhoea and other infectious diseases such as measles. It is, therefore, important to look at other inputs besides food such as water supplies, oral rehydration, immunization programmes, etc. Measles, in particular, kills and debilitates. Wherever possible, immunization for measles should be a priority (OXFAM, WHO and UNHCR are jointly developing an emergency kit for these circumstances). This subject is dealt with in detail in Chapter 18.

Table 19.1. Factors affecting health of famine victim

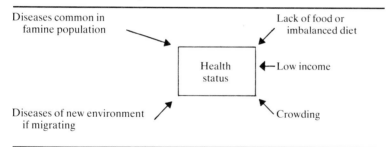

Diseases common in famine population

Lack of food or imbalanced diet

Health status

←Low income

Diseases of new environment if migrating

Crowding

Rehabilitation

Because famine victims have lost most or all their wealth before they begin to starve, the need for relief is a long-term one and the weaning from dependency is usually difficult. Until people are once again able to generate their own income, they must remain dependent on relief supplies. This is in direct contrast to certain other disasters which, while destroying life and sometimes homes, nevertheless leave the community able to continue with its work, albeit in a somewhat hampered manner. After famines the nature of rehabilitation will vary from one situation to another but often seeds, draught animals and culti-vating equipment are needed. Where people have migrated they usually have to be transported back to their villages and some sort of arrangement made so that they can re-establish themselves on the land. Generally they collect food supplies from the centre which are sufficient to last for several weeks. Other inputs may be dams and water systems for irrigation, some form of tree planting to retain moisture and various other systems of water harvesting. It is important that the health and nutritional status is closely monitored during these migrating stages and provision be made so that food will be available in the villages where people work.

In certain circumstances, as when land has become so eroded that it is virtually a desert, there is no hope of people returning to their original locations; consequently, fairly massive resettlement may have to be undertaken. This is often strongly resisted, sometimes with justification, when harsh methods are used. In many drought-prone countries there are few areas left which can be resettled anyway and the problem may seem intractable, with relief needed for long periods. In certain marginalized zones, it is likely to continue almost indefinitely.

Of course, many people will leave the land permanently to swell existing slum populations; for them, the only future lies in paid employment or other forms of income generation.

FURTHER READING

Methodology of Nutritional Surveillance (1976) Report of a Joint FAO/UNICEF/WHO Expert Committee. Geneva, World Health Organization.
Measuring Change in Nutritional Status. Guidelines for Assessing the Nutritional Impact of Supplementary Feeding Programmes for Vulnerable Groups. (1983) Geneva, World Health Organization.

Energy and Protein Requirements. (1985) Report of a Joint FAO/WHO/UNU Expert Consultation. World Health Organization Technical Report Series 724. Geneva, World Health Organization.

Oxfam's Practical Guide to Selective Feeding Programmes. No. 1. (Revised and reprinted 1984.) Oxford, Oxfam.

King M., King F. and Martodipoero S. (1978) Primary Child Care—A manual for health workers. Oxford, Oxford University Press.

de Ville de Goyet C., Seaman J. and Geijer U. (1978) *The Management of Nutritional Emergencies in Large Populations.* Geneva, World Health Organization.

Sen A. K. (1981) *Poverty and Famines—An Essay on Entitlement and Deprivation.* Oxford, Clarendon Press.

APPENDIX TO CHAPTER 19   CHECKLIST FOR FAMINE SITUATIONS

Many of these points are more relevant to situations where communities have migrated into camps.

1. Demography and background
2. Food
3. Water
4. Sanitation
5. Medical care
6. Shelter
7. Logistics
8. Rehabilitation
9. Summary

1. DEMOGRAPHY AND BACKGROUND

Numbers: numbers coming, numbers leaving—forecast?
Proportions: of men, women and children (0–4, 5–14 years)?
    birthrate
    mortality
Is there evidence of migration?
If migrating, where people have come from—previous occupation and environment.
What provisions do they still have?
What is the physical environment like?
Season—rainy or dry—future seasons?
Who administers food distribution—how—what staff are employed?
How well-planned is the siting system?
What degree of community involvement is there—are there committees?
What agencies are working there?
How do they co-operate—tensions?

2. FOOD

What is the general state of nutrition?
Has a simple nutritional survey been done?

Is the situation deteriorating or improving?

Is there any evidence of specific nutritional deficiencies (in xerophthalmia, anaemia etc.)?

What is the population's attitude towards the food provided and the feeding programme in general?

What fuel is used for cooking: if wood, is there an adequate supply close by—will it last?

How is the feeding organized—distribution, preparation and cooking?

What foods are used—where from—how do they relate to the population's normal diet?

How many calories per person?

How are the total food requirements of the population estimated?

Food cooked at community or family level?

Availability of local foods?

Local price of food-stuffs—cattle and staple (maize, sorghum)?

Has this altered recently?

How many meals a day?

Is additional food given to vulnerable groups (selective or supplementary)?
   If so, what, how much and to whom?

How are people selected for this extra food?

Is this food eaten in individual dwellings or 'on the spot' under supervision at a feeding centre?

Who runs it?

Is there any facility for therapeutic feeding of the severely malnourished?
   If so, what, and who runs it?

Is a record kept of those receiving special food?

Is the progress of malnourished individuals monitored?

Is the general nutritional status of the population monitored—how and how frequently?

What are the priority needs in the area of food and nutrition? How can these be met?

3. WATER

How is water supplied to the population (standpipe, river, tanker etc.)?

What is its source (river, well, rain, cistern)?

Is the source relatively clean and likely to remain so?

Is the source adequate at all seasons?

How close is the supply brought to the people's dwelling?

What (approx.) is the consumption rate per head?

Is there evidence of a severe water-related disease problem?
   If so, what (i.e. skin disease, typhoid, diarrhoea etc.)?

Is there any danger of contamination from latrines, livestock or (in the case of rivers) other camps upstream?

Is the water tested regularly?

Is there any system of treatment?

If a pump is used, how is it serviced and what contingency plans are there if it breaks down?

Are washing facilities provided—where?
Where are animals watered?
How is water stored in the shelters or houses—what containers are used?
Does the community understand the concept of contamination of water supplies both at source and in the home?
Is there a health education programme covering water usage?
What is the 'chain' of water supply from source to final utilization?
What are the main problems in the chain?

4. SANITATION

Is there a sanitation problem?
How are excreta and waste disposed of (family or communal, via pit latrines, water-borne system, cartage or random)?
Do they present a health hazard?
How well are existing systems maintained and kept clean?
Is there evidence of a high level of disease which might be related to poor sanitation (i.e. diarrhoea, worms etc.)?
Is there sufficient space to allow for pit latrines to be dug?
How close is the drinking water source to the sewage disposal point?
What is the normal practice of defaecation of the population?
How do they view the existing 'camp' system?
Is the water table high or low?
What is the soil structure (i.e. rocky, sandy etc.)?
How will different seasons affect existing systems (i.e. flooding)?

5. MEDICAL CARE

What basic health facilities exist?
What are the main disease problems of the population?
How are they measured—what records are kept?
Is there any system of surveillance?
Is there an unusually high incidence of communicable diseases (i.e. measles, scabies, TB, diarrhoea)?
What factors may be responsible for the various diseases (i.e. housing, water, crowding etc.)?
What simple preventative measures could be undertaken to alleviate these problems?
What measures are being undertaken already?
What maternal and child health services exist?
What is the existing vaccine coverage, particularly for measles?
Are there effective vaccines against the prevalent diseases, especially measles?
    If so, is there an adequate immunization programme (quality, coverage etc.)?
Are vaccines kept well refrigerated both in transit to camp and in the camp itself?
Is there a need for refrigerators?
Is the curative care simple, cheap and relevant?

Is the drug supply adequate?
Are the drugs relevant to the main diseases?
Is the drug list limited to simple essential drugs—standardization?
Do the health workers know how to use them?
Are there facilities for oral rehydration (where diarrhoea is causing dehydration)?
Who is in charge of health; what agencies are helping?
What evidence is there of community participation in health care?
Is adequate use made of medically trained or trainable members of the community?
Are they trained to do the right things?
Are they supervised?
To what degree is the community involved (health committees etc.)?
Is there a reasonable health education programme?
What records are kept?
Are 'at risk' registers kept (i.e. for TB)?
How are severely sick people referred for more intensive care—where are they sent?

6. SHELTER

What is the normal housing of the population?
How are they housed—individual families or community shelters?
How many people per dwelling?
Is the shelter adequate?
How are the shelters spaced?
Is camp layout organized in small units (e.g. village or tribal groups)?
Is the administration block sufficient?
What cooking facilities are provided?
Are materials for building available locally?
    What are they?
Is there a fire hazard?

7. LOGISTICS

How secure are the deliveries of food?
Are the storage facilities adequate?
How many days' food can be stored?
Are the roads open in all weathers?
Are the stores efficiently run—are they locked?
Is there evidence of rats or other wastage?
Is routine rodent control undertaken?
Is food properly stacked (i.e. away from walls)?
Is there a record system with regular stock-taking?
What form of transport is used, army, government, aid agency, etc.?
What servicing facilities exist for vehicles?
How do the field personnel communicate with the capital?
Is there a regular feed-back of information?

Is this information used in planning intervention and supplies?
What skills are available in the population (i.e. medical, engineering, etc.)?
Are they being employed?
Are local people being trained (i.e. for simple health and nutritional duties)?
What are the priority needs in the area of transport, storage, communication and staffing?

8. REHABILITATION

What are the prospects of the population returning to normal on their own?
   Does the government have detailed plans to help?
How long is it envisaged the problem will last?
What forms of income generation are possible?
What tools are needed?
Is there enough land and livestock?
What other inputs would be needed (i.e. tools, seeds, livestock, advice etc.)?
When is the next harvest?
What is needed to ensure a reasonable crop is sown?
What is the minimum viable herd size?
What is the average herd size at present?
Are there training needs?
What other inputs are needed?
Are there any adult training programmes?
Is there a need for them?
What recreational facilities are there?
How can these be improved?
What are the traditional games and entertainments of the refugees?
What other steps can be taken to raise camp morale?

9. SUMMARY

How serious is the situation?
What are the main problems—list in order of priority?
What is the best way of solving them (alternatives where possible)?
What inputs are needed (cash, supplies, personnel)?
What should be planned for short-, mid- and long-term?
What should be the objectives?
How will progress be monitored?

S. W. A. Gunn

20

Earthquakes

A major earthquake is the most sudden and deadly devastation that can hit society. The seismic-prone areas and countries of the world have been well mapped out, yet preparedness for this kind of emergency remains very poorly developed. Most often the response tends to be improvized, hurried, ad hoc action, after the impact, even in regions where such a disaster can be reasonably expected.

Earthquakes cause massive destruction, a large number of deaths and many casualties, all with frightening suddenness. The emergency creates immediate medical and surgical needs at the site of impact—the epicentre—while new health-related needs may arise in the areas to which the stricken population has moved for safety.

The acute and immediate problems are rescue, triage, evacuation and medical care. These problems of disaster management are dealt with in the relevant chapters; here mainly the characteristics of post-earthquake pathology are outlined. The strains on the general health services and on socio-economic development are not discussed.

Depending on its intensity or magnitude,* the season, the time of the day it occurs, and the population of the area involved, the catastrophe can cause thousands of dead and injured within a few minutes. This was the case on 27 June, 1976 in Tangshan, China, when some 650000 people were killed. Recent studies of the epidemiology of disasters have shed some light on these occurrences and have revealed disease profiles and injury patterns peculiar to each kind of disaster. Thus, it is evident that the health effects, and consequently the medical needs, in an earthquake are very different from those following floods or hurricanes, and call for different approaches.

---

* There exist various scales to express the magnitude or 'size' of an earthquake. As the Richter Scale is the one most commonly encountered, a brief note is given. The Richter Scale is a logarithmic measure calculated from amplitudes of seismic waves, extending from -1 to 8. All tremors measuring 4·5 or over are internationally recorded.

—An earthquake of amplitude 3 on the Richter Scale corresponds to a tremor felt over a limited area
—Amplitude 4·5 can cause light destruction
—Amplitude 6·6 causes considerable destruction
—Amplitudes 7 to 8 cause very great destruction
—Over 8, the amplitude is 100 million times that of 3.

THE EFFECT OF EARTHQUAKES ON HOSPITALS AND OTHER PHYSICAL FACILITIES

Hospitals and clinics are particularly vulnerable to tremors, Even if the principal buildings remain more or less intact, the vital facilities and equipment—electrical installations, X-rays, intensive care service lines, surgical theatres, laboratory glassware and chemicals all tend to become unusable, and this at a time when they are most needed (*see Fig.* 20.1).

Structurally, it is also known that the proportions of deaths and of trapped victims significantly rise according to the number of floors in a building, the

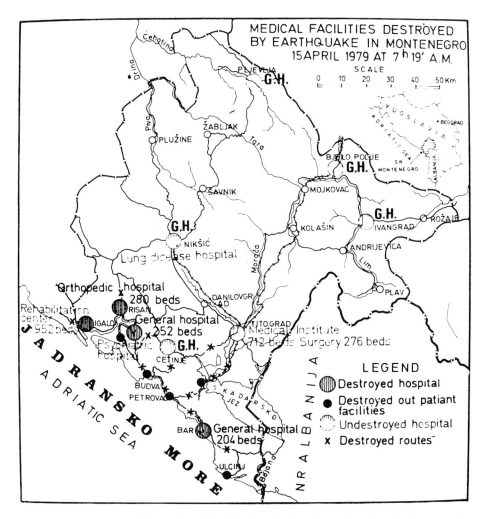

Fig. 20.1. Earthquake in Yugoslavia, 1979. Map showing the destruction of hospitals and health facilities.

(Reproduced by courtesy of WHO.)

ground floor being relatively the least risky (8·5 per cent trapped, 3 per cent dead), with the proportion increasing to 32·5 per cent and 12·3 per cent respectively from the third floor up. Hospitals, of course, tend to be multistorey buildings. In seismically risky areas it is therefore necessary not only to build quake-resistant structures, but also lower, smaller units.

HOSPITAL ADMISSIONS

With the great numbers of casualties it is evident that there will be a large and sudden rush on the outpatient and inpatient facilities, assuming that the hospital has escaped damage. It is, however, significant that, once the initial rush is over, hospital admission patterns revert to normal as early as the 4th–5th day after the earthquake. This has important implications on decision making and also explains why mobile theatres or tent hospitals flown from donor countries almost invariably arrive late and are not to be recommended.

THE DISEASE PROFILE FOLLOWING EARTHQUAKES

In drought situations and floods the risk of infectious diseases and of malnutrition are real and the necessary personnel, medicines and supplies should be geared to these needs. The disease pattern following earthquakes is altogether different. Here the number of dead can be enormous; among those who survive, injuries are the most prevalent (fractures, contusions, cuts, crush syndrome) and there is some momentary panic. The immediate response, therefore, calls for more surgeons than internists—orthopaedic surgeons in particular—for anaesthetists, intensive care and resuscitation teams, stretchers and stretcher-bearers, for splints, traction apparatus, plaster of Paris and bandages rather than antibiotics and antidiarrhoeics. Also needed, of course, are teams to dispose of the large numbers of dead—a task far more difficult than is imagined.

There is quite a strong correlation between the number of dead and the number of injured survivors. The ratio is 3 injured to 1 dead (*Table* 20.1) and De Bruycker has found this to remain quite constant with changing Richter magnitudes and population densities. This has important implications in emergency planning and calculating the casualty load from the number of deaths. From these figures one can deduce the kind and volume of emergency supplies that will be needed, the amount of orthopaedic and other medical help required, and the speed of treatment facilities that must be made available.

Table 20.1. Morbidity/mortality ratios observed after 4 major earthquakes, 1970–80

Earthquake	Injured	Dead	Ratio
Nicaragua, 1972	20 000	6 000	3·3
Pakistan, 1974	15 000	4 700	3·2
Guatemala, 1976	76 500	22 800	3·3
Italy, 1980	8 800	2 614	3·3

INJURY PATTERNS

Major or minor trauma—due to building collapses, flying objects, entrapment, burns and cuts—are the main immediate medical problems in earthquakes. In the 1980 earthquake in Southern Italy, trauma requiring specialized treatment by qualified personnel made up an important proportion of the casualty load. Spinal and multiple fractures (19 per cent) and major crush and tissue injuries (43·5 per cent) needed such care, hence the need for specialized hospitals away from the disaster zone.

The time of the impact is significant: when the earthquake occurs at night, with the population lying in bed, the fractures involve particularly the pelvis, the thorax and the spine. When it occurs during the day, there will be more head injuries and limb fractures. Fractures of the clavicle are a common feature. Such foreknowledge is very useful in mobilizing the right kind of material and personnel.

Entrapment under collapsing buildings is the most common cause of death and causes the most injuries among the surviving casualties. In the above-mentioned Italian earthquake, 35 per cent of those who had been trapped died, while only 0·3 per cent of the non-trapped victims died (*see Fig.* 20.2).

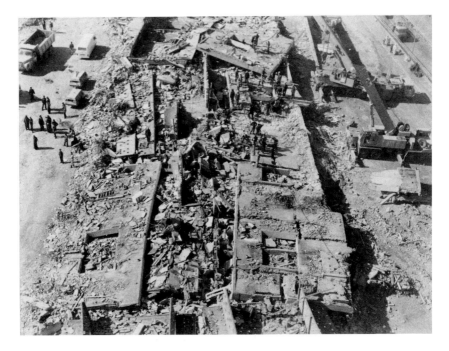

Fig. 20.2. Earthquake at El Asnam, Algeria, 1980. Massive collapse of buildings. (Reproduced by courtesy of UNDRO.)

RESCUE AND IMMEDIATE CARE

Immediate rescue and care are of paramount importance, and it is worth noting that any help coming from outside the area almost invariably arrives too late. Expatriate teams and foreign donors should fashion their assistance accordingly, if they are to be of any effect. Again, in order to make maximum use of local help, it should be realized that in extricating the trapped and the injured, the first helpers come to a large extent (90 per cent) from the same village, and from the inhabitants of the same building (76·2 per cent). Extricating with unsophisticated means, such as hands, shovel, axe, ladder, accounts for the largest number rescued (96·8 per cent) as opposed to the use of sophisticated means, such as tractors or cranes (3·2 per cent).

DELAYED HEALTH EFFECTS

The actual emergency phase after impact is remarkably short—3 to 5 days. Indeed almost all the injuries (97 per cent) occur immediately or within half an hour of the quake, and very rapidly hospital admissions resume the pre-impact pattern.

Among the survivors, however, mass population displacements, crowding in improvized shelters, environmental upheavals, breakdown of garbage disposal and bursting of sewers, shortage of water and temperature extremes may create health hazards and lead to outbreaks of infectious diseases. The risk is real and appropriate countermeasures must be taken. However, field observations and statistics show that such risks and the danger of epidemics are extremely rare and such popular but unproven measures as mass vaccination are quite unnecessary. Indeed they can be counterproductive by diverting much needed help and material away from more urgent tasks. Sensible sanitary measures and hygienic practices will do more to obviate any epidemic.

It is also significant that in investigating the mortality rates among survivors 18 months after the earthquake, De Bruycker found no substantial difference between them and the overall national mortality figures.

Earthquakes are becoming increasingly devastating, not because they are particularly more frequent but mainly because of the increasing concentration of large populations—as illustrated by the 1985 catastrophe which hit Mexico City which has 18 million inhabitants.

This calls for government legislation and disaster planning, at least in the countries known to be on or along seismic faults. The health system must be properly evaluated in the light of possible risks, basic as well as specialized teams must be trained and facilities made available, hospitals (and other buildings) must be tremor-resistant and built according to risk zones, and the population trained and made aware of the land it lives on. For, when disaster strikes, it is these same people who will have to take care of their dead and wounded. Primary health care and basic health education can do more than many experts arriving too late.

FURTHER READING

Cara M. (1982) Effets des tremblements de terre sur la santé des populations. In: Bolt B. C. *Les Tremblements de Terre*, Paris, Pour la Science.

De Bruycker M., Greco D., Lechat M. et al. (1983) The 1980 earthquake in southern Italy: rescue of trapped victims and mortality. *Bull. WHO* **61**, 102.

Gunn S. W. A. (1985) New disease patterns due to disasters and geographical change. In: *Proceedings of the International Federation of Surgical Colleges*, Dublin.

Gunn S. W. A., Murcia M. and Parakatil F. (1984) *Dictionnaire des Secours d'Urgence en Cas de Catastrophe (Dictionary of Emergency Relief and Disasters)* Paris, CILF.

Manni C. and Paderni S. (1983) The earthquake in Italy in 1980. *Disasters* **1**, 413.

21

Floods, Hurricanes and Tsunamis

INTRODUCTION

A disaster is a great, sudden misfortune resulting in loss of life, serious injury, and property destruction. Strictly speaking, if such misfortune befalls even one person it is a disaster. However, in current usage, the term is used to refer to a sudden occurrence which kills and injures relatively large numbers of persons. Disasters are usually classified by the number of lives at risk or lost. In a minor disaster, at least 25 people are killed or injured. In a moderate disaster, 100 or more people are killed or injured. In a major disaster, at least 1000 people are killed or injured.[1] Natural disasters are serious disruptions to life that arise from the forces of nature. Natural catastrophes include floods, tsunamis, hurricanes, earthquakes, forest fires, volcanic eruptions and natural droughts. A natural occurrence or catastrophe becomes a disaster when lives are lost. The basic mission of disaster management is the prevention and minimization of death, disability, suffering and loss. There are eight basic principles of disaster management which need emphasizing in this chapter:

1. To prevent the occurrence of the disaster whenever possible.
2. To minimize the number of casualties if the disaster cannot be prevented.
3. To prevent further casualties from occurring after the initial impact of the disaster.
4. To rescue the victims.
5. To provide first aid to the injured.
6. To evacuate the injured to medical installations.
7. To provide definitive medical care.
8. To promote the reconstruction of the lives of the victims.[2]

The following phases are generally recognized in the chronology of disasters:
—threat
—warning
—impact
—inventory
—rescue
—remedy
—recovery

There are also geographical divisions of the total area concerned with the disaster. The three major divisions are: the impact area, the filter area, and the community aid area.[2] The disaster strikes causing casualties in the impact area. The filter area is the location around the impact area in which notification of the incident is immediate and direct. In general, aid to the impact area usually starts to flow from the filter area immediately without any need for formal notification. Help also flows to the impact area from the community aid area. Notification of the community aid area is apt to be slow and highly selective.

A hurricane is a rotary storm or cyclone involving a wide area with winds exceeding 74 mph or 120 km/h. The winds rotate counterclockwise in the northern hemisphere and clockwise in the southern hemisphere. Hurricanes develop over ocean areas causing maximal destruction when they hit islands or the coastal areas of continents. In the Atlantic and Eastern Pacific, tropical cyclones are called hurricanes from the West Indian word 'huracan' meaning 'big wind'. In the Western Pacific area, the hurricane is usually referred to as a typhoon from the Chinese 'taifong' meaning 'great wind'.

A flood is an overflowing of water beyond its usual confines in lakes, rivers or oceans. Floods of disaster magnitude in coastal areas are usually associated with hurricanes and most of the deaths in hurricanes result from the accompanying floods. A tsunami, or tidal wave, can also cause flooding of a coastal area. Tsunamis are seismic sea waves secondary to earthquakes, sea bottom slides, or volcanic eruptions. Inland floods are usually due to heavy rains, spring thaws or breaks in man-made dams. A Jokulhlaup is the Icelandic term for a flood due to the rupture of glacial ice and the sudden release of water impounded by the glacier (glacial lakes).

Much of the author's experience with hurricanes and floods came in response to hurricanes David and Frederick which struck the Dominican Republic in September of 1979.[3]

HURRICANES

Hurricanes are classified by a disaster potential scale called the Saffir/Simpson Scale which grades them according to their wind velocity and tidal surge.[4] (*See Table* 21.1.)

A storm or tidal surge is a great dome of water 50 to 100 miles wide, that sweeps across the coastline near the area where the hurricane makes landfall. The surge, aided by the hammering effect of breaking waves, acts like a giant bulldozer sweeping away everything in its path. The stronger the hurricane, the higher the storm surge. The combination of storm surge, battering waves and high tide is the hurricane's most deadly weapon. Nine out of ten hurricane fatalities are caused by the storm surge (*Fig.* 21.1).

Table 21.1. The Saffir/Simpson Hurricane Scale

Class	Wind speed		Tidal surge	
	mph	*k/h*	*Feet*	*Meters*
I	74–95	120–150	4–5	1–1·5
II	96–110	150–175	6–8	1·5–2·5
III	111–130	175–210	9–12	2·5–3·5
IV	131–155	210–250	13–18	3·5–5·5
V	>155	>250	>18	>5·5

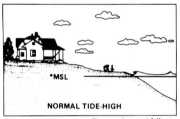

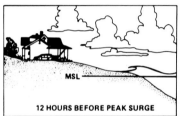

NORMAL TIDE-HIGH

It is a normal beach day. The sea rises and falls predictably with astronomical tidal action. There are the usual small waves. A hurricane has developed and a Hurricane Watch is in effect for the area.

12 HOURS BEFORE PEAK SURGE

The hurricane now poses a serious threat to this beach area and the Watch has been changed to a Hurricane Warning. The hurricane is 12 hours away. The tide is a little above normal; the water moves further up the beach. Swells are beginning to move in from the deep ocean and breaking waves — some as high as five to eight feet — crash ashore and run well up the beach. The wind is picking up.

*MSL: Mean Sea Level

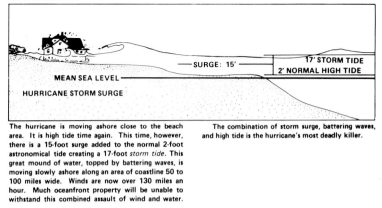

The hurricane is moving ashore close to the beach area. It is high tide time again. This time, however, there is a 15-foot surge added to the normal 2-foot astronomical tide creating a 17-foot *storm tide*. This great mound of water, topped by battering waves, is moving slowly ashore along an area of coastline 50 to 100 miles wide. Winds are now over 130 miles an hour. Much oceanfront property will be unable to withstand this combined assault of wind and water.

The combination of storm surge, battering waves, and high tide is the hurricane's most deadly killer.

Fig. 21.1.   The tidal or storm surge created by a hurricane.

Hurricanes David and Frederick were both Class V hurricanes when they struck the Dominican Republic. As a matter of interest, no hurricane greater than Class III has ever struck the continental United States. The dynamics of hurricanes have been studied and recently described in detail. In brief, temperate trade winds are heated at the surface of the warm, equatorial ocean waters. Storm clouds form and as the air rises, the pressure at the surface drops and the earth's rotation creates a spiral pattern to the clouds with a counterclockwise rotation in the northern hemisphere, or a clockwise rotation in the southern hemisphere.[5] (*See Fig.* 21.2*a*.) If the cycle perpetuates itself to sustained winds of 39 mph (65 km/h), a tropical storm is formed and it is given a name. When sustained winds of 75 mph (120 km/h) are achieved, the storm is upgraded to a hurricane. The usual forward speed of a hurricane circle is 10–15 mph (15–25 km/h) at first, but subsequently may increase to 25 mph or more (40 km/h or more). Like all circular storms, a hurricane, in passing a particular point, seems to have three phases: first, there are high winds in one direction; next, there is a clear phase called the 'eye' which can be several miles wide and quite calm; finally, there is a third phase with high winds blowing in the vector opposite to the initial direction (*Fig.* 21.2*b*).

DYNAMICS OF A HURRICANE

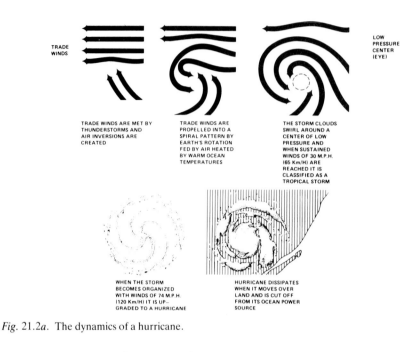

Fig. 21.2*a*. The dynamics of a hurricane.

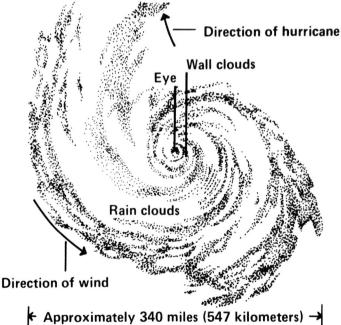

Fig. 21.2*b*. The final phase of a hurricane.

Tropical cyclones originate in the relatively quiet tropics where the primary energy source is the latent heat released when water vapour condenses. Only extremely moist air can supply the energy necessary to spawn and maintain tropical storms and only very warm air contains enough moisture. Tropical cyclones, therefore, form only over oceans with water temperatures of at least 27°C (80°F) (*Fig.* 21.3). The rate of condensation heating resulting from the intense rainfall associated with hurricanes is about 10^{11} kW. In only one day a hurricane produces $2 \cdot 4 \times 10^{12}$ kW or the amount of electrical energy used by the United States in one year.

The causes of hurricanes are just beginning to be understood but, as yet, there are no known ways to prevent the development of a hurricane. The measures for minimizing casualties from the initial impact centre around early warning and efficient evacuation. Since 1966, hurricanes, cyclones and typhoons have been detected and tracked by geosynchronous weather satellites. Early warning of a probable hurricane, together with orderly and efficient evacuation of the population from low-lying coastal areas to inland areas of greater elevation have been shown effectively to save lives. Better training of the public in the importance of early evacuation, however, is still needed. Early recognition activities are carried on by a number of international and national weather tracking bureaux. They can usually recognize the hurricane days before it strikes a coastal region and track it with a fair degree of accuracy. The weather bureaux are able to give timely and adequate warnings in most instances by radio and television. The efficiency of the warning system is such that virtually 100 per cent of hurricane deaths should be preventable at this time. Significant advances are being made in the area of early warning and, in the near future, almost all such natural catastrophes should be reduced potentially to, at most, minor disasters.

The main mechanism of death in hurricanes is from drowning.[6] Hurricane winds drive a wall of water before them which raises the water level to as much as 16 or 18 feet (4·5–5·5 metres) above high tide (tidal or storm surge) (*Fig.* 21.1). In low-lying coastal areas, this rapid rise in the sea level accompanied by even greater waves is capable of causing drownings many miles inland of the usual coast line. Some deaths and injuries also result from the caving-in of houses and still others are caused by trauma from flying or floating objects and debris or from entrapment in mud slides which may accompany the floods. Prevention of further casualties after the initial impact of the hurricane centres

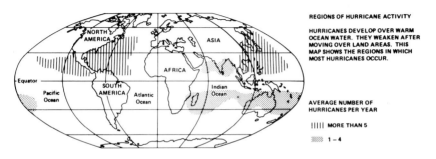

Fig. 21.3. Regions of hurricane activity.

Table 21.2. Moderate and major hurricane disasters

Date	Place	Number of deaths
October 7, 1737	Bengal, India	300 000
October 31, 1876	India	200 000
June 6, 1882	India	100 000
September 8, 1900	US—Galveston Island, Texas	6 000
September 1909	US—Louisiana	350
September 29, 1915	US—Mississippi	275
September 1919	US—Key West, Florida, and Corpus Christi, Texas	500
September 18, 1926	US—Gulf Coast	372
October 20, 1926	Cuba	600
September 12–17, 1928	Lake Okeechobee, Florida, and West Indies	4 000
September 3, 1930	Santo Domingo	2 000
September 1935	Florida Keys	408
September 21, 1938	New England (especially Rhode Island)	600
October 15–16, 1942	Bengal, India	11 000
November 1946	Philippines	500
October 1947	Hong Kong	1 000
February 1948	Reunion Island	300
June 1948	China	200
September 1948	Japan	541
June 1949	Japan	106
August 1949	China	1 000
September 1950	Japan	250
August 1951	Jamaica	154
October 1951	Japan	448
October 21, 1952	Philippines	440
September 25–27, 1953	Vietnam and Japan	1 300
October 12, 1954	Eastern US and Haiti (Hurricane 'Hazel')	347
August 18–19, 1955	Eastern US (Hurricane 'Diane')	400
September 19, 1955	Mexico (Hurricane 'Hilda')	200
September 27–28, 1955	Caribbean (Hurricane 'Janet')	500
June 27–30, 1957	US—Louisiana, Texas and Mississippi (Hurricane 'Audrey')	550
September 27–28, 1958	Japan	615
August 20, 1959	China	720
September 17–19, 1959	Japan and Korea (Typhoon 'Sarah')	2 000
September 26–27, 1959	Honshu, Japan (Typhoon 'Vera')	4 500
October 27, 1959	Mexico	2 000
June 27, 1960	Philippines	100
July 31, 1960	Formosa	100
September 4–12, 1960	Eastern US and Caribbean (Hurricane 'Donna')	148

Table 21.2. (*continued*)

Date	Place	Number of deaths
May 5, 1961	East Pakistan	185
September 12, 1961	Formosa	100
September 17, 1961	Japan	110
October 21, 1961	British Honduras (Hurricane 'Hattie')	400
February 27, 1962	Germany	343
May 28–29, 1963	East Pakistan	22 000
October 6, 1963	Haiti, Cuba, Dominican Republic (Hurricane 'Flora')	7 100
April 10, 1964	East Pakistan	128
June 16, 1964	Pakistan	250
June 3, 1964	Philippines (Typhoon 'Winnie')	107
August 24, 1964	Haiti	100
September 5, 1964	Hong Kong and China (Typhoon 'Ruby')	735
September 13, 1964	Korea	210
November 19–20, 1964	Philippines	580
December 22, 1964	Ceylon (Sri Lanka)	206
December 30, 1964	South India	500
May 11, 1965	East Pakistan	36 000
December 13, 1965	East Pakistan	15 000
September 25, 1966	Japan	174
September 29, 1966	Haiti (Hurricane 'Inez')	480
October 1, 1966	East Pakistan	850
October 9–10, 1966	Caribbean	223
May 16, 1967	Burma	100
July 19, 1967	Japan (Typhoon 'Billie')	200
November 3, 1967	Philippines	107
April 11, 1968	East Pakistan	1 000
May 10–11, 1968	Burma	1 073
August 1969	US—Louisiana, Mississippi, Virginia (Hurricane 'Camille')	256
September 15, 1970	Philippines (Typhoon 'Georgia')	300
October 14, 1970	Philippines (Typhoon 'Seniz')	583
October 15, 1970	Philippines (Typhoon 'Titany')	526
November 13, 1970	East Pakistan (Cyclone)	300 000
August 1, 1971	Hong Kong (Typhoon 'Rose')	130
June 1972	US—Pennsylvania, New York (Hurricane 'Agnes')	122
December 3, 1972	Philippines (Typhoon 'Theresa')	169
September 19–20, 1974	Honduras (Hurricane 'Fifi')	8 000
September 1976	Baja, California and Sur, Mexico (Hurricane 'Liza')	400
September 1979	Dominican Republic (Hurricanes 'David' and 'Frederick')	3 000
August 4–11, 1980	Caribbean (Hurricane 'Allen')	272

around sanitary measures and the repair or demolition of dangerous structures. People evacuated from danger areas should not be allowed to return until a competent official announces that the danger is over. This was one of the major problems which resulted in such a large death toll in the Dominican Republic hurricanes. People began to return to their homes after Hurricane David, only to be met with a second hurricane of equal magnitude (Class V) which took the same path through the Dominican Republic 5 days later.

There is usually extensive damage to sanitary facilities so that rigid measures will need to be instituted to prevent epidemics of disease. These measures must include purification of water and construction of emergency lavatory facilities. Special problems in rescue, first aid, evacuation and definitive medical and nursing care are presented by hurricanes and floods. The major rescue problem is that of locating and bringing to high land persons marooned by the rising waters. For this, special boats and amphibious vehicles with trained crews are often necessary and in some situations, helicopter evacuation may be effective. The evacuation problem may be complicated by flooding of low-lying sections of highways.

Table 21.2 lists some of the moderate and major hurricane disasters by date, place and mortality that are on record.

FLOODS

Floods result from unusual weather conditions, e.g. abnormally large accumulations of snow followed by particularly high spring temperatures and melting snow, or extremely heavy rain over a brief period of time.[6] The latter type, called a flash flood, can develop very quickly and often takes communities by surprise. Flood control is a complex problem. The most effective measures have been the reforestation of watersheds, the construction of reservoirs and flood walls, and the diversion of rivers. In addition, improved techniques for forecasting rising river levels, early warning of potential flood conditions and the rapid evacuation of people from dangerous areas have helped to keep down the number of deaths. A recent review of weather-related disasters from the United States, revealed that floods were the main cause of death and that most fatalities were attributed to flash floods.[7] The highest mortality was associated with four flash floods in which dams broke after heavy rains. Ninety-three per cent of the deaths were due to drowning and 45 per cent of these were car related.[7] Other drownings occurred at homes, campsites or when persons were crossing bridges or streams. Of the automobile-associated deaths, victims had been in cars in low areas, on flooded bridges, or which went off the road into deep water. From these data, it is clear that the involvement of vehicles and driving practices during floods needs to be investigated further, especially in developed nations.[7] Likewise, the high death toll associated with dam breaks from heavy rains deserves special attention. All types of dams should be monitored during periods of heavy rainfall so that sufficient warning of potential dam failures can be issued. The Army Corps of Engineers have identified 68 153 non-federal dams in the United States which were over 2 m high. As of May 1982, only 13 per cent or 8818 of these dams had been inspected by the Army Corps of Engineers and 2925, or one-third, had been found to be unsafe because of various deficiencies particularly due to an inadequate spillway capacity. These unsafe dams pose a public health threat and, therefore, should be closely monitored during periods of heavy rainfall especially when there are large numbers of people immediately downstream. Recently the importance of monitoring dams by personal inspection during heavy rains was demonstrated in Essex, Connecticut. Several dams in the town, which were considered unsafe by the Army Corps of Engineers, were kept under constant vigil during heavy rains on 4 and 5 June, 1982. On the evening of 5 June, water was observed to flow over the top of one of the dams. The fire department evacuated the people in parts of the town that might be affected if the dam failed. Within 1 hour of the evacuation notice, 5 dams in Essex broke. Although most of the area sustained substantial property damage, not a single life was lost.[7]

Surprisingly, in some documented floods, there have been substantial numbers of casualties due to fire. Some of these fires have been due to the floods breaking large oil and gasoline storage tanks with the resultant film of oil and gasoline on the water igniting and spreading the fire through a large area.

Table 21.3 lists some of the recorded moderate and major flood disasters throughout history. The tabulation includes dates, locations, source and the number of deaths in these flood disasters.

Inland floods can be partially prevented, or at least made less severe, by good soil management practices. Inland floods are usually caused by heavy rains or thaws of accumulated snows, or both. These factors may be aggravated by poor land conservation practices. If land is improperly ploughed and farmed, it will not hold as much moisture as if it were properly managed, and floods are likely to be more frequent and more severe. On the other hand, the really great floods which occur at relatively rare intervals are not preventable by land management practices since they involve amounts of water which are much greater than the best managed soil can accommodate. In certain areas the building of dams may help prevent flooding. However, since a broken dam can result in a greater loss of life than most floods, they should be designed with enough strength to make breakage impossible.

Training and education of the population to obey flood warnings are essential to minimize casualties from the initial impact. It is also important to avoid building homes and business premises on the flood plains of rivers.

Floods resulting from heavy rains can usually be predicted. The problem is not the lack of warning, but the tendency of some citizens to ignore the warning because they have experienced other smaller floods in the past.

The major challenge is to rescue stranded inhabitants of the area and trapped motorists. The most practical solution to this problem appears to be the use of special amphibious vehicles and helicopters. Some interesting articles on floods are worth noting here. Coolidge, reporting in 1970 on the medical response to the Rapid City flood, states that the degree of contamination in lacerations was frequently misjudged and the wounds closed primarily.[8] Unfortunately, this was all too common an error in the treatment of mass casualties and virtually all the wounds required re-opening and additional treatment within 24–48 hours. Peavy in 1970 reported that mosquito control after hurricanes and floods is an important risk problem that has not been alluded to in the past.[9] The implications in terms of mosquito-borne diseases is obvious. The problem of mosquito plagues following floods is also reported by I. M. Miles.[10]

Table 21.3. Moderate and major flood disasters

Date	Place	Number of deaths
2300 B.C.	Old Testament Flood	Most of Mankind
1099	England and Netherlands (storm tides)	100 000
1228	Netherlands	100 000
1421	Dort, Netherlands	100 000
1570	Harlingen, Netherlands	100 000
1629	Mexico City, Mexico	100 000
1642	China	900 000
1811	Danube River	500
1824	St Petersburg (Leningrad) USSR (Neva River)	10 000
1852	England (River Thames)	10 000
1869	Hawaiian Islands (Tsunami)	1 000
1883	Java and Sumatra (Tsunami—Krakatoa eruption)	36 000
1887	Honan, China (Hwang Ho River)	900 000
May 3, 1889	US—Johnstown, Pa. (dam collapse)	2 200
1896	Northeast Honshu, Japan (Tsunami)	27 000
September 8, 1900	Galveston, Texas	5 000
June 15, 1903	Heppner, Oregon	325
1911	China (Yangtze River)	100 000
March 25–27, 1913	US—Ohio and Indiana	732
1916	Netherlands	10 000
1927	US—Illinois, Missouri (Mississippi River)	313
March 13, 1928	Santa Paula, California (dam collapse)	450
1931	Shanghai, China (Yangtze River)	200 000
1936	US—Northeast States (ice jam)	107
January 22–23, 1937	US—Ohio and Mississippi Valleys	250
1938	US—New York and New England	137
1939	China, North	500 000
1941	Huarez, Peru (earth slide)	3 000
April 1, 1946	Hilo, Hawaii (Tsunami from underwater quake near Dutch Harbor, Alaska)	200
1946	Honshu and Shikoku Islands, Japan	1 000
July 1947	China	1 000
August 1947	Honshu, Japan	2 000
September 1947	India	1 000
May 1948	China	330
June 1948	China	3 500
September 1948	Japan	858
December 1948	Brazil	600
May 1949	Brazil	200
July 1949	China	57 000
October 1949	Guatamala	500
September 1950	India	270
May 1951	Formosa	300
July 1951	Japan	250
August 1951	Manchuria	4 800
November 1951	Iran	225
November 1951	Italy	150
January 31–February 1, 1953	Netherlands and W. Europe	2 000
June 1953	Japan	1 000
August 1953	Iran	265
July 1954	Tibet	300
August 17, 1954	Farahzad, Iran	2 150
August 1954	Pakistan	300

Table 21.3. (*continued*)

Date	Place	Number of deaths
August 1954	Nepal	1 000
October 1954	Italy	320
August 1955	US—New York and Pennsylvania (rains)	180
October 7–12, 1955	India and Pakistan	1 700
December 1955	India	120
July 24, 1956	Iran	1 200
August 1956	Pakistan	200
August 1956	Turkey	140
July 1957	Philippines	1 000
July 1957	China	550
July 1957	Kyushu, Japan	513
July and August 1957	South Korea	208
September 1957	Iran	120
October 1957	Spain	100
December 1957	Ceylon	300
July 1958	Argentina	350
April 1959	Madagascar	143
June 1959	China	187
June 1959	Columbia	184
July 1959	Pakistan	100
July 1959	India	139
August 1959	Taiwan	1 000
September 1959	India	500
September 1959	Brazil	100
November 1, 1959	Mexico	2 000
December 2, 1959	Frejus, France	323
March 1960	Brazil	100
September 1960	India	256
October 1960	Nicaragua	325
October 10–30, 1960	East Pakistan	10 000
July 1961	India	227
October 1961	India	1 000
November 1961	Somaliland, Africa	100
February 1962	Germany	309
August 1962	Columbia	134
September 1962	South Korea	290
September 1962	Spain	800
April 1963	Afghanistan	107
October 9, 1963	Vaiant, Italy (landslide into reservoir)	2 600
June 1964	West Pakistan	250
July 1964	Japan	106
November–December 1964	South Vietnam	7 000
July 15, 1965	Korea	323
September 16, 1965	Chile	600
January 1966	Brazil	373
March 11, 1966	Jordan	259
March 14–17, 1966	Indonesia	176
May 21–June 14, 1966	Brazil	147
August–September, 1966	Laos	300
November 1966	Florence and Venice, Italy	118
January 18–24, 1967	Brazil	785
March 19, 1967	Rio de Janiero, Brazil	136
August 28–31, 1967	Nigata, Japan	132
November 26, 1967	Portugal	462
July 14, 1968	India and Pakistan	111

Table 21.3. (*continued*)

Date	Place	Number of deaths
August 14, 1968	Gujarat State, India	1 000
October 4–7, 1968	India	2 000
March 17, 1969	Alagoas, Brazil	218
August 1969	St. James Basin, Virginia (Hurricane 'Camille')	153
September 15, 1969	South Korea	250
October 1–8, 1969	Tunisia	500
1970	East Pakistan (Bangladesh) (Ganges River)	300 000
July 22, 1970	Himalayas, India	500
1971	Orissa State, India (sea wave)	10 000
February 1972	Buffalo Creek, W. Virginia (dam collapse)	125
June 9, 1972	Rapid City, South Dakota	238
June 23, 1972	Wilkes-Barre, Pennsylvania and Allegheny County, New York	118
July 1972	Luzon, Philippines	150
August 7, 1972	Philippines	454
1973	Indus River, Pakistan	2 300
1974	Honduras	5 000
July 31, 1976	Big Thompson, Colorado	139
January 1981	Laingsburg, South Africa	100
1981	Szechwan Province, China	753
1981	Hopei, China (Yangtze River)	1 311
1982	Chontayacu River, Peru	600
1983	Saurashtra, India	408
November 1985	Armero, Columbia (volcanic eruption melted icecap resulting in mudslides and flood)	25 000

Both Bennet[11] and Janerich[12] note a significant increase in deaths from cancer following a flood disaster. Janerich specifically noted increases in leukaemia and lymphoma as well as spontaneous abortions.

In 1973, Ussher reported that the most serious problem encountered after a Philippine flood was respiratory infection.[13] He also states that snake bites accounted for 6 deaths and numerous other non-fatal cases. The snakes, the majority of which were cobras, had been driven by the floods to seek higher ground near the towns and villages.

Bouzarth reported in 1974 on some problems encountered after Hurricane Agnes and the resulting floods.[14] He noted that two of the most important elements lacking in the disaster response were command and communication. These deficiencies resulted in unexpected problems such as one doctor in a school first aid station who requested a dozen tetanus booster shots and instead received 1000, and when 10 cots were requested, 100 arrived. Still another enigma was the abuse of sirens by ambulances and medical groups, since there were very few real medical emergencies during the flood. He also noted that dedicated young volunteers who worked around the clock inevitably later became ineffective, disgruntled and disorganized. An important responsibility of medical command is to require workers to sleep 8 hours out of every 24. Another problem of communication was exemplified by the Federal Government's response to the disaster. A member of the United States House of Representatives decided that typhoid inoculations were needed and an appeal was broadcast by radio and television. Public health experts had considered both at the time and in retrospect that typhoid inoculations were unwarranted. It was difficult to persuade the public that radio and television reports were inaccurate. In addition, the military refused to let the people return to their homes after the flood subsided unless they could show proof of recent typhoid inoculation.

Another important aspect is the medico-legal one of victim identification after a major disaster. In two reports on the Big Thompson flood, Schilling[15] and Charney and Wilbur[16] both pointed out the problems of identifying victims of a mass disaster such as a flood. They emphasized that successful identification of bodies is facilitated by the presence of a forensic pathologist, a forensic odontologist and a forensic anthropologist. Their experience after the Big Thompson flood resulted in the establishment of a Centre of Human Identification at Colorado State University. Along similar lines is a report by Koseki[17] in 1970, which discussed the medico-legal aspects of drifted bodies running off into the Japan Sea after the Uetsu flood disaster on 28 August, 1967. He pointed out that in addition to drownings from the overflowing streams, there were as many lives lost in landslides, landfalls and mudflows in the mountain and valley districts. He also described a technique of drift cards to predict where bodies would be found after being washed out to sea.

There have been a number of papers on the emotional and psychological effects of hurricanes and floods.[11,18] One paper reported that women under the age of 65 years had more psychiatric symptoms than men, but that the sex difference disappeared in those over 65 years.[19] Knaus quoted Turchetti as stating that in the immediate post-disaster stage of confusion, disorganization and unstructured routine, most victims simply want to be told what to do. They do not want any further uncertainty and they need a definite routine. There were a number of papers[20-22] surrounding the Slag Dam collapse which inundated Buffalo Creek, West Virginia. Most of this revolved around the successful manoeuvre by the lawyers to gain additional monetary recovery for mental injury and psychic impairment and has been claimed to be a landmark case in terms of compensation for psychological damage.

TSUNAMIS

A tsunami or tidal wave is usually initiated by a sea-bottom slide, earthquake or volcanic eruption. Its dimensions dwarf all of our usual standards of measurement of ordinary sea- or wind-generated waves. Ordinary sea waves are rarely more than a few hundred feet long and travel at less than 60 mph. Tsunamis often extend for hundreds of miles and travel at hundreds of miles per hour. According to Lagrange's Law, their velocity is equal to the square root of the product of the depth of the water multiplied by the acceleration due to gravity.[23] Therefore, the deeper the water, the greater the speed of the wave, and in the deep waters of the Pacific Ocean, tsunamis can reach a speed of 500 mph.

A tsunami is not a single wave, but a series, separated by intervals of 15 minutes to an hour or more because of their great length. The designation 'tidal wave' is a misnomer since the waves have nothing to do with the tidal forces of the moon or sun.

Tsunamis are so shallow in comparison to their length that in the open ocean they are hardly detectable. Their amplitude sometimes is as little as 2 feet from trough to crest. Usually it is only when they approach shallow water or the shore that they build up to their terrifying heights. It is not unusual for fishermen to be at sea and not notice any unusual swells. It is only when they return home at the end of the day that they encounter the havoc and destruction that has resulted.[23]

The giant waves are more dangerous on flat shores than on steep ones. They usually range from 20 to 60 feet in height, but when they pour into a V-shaped inlet or harbour, they may rise to mountainous proportions of 100 to 150 feet.

Generally, the first salvo of a tsunami is a rather sharp swell, not sufficiently different from an ordinary wave to alarm casual observers. This is followed by a tremendous undertow away from the shore as the first great trough arrives. Reefs are left high and dry, and the beaches are covered with stranded fish. This amazing sight may attract curious and unprepared onlookers, fascinated with the denuded beach. Many may pay for their curiosity with their lives, for minutes later the first giant wave will come crashing ashore. Also deceptive is the time gap between the great waves which may be 15 to 60 minutes or more. People may be lulled into thinking the danger is over after the first great wave has crashed ashore and there is a prolonged quiet period. The waves may continue coming for many hours and the third to eighth wave in the series is usually the largest.[23]

The most infamous of all tsunamis was launched by the explosion of the volcanic island of Krakatoa in 1883. The tsunami raced across the Pacific at 300 mph and devastated the coasts of Java and Sumatra with waves 100 to 130 feet high. One of the most damaging tsunamis on record followed the famous Lisbon earthquake of 1 November, 1755. Tsunamis, however, are rare in the Atlantic Ocean and are far more common in the Pacific Ocean. Since 1596, Japan has had 15 destructive tsunamis, of which 8 were major disasters, and the Hawaiian Islands are struck severely on an average of once every 25 years.

A tsunami-warning system has been in existence since 1946 in the Pacific Ocean. The system detects unusual waves with a periodicity of 10 to 40 minutes and sets off alarms warning of an impending tsunami. The centre of the warning system is located in Honolulu, and detection centres are located at Hilo, Midway, Attu and Dutch Harbor. The centre also receives prompt reports on earthquakes from coastal survey stations equipped with seismographs. By means of charts showing wave travel times and ocean depths, it is possible to estimate the rate of approach and probable time of arrival of a tsunami originating from any spot in the Pacific.[23]

A warning system is not enough, however, and in vulnerable areas there should be restrictions on building on exposed coasts or guarantees that the buildings and homes are anchored sufficiently or raised off the ground.

MEDICAL RELIEF

Medical relief will be based on good planning and preparedness. Hurricanes, floods and tsunamis may cause injury and a variety of health problems, such as communicable disease (*see* Chapter 18), psychological problems (*see* Chapter 16), food shortage etc. Emergency supplies of drugs and equipment may be requested and these are considered in Chapter 10.

NATIONAL RESPONSE TO DISASTER

Following a disaster, there is usually a lack of reliable specific information on the extent of damage and the need for medical help. The rapid acquisition of accurate information and estimates are prerequisites both for the planning of a national relief programme and for guiding international assistance.[1] Two broad categories of information are required:

1. General data about the extent of damage, the area and population affected, the functional damage to public services, including telecommunications, roads, power and other utilities.
2. Specific medical, epidemiological and administrative information on health problems and available resources.

The number and proportions or rates of injuries need to be specified. A quick survey of the site of impact will provide baseline data and should lead to the establishment of an epidemiological surveillance system based on reporting of suspected cases of selected diseases. A detailed inventory of functional undamaged health facilities and a quick survey of medical supplies available already at the site of the disaster is requested. This quick survey may indicate that urgently needed drugs or material can be easily salvaged and used from the immediate disaster site or from areas immediately adjacent to the disaster area.

The health problems are not limited to the management of mass casualties. A clean water supply and sanitation system is important and a survey of the facilities should be included in the early assessment to determine which human or material resources will be required to cope with the emergency. Time is of the essence because, unless these resources are made available, readily and promptly, it may be too late for them to be useful. The responsibility and authority for conducting these assessments lies with the government of the affected country. Should the national resources be found insufficient for relief, external assistance from international sources will have to be sought. However, when a disaster is of such magnitude as to make extensive international aid necessary, it often happens that nationals with the necessary expertise are too scarce to conduct an adequate assessment of the extent of the damage and the needs. Consequently, teams or individuals are frequently sent to the affected area by each organization involved to carry out an independent survey and provide first-hand data on the requirements. The participation of the international community, and the joint assessment of disaster situations under the authority of the affected country, could greatly contribute to a better and more efficient response to the challenge of natural disasters. After an adequate assessment is made, appropriate measures must be initiated in different areas.

In a recent well-performed and well-conducted study, Bissell demonstrated a significant increase in post-disaster infectious diseases following hurricanes David and Frederick in the Dominican Republic.[24] He had obtained approximately 44 months of pre-disaster epidemiologic data on the endemic rates of various infectious diseases in the Dominican Republic and then compared these results with 16 months of epidemiologic data accumulated after the twin hurricanes. Of the 5 diseases examined—malaria, typhoid and paratyphoid fevers, hepatitis, gastroenteritis and measles (rubeola)—he noted statistically significant increases in hepatitis, infectious gastroenteritis, and measles occurring several months after the disaster. He also noted an increase in malaria, although the increase did not reach statistical significance and may have been due to the termination of malaria control programmes in that country several years prior to the hurricanes. There was also a statistically significant increase in typhoid and paratyphoid fever, but only in the single province most remote from the centre of the hurricane's destructive impact.

The likely reasons for the increases in infectious diseases were:

a. overcrowding of makeshift refugee centres with insufficient sanitary facilities;

b. flood-caused water transmission of pathogens.

The extreme crowding which we all witnessed clearly increased the probability of disease transmission, particularly when sanitary facilities were insufficient. There was also low population compliance with the government-supported campaigns to convince the populace to boil their water in the post-disaster period. Measles dramatically increased under the conditions of the sudden extreme population crowding after the hurricanes and took an extremely heavy toll in the malnourished or borderline-nourished paediatric population. The overcrowding increased and facilitated the airborne droplet transmission of the measles virus. The disease was already highly endemic in the Dominican Republic with a 1978 rate of more than 113 cases per 100 000 population. Vaccination campaigns had proved ineffective in stemming a generalized increase in the disease nationwide, probably due to poor cold-chain maintenance during vaccine distribution and administration. The dramatic increase in measles which occurred for the 2–3 months immediately after the hurricane provided further evidence that an insufficient portion of the vulnerable population had been provided with immunity by the previous year's vaccination campaigns.

REFERENCES

1. Champion H. R. (1984) The response to disasters. In: Shoemaker W. L., Thompson W. L. and Holbrook P. R. (eds.) *Textbook for Critical Care*. Philadelphia, Saunders, pp 93–100.
2. Garb S. and Eng E. (1969) *Disaster Handbook*. 2nd Edition. New York, Springer, pp 195–200 and 207–11.
3. Orlowski J. P. (1985) Experience with a medical disaster team in response to Hurricanes David and Frederick. *Abs. World Assoc. Emerg. and Disaster Med.* (Brighton) p 9.
4. Longmire A. W. and Ten Eyck R. P. (1984) Morbidity of Hurricane Frederick. *Ann. Emerg. Med.* 13, 334–8.
5. Eliot J. L. (1980) Into the eye of David. *National Geographic* 158, 368–71.
6. Mortality from tornadoes, hurricanes, and floods. (1974) *Statistical Bulletin, Metropolitan Life Insurance Co.* 55, 4–7.
7. French J., Ing R., Von Allmen S. et al. (1983) Mortality from flash flood: a review of National Weather Reports, 1969–1981. *Public Health Report* 98, 584–8.
8. Coolidge T. T. (1973) Rapid City Flood: Medical response. *Arch. Surg.* 106, 770–2.
9. Peavy J. E. (1970) Hurricane Beulah. *Am. J. Public Health* 60, 481–4.
10. Miles I. B. (1976) The role of the nurse in floods and earthquakes. *S. Afr. Nurs. J.* 43, 27–29.
11. Bennet G. (1970) Bristol Floods 1968. Controlled survey of effects on health of local community disaster. *Br. Med. J.* 3, 454–8.

12. Janerich D. T., Stark A. D., Greenwuald P. et al. (1981) Increased leukemia, lymphoma and spontaneous abortion in Western New York following a flood disaster. *Public Health Reports* **96**, 350–6.
13. Ussher J. H. (1973) Philippine flood disaster. *J. R. Nav. Med. Serv.* **59**, 81–3.
14. Bouzarth W. F. (1974) Flood revisited: lessons 'unlearned' from Hurricane Agnes. *Pennsylvania Med.* **77**, 61–2.
15. Schilling R. J. (1977) Victim identification in the Big Thompson flood. *J. Colo. Dent. Assoc.* **65**, 23–4.
16. Charney M. and Wilbur C. G. (1980) The Big Thompson Flood. *Am. J. Med. Pathol.* **1**, 139–44.
17. Koseki T. (1970) Medical/legal and oceanographic notes on the drifted bodies run off into the Japan Sea at the Uetsu flood disaster, August 28, 1967. *Acta Med. Biol.* **17**, 277–84.
18. Abrahams M. J., Price J., Whitlock F. A. et al. (1976) The Brisbane Floods, January 1974: their impact on health. *Med. J. Aust.* **2**, 936–9.
19. Price J. (1978) Some age-related effects of the 1974 Brisbane floods. *Aust. NZ J. Psychiatry* **12**, 55–8.
20. Newman C. J. (1976) Children of disaster: clinical observations at Buffalo Creek. *Am. J. Psychiatry* **133**, 306–12.
21. Rangell L. (1976) Discussion of the Buffalo Creek disaster: the course of psychic trauma. *Am. J. Psychiatry* **133**, 313–16.
22. The Medical Letter: Drugs for parasitic infections. January 31, 1986; **28** (issue 706): 9–16.
23. Bernstein J. (1954) Tsunamis. *Sci. Am.* **191**, 60–4.
24. Bissell R. A. (1983) Delayed impact infectious disease after a natural disaster. *J. Emerg. Med.* **1**, 59–66.

FURTHER READING

Centers for Disease Control: flood disasters and immunization—California. (1983) *MMWR* **32**, 171–2, 178.
Cervenka J. (1976) Health aspects of Danube River floods. *Ann. Soc. Belg. Med. Trop.* **56**, 217–20.
DeMan A., Simpson Housley P., Curtis F. et al. (1984) Trait anxiety and response to potential flood disaster. *Psychol. Rep.* **54**, 507–12.
Knaus R. L. (1975) Crisis intervention in a disaster area: the Pennsylvania flood in Wilkes-Barre. *J. Am. Oesteopath Assoc.* **75**, 297–301.
Logue J. N., Hansen H. and Struening E. (1979) Emotional and physical distress following Hurricane Agnes in Wyoming Valley of Pennsylvania. *Public Health Rep.* **94**, 495–502.
MacMahon A. G. and Swart J. P. (1983) The Laingsburg flood disaster. *S. Afr. Med. J.* **63**, 865–6.
Schmitt N., Catlin H. B., Bowmer E. J. et al. (1970) Flash flooded trail, British Columbia, 1969. *Can. J. Public Health* **61**, 104–11.
Titschener J. L. and Kapp F. T. (1976) Family and character change at Buffalo Creek. *Am. J. Psychiatry* **133**, 295–9.
World Health Organization (1980) Emergency care in natural disasters: views of an international seminar. *WHO Chronicle* **34**, 96–100.
World Health Organization (1979) The selection of essential drugs: second report of a WHO expert committee. *WHO Technical Report Series* **641**, 7–44.

C. Manni, S. Magalini and R. Proietti

22

Volcanoes

Interim e Vesuvio monte pluribus locis latissimae flammae altaque incendia relucebant, quorum fulgor et claritas tenebris noctis excitabatur.

From *The Letters of Pliny Book VI. 16*

VOLCANIC PHENOMENA

Volcanic events have had a considerable importance in the geological history of our planet and their enormous destructive power is referred to in many stories and legends which have been handed down through the ages.

These processes continue today, although with less frequency than in ancient times, and often produce profound effects on human life. There are about 500 volcanoes in which recent activity is recorded. There are many other inactive volcanoes, considered to be extinct, but some of them could become active again in the future.

The molten material which is expelled by the volcano is called magma or lava and is made up of a mixture of siliceous and other material containing dissolved gases. The force which drives the magma towards the surface of the volcano is produced by the dissolved gases. The degree of violence of the eruption is directly proportional to the quantity and effervescence of the gases as well as the viscosity of the magma.

Normally, the basaltic lavas are less viscous and contain less gas than the siliceous ones. Their eruptions are thus quieter and produce currents of lava compared with the siliceous lava volcanoes which are explosive and produce abundant pyroclastic material. Pyroclastic material is classified as lapilli if roundish in shape with little liquid content. If, instead, it appears as irregular fragments of magma foam it is called ash, and the even smaller fragments (about 1–4 mm) make up the dust.

Volcanic activity is not continuous. There may be long periods of dormancy and eruptions can vary greatly in duration and magnitude, not only from one volcano to another but even in the same volcano. An eruption manifests itself in different ways. These may follow each other as sequential stages of one eruption, with the expulsion of different types of material. Moreover, other geological events can be associated with the eruption, such as earthquakes or seaquakes, which aggravate the effects of the eruption itself. The different ways in which a volcanic eruption can manifest itself include:

Ashfall
Pyroclastic flow
Mud flow
Lava flow
Volcanic gases
Tsunami

Ashfall

In explosive eruptions the magma is fragmented into liquid and solid parts and is projected by the gases to form a column of material which extends from the mouth of the volcano upwards. Pliny, describing the eruption of Vesuvius in 79 AD, said that '. . . its general appearance can best be expressed as being like an umbrella pine, for it rose to a great height on a sort of trunk and then split off into branches . . .'. The larger fragments rapidly fall in an area adjacent to the volcano, while the smaller ones and the ashes can be taken many kilometres away by the wind. The volume of ash erupted can be very large and usually amounts to a cubic kilometre of material. Ashfall is the most common eruptive phenomena and is produced in virtually every eruption.

The effect of ashfall is dependent on its volume and the duration and intensity of the eruption and can accumulate in considerable depth around the volcano. Pliny tells us that, '. . . the courtyard giving access to his room was full of ashes mixed with pumice stones . . .'.

The weight of ash on roofs can make them cave in. Fine ash dispersed in the air can cause respiratory problems for humans and animals, and in high concentration can cause fatal asphyxia. Furthermore, the ash contains toxic substances such as fluorine which can contaminate water sources and stores.

High concentrations of ash make traffic circulation difficult by causing a cloud which obscures visibility, hindering the evacuation of the disaster areas and the arrival of help by air and by land. Engines often break down because of air filter obstruction, radio communications become impossible, and short circuits in aerial electrical systems occur, causing interruption in the supply of electricity.

Pyroclastic Flow

Some explosive eruptions produce currents of gases containing ashes and lapilli in direct suspension. This phenomenon is called a pyroclastic current or a glowing avalanche and can be compared to the rings of an atomic mushroom. They move at great speed and have an enormous destructive power. Due to the weight of the ashes and the larger fragments of lava, these pyroclastic currents are denser than the surrounding air and slip down the sides of the mountain, behaving like avalanches of snow or rocks. The main features of this type of eruption are the high velocity (up to 500–700 km/h), the horizontal direction of spread, and the very high temperature (more than 1000°C).

Pyroclastic flows represent the most lethal and destructive volcanic phenomena; they burn and destroy everything in their path. There is practically no chance of survival. Direct contact, suffocation by the enormous quantity of ash and the intense heat cause the death of all animal and vegetable life. The effect is also devastating on buildings which are burnt, destroyed and buried by the pyroclastic material. The city of St Pierre in Martinique was devastated by this type of eruption in 1902, causing the deaths of 29 000 people.

Mudflow

The pyroclastic material produced by volcanic eruptions accumulates on the sides of the mountain and in the adjacent valleys and in some cases can form enormous deposits, many metres thick.

When heavy rain falls on these deposits, they are transformed into a dense fluid mixture with a consistency like that of fresh cement which can easily flow down the flanks of the mountains towards the valley. The phenomenon particularly occurs in volcanoes situated in humid, tropical regions with heavy atmospheric precipitations, as in Indonesia, where they are called 'lahars'. The rate of flow depends on the volume and viscosity of the mud as well as the slope of the terrain; it usually reaches 50 km/h, but in exceptional cases it can even reach 100 km/h. Many mudflows are formed when heavy rainfall occurs after an eruption, but any condition which causes water to mix with the pyroclastic material can be the cause.

Like pyroclastic flows, mudflows are very dangerous and their high density makes them capable of destroying everything in their path. When the flow stops, it is possible to see deposits of material several metres thick. These deposits are too soft to be crossed and so the population remains trapped as if by quicksands and rescue is rendered very difficult. In the recent eruption of the Nevado del Ruiz in Columbia (November, 1985), the eruption had melted the glaciers and the mudflow buried the town of Armero causing the death of about 23 000 people.[1]

Lava Flows

Lava flows are formed by melted magma which escapes from the volcano in a non-explosive manner and spreads over the surrounding land. The flow rate depends on several factors, such as the emission rate, the slope of the land and the viscosity and volume of the lava.

Viscous lava advances very slowly and its surface often assumes a solid aspect as in the case of Etna and Vesuvius. In the Hawaiian volcanoes, by contrast, eruptions of very fluid lava occur and are emitted in torrents which travel for a distance of several kilometres from the volcanic orifice. Lava flow, however, independently of its viscosity, destroys practically everything in its path. Furthermore, surfaces covered by lava cannot be used for cultivation for many years. On the other hand, the speed of flow is in general sufficiently low to permit humans and animals to be saved.

Volcanic Gases

The emission of volcanic gases always accompanies an eruption. The chemical composition of these gases varies from volcano to volcano and can also undergo changes, over time, in the same volcano.

The most common gases are: steam, carbon dioxide, sulphur dioxide, carbon monoxide, hydrogen, hydrocyanic, hydrochloric and hydrofluoric acids and methane. They represent a danger for all forms of life and since they can continue to be emitted even during periods of quiescence they constitute a constant risk in the neighbourhood of an active volcano.

Tsunami

Tsunami is a Japanese word which describes a gigantic wave caused by a collapse of the ocean bed. It can be caused by subsidence of the wall of a volcano's crater located at sea level. The agitation of water can cause waves up to 30 m high, which can have disastrous effects on coastal areas. The eruption of Krakatoa in 1883 produced a wave that hit the coast of Java and Sumatra and caused the deaths of 36 000 people.

PRECURSORY PHENOMENA

The degree of danger due to an eruption is determined by the type of volcanic event and its violence. Eruptions with pyroclastic flow and mudflow offer no hope at all of salvation for individuals who have been hit by the eruption. In these cases the only hope is to predict the eruptive event in time to arrange for the population to be evacuated to a safe place. Even with current technology it is still not possible to 'look inside' the volcano to follow all the reactions which precede the start of an eruption. However, some physical and chemical phenomena have been observed before volcanic eruptions which can be considered as premonitory. These include:

Seismic activity
Ground deformation
Hydrothermal phenomena
Chemical changes

The presence of these phenomena cannot predict with certainty how and when an eruption will occur, but it can indicate the probability that within a certain period there is the possibility of an eruption.

Seismic Activity

One of the earliest and most common precursory phenomena of an eruption is an increase in seismic activity around the volcano. It has been noted that almost all the major eruptions have been preceded by local earthquakes days or months before, often with a dramatic increase in the hours before the beginning of the eruption.

Ground Deformation

As the magma is projected towards the mouth of the volcano, the earth on the slopes of the volcano or in the immediate neighbourhood sometimes is elevated. In some cases these deformations can be spectacular and visible to the naked eye; at other times sensitive instrumentation is necessary to check the vertical and horizontal movements of the earth.

Hydrothermal Phenomena

Changes in temperature and discharge intensity in fumaroles and springs around a volcano have been observed, and although these phenomena are not easy to interpret they can give indications of the imminence of eruptive phenomena.

Chemical Modifications

Even in periods of inactivity volcanoes emit gases from the underlying magma. Variations in the relative concentration of the main constituents, and in particular an increase in the relative content of sulphur compared with chlorine, can be considered as signs that the magma is approaching the surface.

Although the science of predicting volcanic eruptions is still in its early days, by analysing various signs together with the history of the volcano, it is possible to forecast its future behaviour in order to take appropriate precautionary measures. These measures can only consist of the evacuation of the potentially affected areas. In 1976 at La Souvrière in the French Antilles, 72 000 people living around a volcano were evacuated in the expectation of an imminent eruption which then actually did not take place. In 1980, before the eruption of Mount St Helens in the USA, the surrounding zone was evacuated and this meant that there were only 52 victims when it occurred.

PREPARATION OF EMERGENCY PLANS

Every populated area situated in the neighbourhood of an active volcano exposed to the risk of a volcanic event should have an emergency plan for tackling a possible eruption. Emergency plans of this type must encompass:
1. Identification and delineation of the areas at risk.
2. Identification of adjacent areas to where the population can be evacuated in case of a dangerous eruption.
3. Identification of collecting points and roads to use in case of evacuation.
4. Training and instruction of personnel who will conduct the rescue and evacuation of the population affected by the eruptive phenomenon.
5. Identification of hospitals and medical services situated in the nearby areas.
6. Arranging procedures for alerting the population (sirens, radio warnings, etc.).
7. Periodic exercises.

RULES OF BEHAVIOUR IN CASE OF ERUPTIONS

The danger areas must be totally evacuated if eruption is forecast. All the inhabitants of such zones should know about the evacuation plans which directly involve them. Thus, at the alarm signal, they ought to leave their houses calmly, turning off electricity, gas and water as they depart.

In the areas which can be affected by secondary phenomena, such as ashfall, the inhabitants should:
1. Remain inside with doors and windows closed.
2. Outside, wear heavy, non-inflammable woollen garments and place masks

or gauze soaked in water over the nose.
3. Not attempt to escape by car since the engine could break down due to ash aspiration.
4. Keep informed by the radio, without overloading the telephone lines.
5. Extinguish any fires due to the fall of lapilli.
6. As soon as possible remove ash from the roof to avert the danger of collapse.

MEDICAL PROBLEMS

Very few data exist in the literature concerning the type of lesions caused by a volcanic event. Almost all the data at our disposal relates to the eruption of Mount St Helens which occurred in May 1980 in the USA. In the major volcanic eruptions recorded in history, the disasters of 79 AD in Pompeii or at St Pierre in Martinique in 1902, the entire population was wiped out in the space of a few minutes. Death, or survival without serious lesions, seems to be the general rule on such occasions. However, it is sometimes possible to find a few, seriously wounded survivors, who were on the margins of the destructive flow of the volcanic eruption.

As for the other types of major disasters, it is necessary to prepare a plan for evacuating the wounded and the homeless to safe zones, where emergency services will be provided. From the medical point of view, there are basically three problems which have to be tackled:
1. Polytrauma and fractures caused by impact with fragments of solidified lava or from the collapse of buildings.
2. Skin burns.
3. Respiratory problems in victims exposed to air with a high ash content, together with thermal damage to the respiratory tract, caused by exposure to hot vapours.

In addition, individuals may be asphyxiated by toxic gases such as carbon dioxide, accumulating in low-lying places such as house cellars or valleys. Later on, problems caused by drinking water contaminated by toxic substances of volcanic origin may occur.

The diagnostic and therapeutic aspects concerning multiple injuries and burns are dealt with in Chapter 2, so only the respiratory problems which have particular importance in a volcanic event will be considered in greater detail.

RESPIRATORY PROBLEMS

Inhalation of Ash

The most frequent cause of death in volcanic eruptions is by asphyxia from inhaling ash. After the eruption of Mount St Helen in 1980, 23 autopsies were carried out on the bodies found and 18 of these had died from asphyxia.[2] In the majority, the ash had mixed with mucus and formed plugs which had obstructed the principal airways (trachea and main bronchi). According to Thorarinsson,[3] in the eruption of Vesuvius in 79 AD the main cause of death, similarly, was the inhalation of great quantities of very fine ash. This phenomenon was already noted by Pliny who in his letter reports: '. . . I imagine because the dense fumes choked his breathing by blocking his windpipe . . .'.

In victims exposed to a lesser degree, the inhalation of volcanic ash can result in the adult respiratory distress syndrome (ARDS). Two patients who were struck by the edges of a pyroclastic flow during the eruption of Mount St Helen were admitted with extensive burns and rapidly developed fatal ARDS.[4] The autopsy revealed the presence of volcanic ash in the lungs. Ashfall can spread a great distance from the volcano, and this can cause mild respiratory disturbances in wide sections of the population. After the ashfall following the eruption of Mount St Helen there was a considerable increase in admissions for respiratory disease, mainly consisting of asthma, bronchitis and resurgence of chronic respiratory failure, over a radius of about 200 km.[5]

In the patients affected by asthma, the symptoms most frequently observed were dyspnoea, wheezing and irritating cough. In patients with acute bronchitis there was a cough with abundant sputum, congestion of the nose and upper airway and chest pains. The most serious cases were naturally in patients already suffering from chronic respiratory failure. The presence of ash also caused an increase in eye disturbances, mainly consisting of conjunctivitis and corneal abrasion.

At the time of the Mount St Helen eruption, studies were undertaken to assess the effects of volcanic ash on the lungs and the potential risk of inducing pneumoconiosis.[6] Laboratory tests carried out on the ash from the eruption of 18 May showed that it did not have an acute toxicity. It contained 3–7 per cent silica crystals but the fluorine and heavy metals content was not high and, moreover, the sample was not radioactive. Research carried out *in vivo* also demonstrates that volcanic ash has little fibrogenic power and, therefore, the risk of pneumoconiosis arising is only likely in people exposed for a long time. Furthermore, these substances induce a marked inflammatory reaction at pulmonary level. This data has also been confirmed by the post mortem examination of the lungs of the two people who died from ARDS, which showed an acute interstitial reaction with the presence of giant cells and macrophages containing ash.

For patients with respiratory problems which might lead to ARDS, it is advisable to arrange admission to an intensive care unit where appropriate respiratory support measures are available, ranging from CPAP to mechanical ventilation with PEEP.

As far as asthmatic crises are concerned, it is advisable to administer bronchodilators such as aminophylline and corticosteroids intravenously or by aerosol combined with O_2 therapy as required.

Inhalation of Volcanic Gases

The inhalation of volcanic gases can give rise to respiratory disturbances which can be of a serious nature. Various volcanic gases produce toxic effects in man.

Carbon Monoxide

This gas binds with haemoglobin through a bond 200 times more tenacious than that of oxygen and haemoglobin and thus reduces the amount of oxygen carried to the tissues, causing hypoxic damage to the nervous system, heart, kidneys and liver. The toxic effect is directly proportional to the inspired concentration of the gas and to the length of exposure.[7] The signs and symptoms of intoxication from carbon monoxide (CO) relate well with the blood levels of carboxyhaemoglobin. Concentrations of carboxyhaemoglobin up to 20 per cent do not usually cause symptoms; headache, nausea, vomiting and psychomotor agitation appear from 20–40 per cent; hyporeflexia and hypotonia associated with a soporific state or light coma develop at 40–60 per cent and levels above 60 per cent are generally fatal.

The first therapeutic measure for CO intoxication is to administer oxygen for at least 2 hours, until the carboxyhaemoglobin level has fallen to 15 per cent. Hyperbaric oxygen therapy reduces the half-life of the carboxyhaemoglobin and results in a conspicuous rise in the quantity of oxygen dissolved in the blood. This is usually sufficient to ensure adequate tissue oxygenation. Subsequently, neurological tests should be carried out to assess the degree of hypoxic damage to the central nervous system.

Hydrofluoric Acid

This substance inhibits enzymatic processes by capturing calcium. A lethal dose corresponds to $0\cdot03–0\cdot06$ per cent concentration in the blood. Symptoms include coughing, oedema of the glottis, dyspnoea, pulmonary oedema and hypo-calcaemia. Therapy consists of respiratory assistance, corticosteroids and calcium.

Sulphur Dioxide

This is colourless gas with an irritant and suffocating effect, produced by the combustion of sulphur and carbon. The maximum acceptable dose is 5 ppm; at 3 ppm the odour is perceived and at 20 ppm there is irritation of the upper airways, coughing and inflammation of the eyes. At 400–500 ppm inhalation can be lethal. Symptoms are irritation of the larynx, coughing, difficulty in speaking, dyspnoea, broncho-constriction, and respiratory arrest. After a few days, pulmonary oedema, pneumonitis, conjunctivitis and corneal lesions can appear. The therapy consists of the administration of steroids and bronchodilators, intravenously or by aerosol, associated with appropriate fluid therapy and respiratory support.

Thermal Airway Damage

The inhalation of superheated air can cause burns of the respiratory tract. The lesions are usually located on the face, oropharynx and in the upper airways (above the vocal cords); lower burns (trachea and pulmonary parenchyma) are rare since before arriving at this level the air is effectively cooled in the oropharynx and nasopharynx.[8]

However, the inhalation of steam, which has a latent heat capacity 4000 times greater than air, can cause burns down to the level of the bronchioli and pulmonary alveoli. This can lead to pneumonitis with an increase in the capillary permeability and pulmonary oedema, which may progress to ARDS.

Thermal lesions may be combined with those caused by inhaled toxic gases. The type and location of these lesions will depend on the substance inhaled, its concentration and the length of exposure. Those agents of volcanic origin generally cause inflammatory lesions in the upper respiratory tract, which may progress to ulceration. When the lower portion of the respiratory tract (trachea and bronchi) is damaged, the ciliary apparatus ceases to function, preventing the expulsion of secretions. The tracheal and bronchial mucous membranes become inflamed and oedematous and this may progress to necrosis, with the formation of pseudomembranes. The chemical irritation can also cause bronchial spasm.

Treatment consists of maintaining the patency of the airway by endotracheal intubation or tracheostomy, correcting the hypoxemia, and aspiration of secretions from the respiratory tract.

Burns of the upper airway may cause acute obstruction, so when there is stridor present or considerable oedema of the lips, tongue, palate and oropharynx, it is advisable to intubate the patient as soon as possible and, in cases where the lesions are particularly serious and extensive, it is better to carry out a tracheostomy at an early stage.

Hypoxemia represents one of the greatest dangers and oxygen must be administered as soon as possible and continued with artificial ventilation if necessary.

Bronchospasm and retained bronchial secretions should be treated with bronchodilators and careful bronchial toilet.

Finally, there is a strong likelihood of secondary infection which should be treated with appropriate antibiotics, based on the results of sputum and blood culture.

CONTAMINATION OF THE ENVIRONMENT

The zones covered by ashfall can be very extensive. The ashes can contain toxic substances such as fluorine and sulphur which can contaminate the water supply used for drinking or irrigation. Chemical analysis should be carried out to ensure that the water is drinkable, and the population should be kept informed of the situation until it has returned to normal.

The same procedure should be followed before authorizing the sale of vegetable products which have been contaminated by ash.

REFERENCES

1. Editorial (1986) Columbia Nevado del Ruiz volcano erupts. *Disaster Preparedness in the Americas* Issue 26.
2. Eisele J. W., O'Halloran R., Reay D. et al. (1981) Death during the May 18, 1980, eruptions of Mount St Helens. *N. Engl. J. Med.* **305**(16), 931–6.
3. Thorarinsson S. (1979) On the damage caused by volcanic eruption with special reference to tephre and gases. In: Sheets P. D. and Graison D. K. (eds.) *Volcanic Activity and Human Ecology.* New York, Academic Press, 133.

4. Porsley P. F., Kiessling P. S., Antonius J. et al. (1982) Piroclastic flow injury. Mount St Helens, May 18, 1980. *Am. J. Surg.* **143**(5), 565–8.
5. Baxter P. J., Roy I., Falk H. et al. (1981) Mount St Helens eruptions May 18 to June 12, 1980. An overview of the acute health impact. *JAMA* **246**(22), 2585–9.
6. Green F. M., Vallyathon V., Hentroch M. et al. (1981) Is volcanic ash a pneumoconiosis risk? *Nature* **293**, 216–17.
7. Jackson D. L. and Menges H. M. (1980) Accidental carbon monoxide poisoning. *JAMA* **243**, 772–4.
8. Chu C. (1981) New concept of pulmonary burn injury. *J. Trauma* **21**, 958–62.

FURTHER READING

Tomblin J. F. Managing volcanic emergencies. *UNDRO News*, Jan. 82.
Volcanic Emergency Management (1985) Office of the United Nations Disaster Relief Co-ordinator (UNDRO), Geneva.

Man-made Disasters

Judith Fisher

23

Road Traffic Accidents

INTRODUCTION AND HISTORICAL REVIEW

To many people road accidents simply happen. Society is complacent about road traffic accidents until they or their family become an accident statistic. The very term 'accident' suggests the event is beyond control. In the European Community one and a half million people are injured and 55000 killed every year in road traffic accidents.[1] (*Fig. 23.1.*)

Statistics show that lives are lost needlessly, frequently from simple causes such as a blocked airway or fluid depletion. The mortality increases with increasing delay before definitive medical therapy is given to the patient.[2] Trauma care systems must continue to develop throughout the world in an attempt to reduce this carnage which is sometimes described as the biggest epidemic of our time.

Accidents have happened in relation to moving vehicles since the invention of the wheel (*Fig. 23.2*). In the USA it took just 52 years to kill 1000000 people as a result of road traffic accidents. The first fatal accident according to Baldwin[3] occurred in New York City in 1899; the millionth occurred in December, 1951.

With increasing power and speed has come an increase in injury and death. Road accident statistics in the United Kingdom were first recorded in 1909 but injuries were not included until 1926. In 1909 there were 101000 motor vehicles on the roads and 1070 associated fatal accidents.[4] By 1985, there were over 21000000 vehicles and around 5000 fatal accidents.[5] Road deaths did not follow a steady upward trend. The peak in 1941 (9169) may have been influenced by the prevalent war time conditions including blackout, inexperienced drivers and absent road signs (*Fig. 23.3*).

318

The worst recorded road traffic accident occurred in Afghanistan in November, 1982 when a petrol tanker exploded in the Salang Tunnel. Accurate figures for fatalities were unobtainable but estimates ranged from 1100 to 2700, most deaths being due to carbon monoxide inhalation.[6]

In 1949, Smeed[7] examined road traffic accident statistics from 20 countries in various stages of development and observed that deaths declined as vehicle ownership increased. He supported this observation with a complicated mathematical formula which, although not totally matching the figures for every country world wide, approximately reflected the psychological and social pressures keeping accidents in check. This hypothesis is reinforced by the declining deaths per 100 million vehicle kilometres travelled per annum.[8] These figures for the United Kingdom were 318 in 1955 compared with 88 in 1983. Declining figures were also seen in Europe and the bulk of the 'developed' nations. However, an increase in these figures was noted not only in countries where the petrol engine and sophisticated road technology are comparatively recent innovations (such as Chile and Korea), but also in New Zealand, South Africa, Hong Kong and Japan. It is postulated that these countries may have reached the limit where no further improvement can be obtained because legislation, engineering and improvements in attitude can no longer hold back the tide.

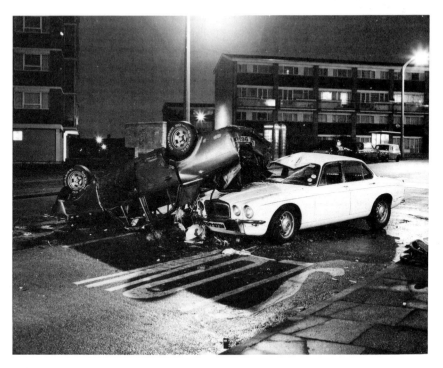

Fig. 23.1. Two-car collision: Jaguar with second car overriding its bonnet.

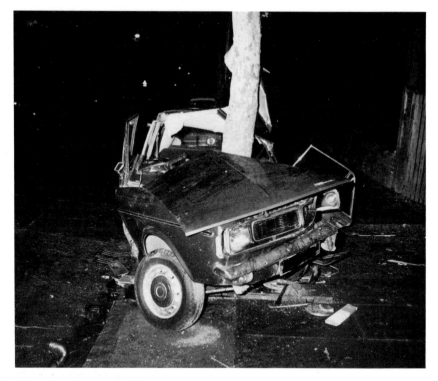

Fig. 23.2. The side of the car is its weakest point.

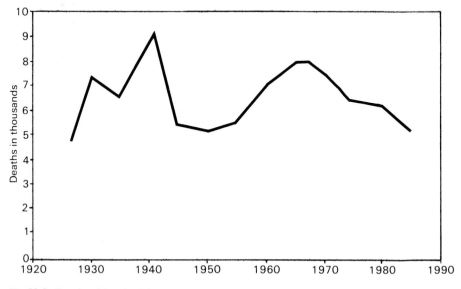

Fig. 23.3. Road accident fatalities in the United Kingdom, 1926–1985.

AETIOLOGY AND PREVENTION

The much neglected pandemic of road accidents does not follow the expected pattern of increasing accidents with increasing density of road traffic. The figures are influenced by various fluctuating human and socio-economic factors. However, certain trends emerge:

a. The vulnerability of travel by two-wheeled transport.
b. The role of alcohol, vehicle and road engineering, legislation and driver's age.
c. The increasing ability of road users to avoid accidents and perceive risks.

Various national and international organizations have studied this epidemic. One of the most comprehensive reports reflecting international opinion is that by Dr Werner Dollinger, West German Minister of Transport, in his 1984 Road Safety Programme for the Federal Government.[9] This states that traffic safety must be a common concern and ends with an appeal for co-ordinated action to fight death and injury on the roads. The West German report highlights the following trends in the period under review (1970–82):

1. The total number of accidents did not fall but the number of fatalities was markedly reduced with a moderate fall in total casualties.
2. The risk of becoming involved in an accident decreased, despite the large increase in traffic.
3. Motorways (autobahns/autoroutes/autostradas/freeways) are the safest roads per vehicle kilometre.
4. The risk of injury to car passengers and pedestrians decreased.
5. The number of accidents involving cyclists increased.
6. Accidents involving motorcycles and mopeds has increased to alarming levels.
7. Overall, the number of children involved in accidents has decreased; they are less endangered as pedestrians but as cyclists the chance of injury has increased.
8. Learner and inexperienced drivers are a danger both to themselves and to other road users.
9. Excessive speed, together with alcohol, are still the major causes of accidents.

Following these findings, Dollinger proposed a comprehensive accident prevention plan together with steps to reduce the time between an accident and the provision of medical care. Mortality and morbidity can be reduced by this decreased response time.

A pilot study of earlier accident detection was held in the Darmstadt area of West Germany from 1982–4.[10] It showed that it was cost-effective to reduce the time from accident to mobilization of the rescue services (Period A, *Fig.* 23.4), rather than increase the number of vehicles deployed to reduce the response time (Period B, *Fig.* 23.4). This reduction was achieved by fitting small transceivers in passenger vehicles which were either manually or automatically triggered by an accident. A series of relay stations throughout the region transmitted the signal to the central control based at the ambulance HQ. The central control could locate the signals on a computerized map and despatch rescue vehicles to the correct location. Two-way transmission, with a conscious accident victim on site, allowed assessment of the situation and, if necessary, first aid instruction. This *Autonotfunk* system cost about £120 per vehicle but it was estimated that not all vehicles needed to be fitted as, during the trial, accidents tended to be reported by passing vehicles. It has been estimated that if the system was fitted to 1 in 20 vehicles it would markedly reduce response time— much less expensive than employing extra highly trained staff with sophisticated vehicles.

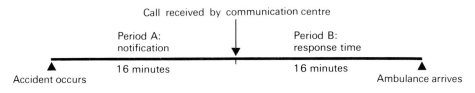

Fig. 23.4. Reporting and response times in Darmstadt, FRG.

TRAINING

Resuscitative procedures are poorly dealt with in medical schools in the UK despite industry producing increasingly life-like training aids. In the USA CPR is compulsory for licensure in most states but training in arresting haemorrhage and coping with fractures is sporadic. Postgraduate experience is variable but increasingly more hospitals are running joint disaster exercises with their colleagues who work in the community. These may be table top exercises or simulated accidents on newly completed but unopened stretches of motorways.

Improvement in pre-hospital morbidity depends as much upon the doctor working alongside other medical, paramedical and rescue personnel as on the individual skills and techniques he needs to master. These techniques can be learnt in formal advanced trauma courses but it is also essential to acquire the skills of intubation and intravenous cannulation at regular intervals in the operating room rather than relying on the intermittent practice obtained at poorly lit roadsides, frequently in the wind and rain. Studies have shown that advanced life support skills decay within months[11] if not regularly used.

An imaginative course on principles of field extrication covering immediate care for medical personnel has been pioneered by the Emergency Medical Services at Burbank together with the Los Angeles County Department of Health Services.[12] Hospital-based doctors responsible for monitoring the progress of an incident and the performance of the paramedics, together with the paramedics themselves, spend a weekend obtaining 'hands on' experience and having seminars on incident management. At the Maryland Institute for Emergency Medical Services the first bachelors degree in EMS management was instituted in 1981 after an initial assessment of need.[13] In the UK the Royal College of Surgeons of Edinburgh, after running a successful course in pre-hospital medicine, has decided to establish a Diploma in Immediate Care. Such courses are helping establish immediate care as a specialty in its own right.

PREPARATION

A family practitioner interested in practising road traffic accident medicine needs to have not only his medical skills kept sharp but also a special understanding of and attitude towards the hostile environment of the accident scene. He and his family must be prepared for sudden unscheduled interruptions to their daily life, not to mention sharing the family car with a wide selection of equipment. The equipment required can be divided into:

Transport
Communication
Protection
Medical
Documentation

Transport

A reliable vehicle suitably adapted to regional weather and geographical variations should be immediately available. It should have adequate storage space for equipment and suitable emergency lights and markings. In the UK a green rotating beacon is used exclusively by doctors. In Hong Kong emergency motorcycles are used and it has been suggested that an ordinary bicycle can be fitted with sufficient equipment to cope with a cardiac arrest and circumvent traffic jams. A spare set of car keys should always be carried to allow the police to remove or secure the car when necessary.

Communication

At the simplest level call-out can be by telephone. The ambulance service and, if appropriate, the police service, must have current telephone numbers and locations for each doctor at all times. A portable radio telephone makes this easier. Doctors may be more willing to be involved in immediate care schemes if they have pagers or two-way radio to give more freedom. The two-way radio, particularly if linked to the local ambulance service, will allow monitoring of the incident on the way to the call as well as providing a facility for radio advice. If the attending doctor is no longer required at the scene he can also be informed while *en route*.

Protection

It is of course foolish for the doctor to become a casualty statistic. He must remember at all times the rule to protect himself as a first priority. This will include an attitude of mind as he drives rapidly but safely to the scene of the incident. To have an accident will only create more work for the other emergency services and cause embarrassment all round. The doctor is no use to anyone unless he arrives. Driving must only be at speeds compatible with the prevailing conditions. A wide variety of hazards, including weather, toxic substances, petrol, glass and electricity, may make the scene even more hostile. A variety of protective equipment is therefore necessary to meet all possible situations and these must include (*Fig.* 23.5):

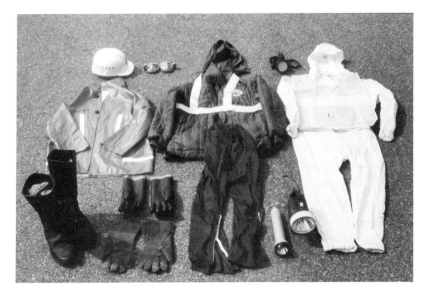

Fig. 23.5. Protective clothing.

Waterproof/windproof jacket and trousers
Fluorescent tabard inscribed 'DOCTOR' front and back
Protective helmet and goggles
Oil- and acid-resistant boots
Respirator (if the situation demands)
Protective gloves

Hazards from blood are increasingly a problem. The doctor must be alert to this and take appropriate precautions, including having hepatitis B vaccine to minimize the risks.

Medical

Medical equipment should be familiar to the user and packed in sturdy, easily portable containers, each clearly marked.

Airway

A range of Guedel airways.
A laryngoscope with adult and paediatric blades, spare batteries and bulb.
A selection of endotracheal tubes ready cut to size and with appropriate connectors. Magill forceps. Syringe to inflate the cuff of the endotracheal tube. Small artery forceps, tape and bandage to secure the tube.
Aspirator and catheters.
Self-inflating bag and a selection of face masks of different sizes. A paediatric/ neonatal bag is also advisable.
Oxygen cylinder connected to a suitable automatic ventilator.
Chest drains and Heimlich valves (or urine bag with flap valve).

Intravenous Infusion

Giving sets suitable for blood transfusion later.
Selection of cannulae.
Fluids, e.g. normal saline, Hartmann's solution and Haemaccel or Gelofusine.
Blood tubes and syringes for cross-matching.
Arm splints, tape and bandages to secure the i.v. line.
Hot packs to enhance venous dilation.

Surgical Equipment

Scissors, artery forceps.
Cut down set.
Amputation set.
Cricothyrotomy set.
Esmarch bandage.

Splints

Box splints.
Inflatable splints.
Traction splint.
Cervical splint.

Dressings

Selection of field wound dressings.
Triangular bandages.
Crêpe bandages.
Burns dressings.
Tape and strapping.
Safety pins.

Diagnostic

Stethoscope.
Sphygmomanometer.
Auroscope/ophthalmoscope.
Pen torch.

Miscellaneous

Shears or strong scissors.
Waterproof torch.
Reflective foil blankets.
Accident report forms.
Triage cards.
Blood forms.
Note pad.
Camera.

Drugs
Entonox (50% nitrous oxide/oxygen).
Sterile water.
Diamorphine or morphine.
Nalbuphine.
Naloxone hydrochloride.   Preferably in pre-loaded syringes.
Ketamine.
Diazepam.
Phenytoin.

		score
1.	Measure 'Capillary Return'	
	Normal	2
	Delayed	0
2.	Measure Respiratory Effort	
	Normal	3
	Shallow	2
	Retractive	1
	None	0
3.	Eye Opening	
	Spontaneous	3
	To voice	2
	To pain	1
	None	0
4.	Verbal Response	
	Orientated	4
	Confused	3
	Inappropriate words	2
	Incomprehensible words	1
	None	0
5.	Motor Responses	
	Obey commands	4
	Withdraws	3
	Flexion	2
	Extension	1
	None	0
	The Trauma Index =	
	Sum of scores for functions 1 − 5	

Fig. 23.6. Trauma Index.

Medical problems may have precipitated the accident, so drugs for medical emergencies are useful:

Dextrose (50% sol. in 50ml).
Glucagon.
Adrenaline 1:10000.
Hydrocortisone hemisuccinate.
Lignocaine hydrochloride.
Atropine.
Salbutamol sulphate for i.v. administration or as nebules for use with nebulizer.

GLASGOW COMA SCALE

Eyes	Open	Spontaneously	4
		To verbal command	3
		To pain	2
	No response		1
Best motor response	To verbal command	Obeys	6
	To painful stimulus	Localizes pain	5
		Flexion - withdrawal	4
		Flexion - abnormal (decorticate rigidity)	3
		Extension (decerebrate rigidity)	2
		No response	1
Best verbal response		Orientated and converses	5
		Disorientated and converses	4
		Inappropriate words	3
		Incomprehensible sounds	2
		No response	1
Total			3-15

Fig. 23.7. Glasgow Coma Scale.

Documentation

The clinical state of a person involved in a road accident is constantly changing and this altering pattern of signs and symptoms is critical in diagnosis, particularly in the case of closed head injury and, to a lesser extent, in the case of chest and abdominal injuries. In the chaos of the initial event it is essential that observations are recorded and the doctor is more likely to do so if he only has to complete a simple form with boxes to tick. Various accident report forms have been devised; the important thing is to be familiar with the form, have it produced with non-carbon duplicating paper so that a copy can go with the patient and allow enough space for repeated observations to be recorded. Three copies are useful as the third can be used for statistical analysis and research.

When there are several casualties, triage labels are useful. There are several international systems available such as that used by British immediate care doctors. These are sturdy cards enclosed in a waterproof polythene envelope attached to the patient with a large safety pin. These are colour-coded and read:

1. Immediate priority—RED
2. Urgent priority—YELLOW
3. Delayed priority—GREEN
4. Dead—WHITE
5. Patient report form

The uppermost card shows the priority category. This is easily changed by displaying a new priority card. The 5th card is visible on the reverse. Various scoring systems have been devised to enable information to be passed in numerical form and predictive values have been given to these scores in some systems, such as the Trauma Index (*Fig.* 23.6). This score is also used as a triage index with the lowest score, less than 7, being given immediate priority. Intermediate priority is given to scores of 7–15 and those of 15–16 get a low priority (*see* Chapter 2).

Scales have been devised for levels of consciousness, the most well known being the Glasgow Coma Scale (*Fig.* 23.7), which is simple but reliable, providing the observer is aware of the complicating effects of drugs and alcohol. Any form is only of value if properly and clearly completed. A hard-backed clipboard with a waterproof cover makes the task simpler.

APPROACH TO THE ACCIDENT

It is important to arrive at the scene and park in a safe and effective position. The position of vehicles at the scene of an accident is extremely important. On motorways there is a standard procedure with parking positions to be adopted by the arriving emergency services. It is normal for the doctor's vehicle to be driven in front of the incident and parked to leave space for the ambulances between the accident and the doctor's vehicle (*Figs.* 23.8 and 23.9). The keys should be left in the vehicle with the engine running and warning lights and beacons flashing. The police are acquainted with the vehicle and advised that it may be moved, if necessary. On other main roads the emergency vehicles arriving must plan to park themselves in a manner to protect the accident from both directions and the ambulance should park so that the loading of passengers is made as easy as possible, with the minimum carrying distance. The area protected by emergency vehicles should be a safety zone in which the personnel can work (*Fig.* 23.10).

On arrival the doctor needs to look, listen/talk, smell and observe the situation:

Look

- —Clock
- —Scene
- —Casualties and their numbers
- —Vehicles
- —Trail of damage
- —Steering wheel—the chest
- —Vehicles—the abdomen
- —Contents of cars
- —Blood stains

Listen/Talk

- —Respiration
- —Speech
- —Consciousness
- —Intoxication
- —Amnesia
- —Pain
- —Story of accident
- —All accounted for
- —Reassurance

Smell

- —Petrol
- —Fire
- —Vomitus
- —Acetone
- —Alcohol
- —Gas

Observe

- —Colour
- —Respiration
- —Vomitus
- —Bleeding
- —Deformity
- —Movements—normal and abnormal
- —Response to stimuli
- —Pupils
- —Pulse

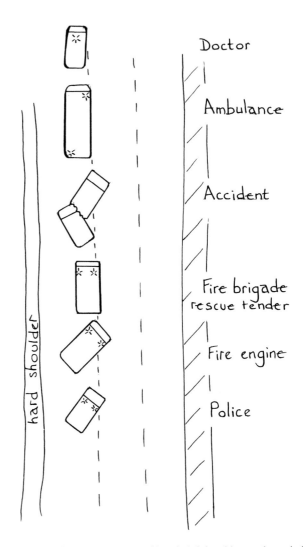

Fig. 23.8. Parking plan for emergency vehicles: motorway accident in left-hand lane only, or in left and centre lanes.

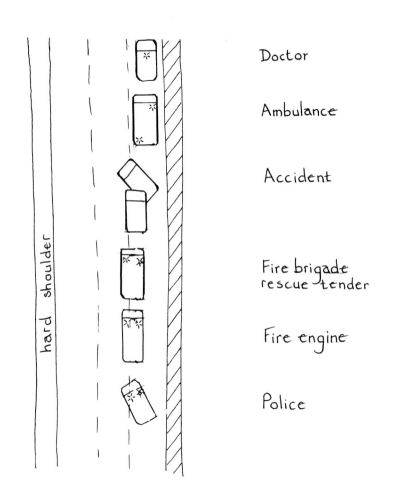

Fig. 23.9. Parking plan for emergency vehicles: motorway accident in right-hand lane, or in right and centre lanes.

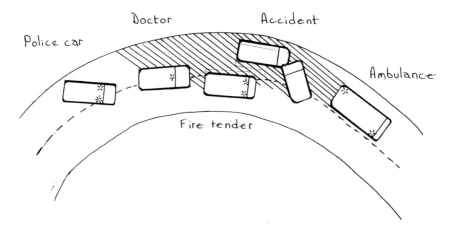

Fig. 23.10. Emergency vehicle positions at a road accident on a normal British road (hatching indicates safe area).

The doctor is then able to make a quick assessment of casualties—they may be being attended to by members of the public or emergency services or left entirely on their own. The golden rule is to look at the quiet ones first; those making most noise are at least breathing and, therefore, can initially be ignored in favour of those who are quietly dying in a corner.

THE MANAGEMENT OF CASUALTIES

Having identified the priority casualties, the doctor must ensure an airway and ventilation in each casualty. Major haemorrhage should be adequately and appropriately controlled and an intravenous infusion started on patients with multiple injuries or entrapment with associated injuries.

Having dealt with the problems associated with the airway and fluid loss, the next priorities are pain control and management of fractures and burns. Pain relief is normally achieved by inhaling Entonox, a 50 per cent mixture of oxygen and nitrous oxide (*Fig.* 23.11). It can be self-administered by the casualty, using a demand system, or by the attending medical or ambulance personnel using an override valve. Entonox should not be used in the presence of a major head injury but if the patient is conscious and in pain, then it can be safely used.[14] If Entonox proves ineffective, further analgesia can be obtained by using small titrated amounts of intravenous morphine, diamorphine, ketamine or nalbuphine. It is important that the drug is given intravenously because it is not absorbed from an intramuscular site in a shocked patient. As a result further injections may be given and it is not until the patient is recovering from shock in hospital that a large amount of the drug is suddenly absorbed and signs of overdose, or even respiratory arrest, develop. If analgesia needs to be extended to the point of anaesthesia, then ketamine is the drug of choice.

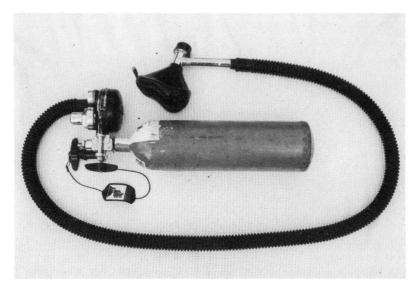

Fig. 23.11. Entonox equipment.

Fractures should be dealt with by immobilization and this in itself will reduce pain. There are a variety of devices available to immobilize fractures. Fractures of the cervical spine are probably the most critical fractures to stabilize and wherever possible the patient should have his neck immobilized with a cervical splint, such as the Hines cervical splint, before being extracted from the vehicle[15] (*Fig.* 23.12). Any unconscious patient with a head injury should be assumed to have a cervical spine injury until proved otherwise. Fractures of the arms and legs are best dealt with by immobilization, using box splints, inflatable splints and even triangular bandages. Once the patient is released onto an ambulance stretcher trolley, it is desirable to use traction splints for fractures of the femur since these are not easily stabilized by other methods.[16] The value of early effective splinting is in reducing pain, blood loss, subsequent shock and other complications.

Burns occurring as a result of a road traffic accident are relatively rare and occur only in about 1 in 500 accidents. Burns should normally be dealt with by cooling with cold water and by covering to protect from secondary contamination. Intravenous fluid replacement is mandatory if the burn is more than 10 per cent of the surface area, particularly if it is associated with other injuries.

Chest injuries require skilled assessment by an immediate care physician who can identify a developing tension pneumothorax. In such circumstances, a chest drain inserted in the second intercostal space in the midclavicular line, may be life-saving. The drain is then attached to a Heimlich valve or urine bag with a flap valve or purpose-designed chest drainage bag. Penetrating wounds of the chest are best covered by waterproof and airproof dressings, sealed on 3 sides only to prevent intrapleural tension rising. Any developing surgical emphysema should be noted.

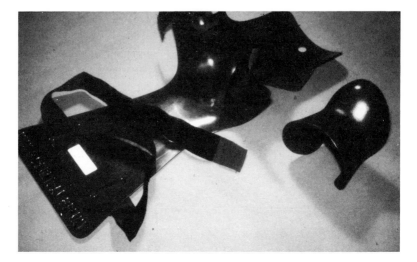

Fig. 23.12. Hines Cervical Splint.

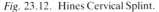

Cricothyrotomy, and other similar procedures to preserve the airway, are very rarely necessary at the roadside but the physician should have the equipment available to perform these should the situation arise. Modern cutting and rescue equipment mean that amputations are virtually never necessary at the roadside, although they are required, from time to time, at accidents involving trains. If an amputation is considered, it is normal policy to have two doctors agree that the procedure is needed to save the patient's life. The amputation is done quickly and as low as possible, using ketamine/diazepam anaesthesia, if required. The amputation can be revised in hospital later.

Where there are multiple casualties, the immediate care doctor, together with a senior ambulance officer, should make evacuation arrangements. Where there is a large number of critically injured casualties it seems appropriate to distribute them to more than one hospital, if at all possible (*see* Chapter 11).

READING THE WRECKAGE

The experienced immediate care doctor becomes able to read the wreckage of a road accident and anticipate the types of injuries he will find in the casualties. Rear end collisions cause a whiplash injury to the driver of the car in front and also to his front seat passenger.

The head-on collision, with a distorted steering wheel, suggests the driver of that car will have chest injuries. Bodies are softer than metal and where there is major distortion of the car frame, one should also anticipate even greater degrees of distortion to the passengers. The weakest parts of a car are the side doors and a side collision on the left side should alert the attending doctor to the possibilities of a ruptured spleen, ruptured left kidney, or ruptured left lung, with associated rib fractures. Similar left-sided limb or pelvic fractures may occur. If the collision is on the right side of the vehicle, the right-hand passengers are likely to suffer right-sided injuries, including the possibility of a ruptured liver. The dashboard and parcel shelf are another common cause of injury (*Fig.* 23.13). Fractures of the hip are commonly caused by the passenger's knees coming into contact with the dashboard. Similarly, the internal vehicle mirror may be responsible for lacerations to the head. Windscreen injuries have become rare since the introduction of safety belts. A quick examination of the seat belts should indicate whether or not they were being worn at the time. The windscreen can be broken both from within, by the passenger's head, or from without, as a result of the collision. The distribution of glass and the direction of the dent in the screen should give this clue.

Fractures of the ankle and lower leg, associated with entanglement in the pedals, is also common. The injuries observed and the pattern of the vehicle damage is often enough to confirm who was the driver in situations where it is subsequently disputed.

When pedestrians are involved in collisions there may be impact marks on the vehicle and it is possible to correlate these with the injuries the pedestrian has sustained. Eye witness accounts of the direction in which the pedestrian was

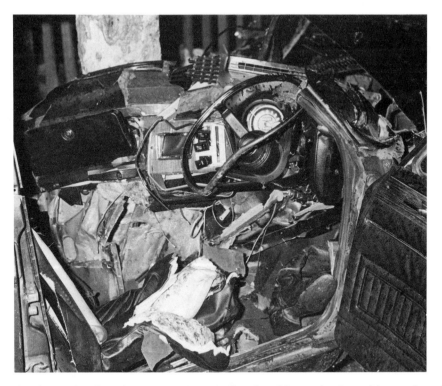

Fig. 23.13. Interior of car after RTA showing gross distortion of the metalwork—anticipate reciprocal injuries in the passengers.

going and how he was thrown, perhaps onto the bonnet or roof, will also be of help in assessing the likely injuries sustained.

This information about the scene of the accident and the state of the wreckage is rarely available to the doctors at the hospital. It is important that the suspicions of the doctor on site should be relayed to the emergency department who will treat the patient later, using the agreed report forms. On occasions, polaroid photographs of the accident are of enormous assistance to the hospital staff in understanding more clearly what happened in the accident.

ENTRAPMENT

The fire brigade provide the manpower and the equipment for extricating trapped casualties. Once the first risk is minimized, they work with the ambulance service and the doctor to remove the patient safely, without further injury or delay. The ambulance crew and doctor stabilize the patient's condition by maintaining an adequate airway, commencing an intravenous infusion, stabilizing fractures, where possible, and providing adequate analgesia prior to the release of the patient.

There are certain common types of entrapment seen at the roadside and some simple techniques which may enable the patient to be released with the minimum of difficulty. Where possible at least one ambulanceman should be in the vehicle with the victim whilst he is being released to monitor progress, to offer reassurance, observe the casualty's vital signs and protect him from further damage. It is quite common for the door nearest the trapped casualty to be jammed, but often the other doors are undamaged and may offer access. The front seats can often be slid back to give better access to patients trapped in a folded floor panel, or around the pedals. The seats of some modern cars can be tipped back into the horizontal position and this is particularly helpful if the casualty is shocked. The principle involved when dealing with entrapment is to create a big enough hole to release the patient without any risk of further damage or unnecessary aggravation of pain (*Fig.* 23.14). It is quite simple to cut the A and B posts on the side of the car and remove the whole of one side of the car or the roof. It is also possible to cut the steering column or pedals if these are obstructing the patient's removal. Spreader bars and jacks can be used to separate folds of buckled metal to release a limb that is tangled between them. A useful technique is to release the shoe of the patient by cutting and removing the shoe lace. If necessary, a sharp pair of shears can be used to cut the shoe itself allowing the foot to be released, leaving the trapped shoe behind.

Occasionally, entrapment is complicated by impalement on roadside furniture such as road signs, scaffold poles, wooden fences or stakes or pieces of metal from other vehicles such as the bumper (fender), pedals or door handles. The golden rule is to leave any object impaled in the victim until he is in the operating room. This means that the impaling object needs to be cut to a reasonable size, packed, padded and supported during transport to hospital. Caution is required with hot cutting of metal since heat is conducted to the victim. Heat retarding putty may prevent heat transmission. With wooden objects a saw is usually best, provided it is adequately supported and does not cause undue movement of the impaling object (*Fig.* 23.15).

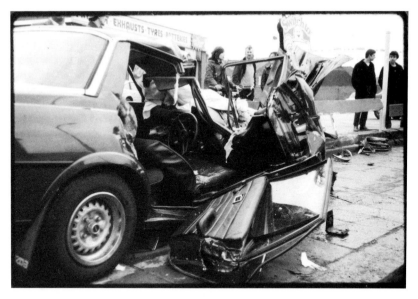

Fig. 23.14. Make a large enough hole to remove the trapped casualty without increasing his injuries.

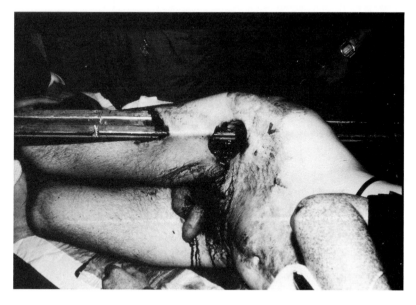

Fig. 23.15. Penetrating wound—a piece of lorry trim causing penetrating injury to car driver.

CONFIRMATION OF DEATH

An important role of the immediate care doctor is to confirm death at the scene of the accident. This enables the rescue services to spend time with those patients who are likely to have a chance of survival rather than attempting resuscitation of those who are beyond hope. Photographs of the deceased can be taken *in situ* by the investigating police officers and the bodies can be removed directly to the nearest public mortuary, without crossing local authority boundaries, so that they can be dealt with by the coroner or equivalent officer in whose area the death was confirmed. Attending doctors can prepare statements for police officers investigating the accident while still at the scene, so avoiding considerable delays later on. In the accident and emergency department, staff who would be involved in confirming death and making statements can concentrate on attending to the injured. It is important, where live casualties are admitted, that the hospital is made aware of the number and identity of victims confirmed dead and delivered to the public mortuary so that enquiries can be handled effectively and sympathetically.

SUMMARY

The concept of 'snatch and run' which used to get the patient to hospital as quickly as possible with minimum care at the scene has now largely been replaced internationally by a philosophy involving a reasonable period of 'stay and stabilize'. This stabilizing policy has been shown effectively to reduce morbidity and mortality both in war and in peace. The benefits of extended ambulance training to paramedic level and the provision of skilled medical aid at the scene of road accidents has been studied by Dooley,[17] and others, and all report the value of aggressive pre-hospital resuscitation as long as unnecessary delay is not incurred.

Accident statistics remain appalling. In the UK there are still some 5000 deaths from road accidents each year. This epidemic of carnage and injury is a major challenge to the emergency services. In many countries the ambulance services are progressing towards training which will include intravenous cannulation and infusion, intubation and defibrillation. There will, however, still be a need for doctors to work alongside these professional ambulancemen. Techniques using chest drains, amputations, intravenous analgesia and cricothyrotomies almost always require a doctor's presence. In the USA it has been rare to have a doctor on site, but paramedics work according to protocols or are advised or directed by radio. In the UK the integrated team approach using doctors and highly trained ambulancemen has been a successful model to work from. A recent report from San Francisco, assessing quality assurance in pre-hospital care, raised the question of medical involvement in the prospective, immediate and retrospective aspects of emergency work.[18] In the pre-hospital care of road traffic accident victims, the ambulanceman and the doctor have an excellent opportunity of working together and establishing a combined, highly skilled, efficient service for the multiply injured victim.

REFERENCES

1. *Road Accidents Great Britain, 1985*. (1986) London, HMSO.
2. Mackenzie C. F., Shin B. and Cowley R. A. (1986) Comparison of deaths, clinical status and duration of helicopter or ambulance transport following motor vehicle accidents. *J. World Assoc. Emerg. Disaster Med.* **1–4**, 199.
3. Baldwin D. M. (ed.) (1955) *Motor Vehicle Traffic Accident Facts 1955*. Sun Life Assurance Co. of Canada, p. 41.
4. *Transport Statistics Great Britain, 1974–84*. (1985) London, HMSO.
5. *Basic Road Statistics*. (1985) British Road Federation.
6. McWhirter N. (1985) *Guinness Book of Records*. Enfield, Guinness Superlatives.
7. Smeed J. R. (1949) Some statistical aspects of road safety research. *J. R. Stat. Soc.* Series A, Part I.
8. International Road Federation *World Road Statistics, 1979–83*.
9. The Federal Ministry of Transport (1985) *Road Safety Programme 1984*. Bonn.
10. Fisher J. M. (1985) What price earlier accident detection? *J. Br. Assoc. Immed. Care* **8**, 37–8.
11. Kaye W. and Mancini M. E. (1985) A tool for evaluating actual advanced life support performance. (Paper presented at the 4th World Congress on Emergency and Disaster Medicine.)
12. Rottman S. J., Rasumoff D. et al. (1986) Principles of field extraction for medical personnel. *J. World Assoc. Emerg. Disaster Med.* **1–4**, 175–7.
13. Gordon D. L. and Cowley R. A. (1986) Educating for the future of emergency medical systems. *J. World Assoc. Emerg. Disaster Med.* **1–4**, 171–4.
14. Baskett P. J. F. and Withnell A. (1970) Use of Entonox in the ambulance service. *Br. Med. J.* **2**, 41–3.
15. Hines K. C. (1980) The Hines Cervical Splint. *J. Br. Assoc. Immed. Care* **3**(1), 23.
16. Robertson B. (1986) Sager Traction Splint. *J. Br. Assoc. Immed. Care* **9**(3), 61–2.
17. Dooley A. (1979) Co-ordination. *J. Br. Assoc. Immed. Care* **2**, 20–5.
18. Holroyd B. R., Knapp R. and Kallsen G. (1986) Medical control—quality control in pre-hospital care. *JAMA* **256**, 1027–31.

Railway Accidents

It was an awful sight
Amid the pouring rain,
The dead and dying lying there
Beneath that mighty train.
No tongues can ever tell,
No pen can ever write,
No one will know but those who saw
The horrors of that night.

From: *The Wreck of the Royal Palm* by Rev. Andy Jenkins, 1926. In: K. L. Lyle
(1985) *Scalded to Death by the Steam*. London, W. H. Allen.

INTRODUCTION

Ever since the beginning of railways in the early 19th century accidents have
occurred all over the world as a result of mechanical failure, human error or
environmental disaster. The latter, such as landslips, floods, bridge or tunnel
collapses, can and have overtaken trains and their passengers with disastrous
consequences. Railway accidents can also result from malicious acts of vandalism
as well as livestock straying onto the track.

Generally, however, railways remain a relatively safe form of travel. In 1984,
415 people died and 9228 were injured on the railways of the United Kingdom.
Of the fatalities only 76 were killed in accidents related to actual train operation,
the remaining 339 being trespassers and suicides. Those killed in relation to
railway operation were approximately equally divided between passengers and
railway staff and the figures include the occupants of vehicles involved in
accidents at level crossings.[1]

HISTORICAL REVIEW

The earliest fatality on the UK railways is traditionally considered to be William
Huskisson, the Member of Parliament for Liverpool, who was hit by Stephenson's *Rocket* and sustained a fractured femur at the opening ceremony of the
Liverpool and Manchester Railway on 15 September, 1830 (*Fig.* 24.1). He was
then taken to Eccles, riding on the engine *Northumbrian* which established a
world speed record on that journey of 36mph (57kmph)! In fact Huskisson was

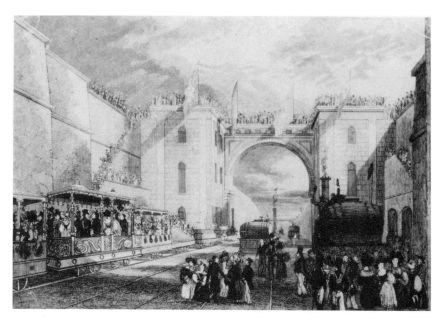

Fig. 24.1. The opening ceremony of the Liverpool and Manchester Railway, 15 September, 1830.
(Reproduced by courtesy of National Railway Museum.)

not the first railway fatality. That dubious honour goes to one David Brook who
was killed by a Blenkinsop engine on 5 December, 1821 while walking home
along the track.[2] One hundred and sixty-three years later in 1984, 179 people
were killed or injured trespassing on UK railways walking along the track and
being struck by trains.[3] Nothing ever changes and people rarely learn from
history.

Historically, the worst railway disaster in the world occurred as recently as 6
June, 1981 when over 800 died after a train plunged into the Bagmati river in the
Bihar State of India. The high death toll was largely due to the local custom of
riding on the roof of the rolling stock, something which would certainly not be
encouraged by western railway operators (*Fig.* 24.2).

The worst railway accident in the United Kingdom occurred at 06.50 h on 22
May, 1915, at Quintinshill in Dumfrieshire. It involved 5 trains, and 227 people,
mostly troops on their way to the ill-fated Dardanelles, met their deaths, with a
further 246 injured in the conflagration that followed the collision of 3 of the
trains (*Fig.* 24.3). The cause was human error, in that a signalman forgot where
he had shunted a local train and, to quote from a book on the disaster, 'other
great accidents may yet occur, but there will never be another Quintinshill.
It belongs to a vanished era—the era of steam. Never again will live coals from a
locomotive firebox set ablaze wooden carriages lit by gas.'[4] In the days before
motor ambulances were common and when it took the Carlisle fire brigade over
3 hours actually to bring hoses to play on the burning coaches, contemporary
accounts describe horrendous injuries. Local doctors were on the scene then and
with the help of joiners' saws were amputating limbs of hopelessly trapped

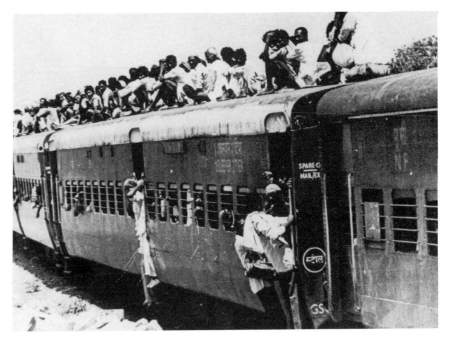

Fig. 24.2. The local custom of riding on the roof of the rolling stock contributed to the high death toll in the Bagmati River railway accident.
(Reproduced by courtesy of Popperfoto.)

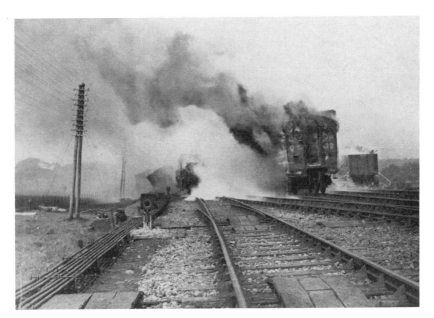

Fig. 24.3. The Quintinshill rail disaster, 22 May, 1915.
(Reproduced by courtesy of *Illustrated London News* Picture Library.)

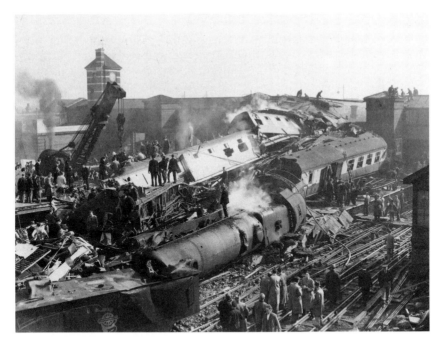

Fig. 24.4. The Harrow railway accident, 8 October, 1952.
(Reproduced by courtesy of Fox Photos Ltd.)

victims to free them from the blazing inferno. There is even an account of soldiers being shot by their own officers as an act of mercy as they lay trapped and burning helplessly.

England's worst rail accident occurred on 8 October, 1952 at Harrow, North London, when 112 died in a triple train accident (*Fig.* 24.4). Like Quintinshill, these types of accident should now be a thing of the past as they ought to be prevented by the modern type of automatic train control and warning systems.

CLASSIFICATION OF RAILWAY ACCIDENTS

All involved in medical rescue services should be aware of the specialized situations in which they may have to work when called to incidents on the railways. It is worth remembering, therefore, the UK classification of railway accidents because they can all give rise to casualties. The current classification is:

1. *Train accidents,* such as derailments.
2. *Movement accidents* caused by the movement of railway vehicles killing or injuring staff working on the railway or passengers falling from trains or platforms.
3. *Non-movement accidents* to people on railway premises.
4. *Failure* of railway stock, track or structures.

THE APPROACH TO A RAILWAY INCIDENT

In all railway incidents safety of all personnel must be paramount. Electrification, be it by overhead cables or a third rail, presents a constant hazard, particularly if the accident has brought down overhead power lines. The voltages used for railway traction vary around the world, although an international standard of 25kV 50Hz has been adopted for new electrification work. Within the UK other voltages will be found, ranging from 1500V d.c. overhead to 750V d.c. in a third rail system. A small amount of third rail system is operated at 1200V d.c. The London Underground operates by a third rail at 600V d.c. outside the running rails and has a fourth rail between them which is part of the return circuit and can carry up to 250V d.c.

Although it is assumed that the medical presence at the scene of a railway incident is part of an organized emergency service response, there are some

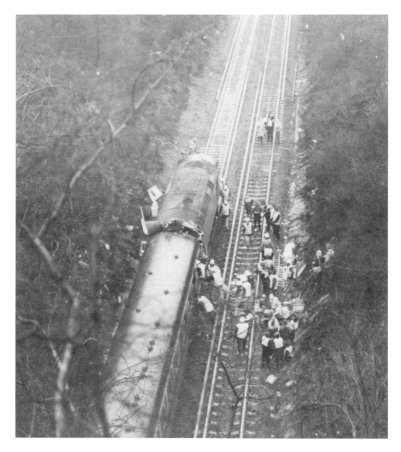

Fig. 24.5. The problems of access to the scene of a collision at the mouth of a tunnel near Micheldever, Hampshire.
(Reproduced by courtesy of *Basingstoke Gazette*.)

important rules to be observed by all involved to ensure everyone's safety. All rescue personnel should wear high visibility protective clothing, including a hard hat when working on the permanent way.

Following any incident the train crew, if capable, will safeguard the train by warning the nearest signalman, thus raising the alarm. Detonators will be placed on the track to warn following drivers. If the incident occurs on third rail electrified track a short-circuiting bar, which is carried on the train, can be used by the train crew to short-circuit the current.

Never assume that the electric current is off until confirmed by railway staff either present at the scene or via one of the emergency service controls who will be in contact with the appropriate railway control room. It is important to remember that electric trains can coast over dead track for some considerable distance and diesel units will, of course, be able to run normally over electrified track even when the current is off. If the incident is confined to a single track, as may be the case with a suicide, then trains may well continue to operate, albeit under caution, on the adjacent track or tracks and it is important to remember that the third rail, if present, will still be live.

Most modern railway systems have some form of trackside communications for the use of railway staff. Should it prove necessary to use railway trackside telephones, two types are available in the United Kingdom. Signal telephones will be found at intervals on a lineside structure and are clearly marked with

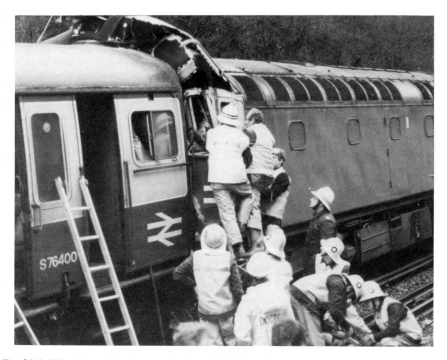

Fig. 24.6. The driver of the locomotive that collided into the rear of a staff train near Micheldever, Hampshire, remained trapped in the wreckage of his cab for some 4 hours.
(Reproduced by courtesy of *Basingstoke Gazette*.)

black and white diagonal stripes. Electrification telephones are identified by a red telephone motif on a white background and the word electrification. If used by non-railway personnel it is important to state clearly what the problem is; your name and the service or organization to which you belong; the telephone box number you are using and the name of the nearest railway station, if known.

One feature often differentiates railway accidents from other types of incident. The inaccessibility of the scene of the accident often leads to both equipment and casualties needing to be carried for considerable distances. A typical example of this occurred at Micheldever in Hampshire, where a free-running locomotive ran into the back of a staff train (*Fig.* 24.5). This occurred at the mouth of a tunnel and the entire initial emergency service response had to descend down the side of the cutting with many attendant hazards. The driver in this case was trapped by his leg and intravenous resuscitation was commenced during a prolonged 4-hour release operation. The major rescue problem here was the difficulty for the fire brigade of cutting the heavy metal of the locomotive (*Fig.* 24.6).

Railway incidents may also be spread over a large area and therefore access points, emergency service rendezvous points, casualty collecting points and equipment dumps may all need to be established. The access and emergency service rendezvous points will usually be controlled by the police. They will undertake a co-ordination role in liaison with all the other services present as they would at any major incident. It is important to remember that in addition to the local police force in whose area the accident has occurred, the transport police will be involved in the investigation, so their officers will arrive at the scene in due course. In addition, the railway's own engineering, maintenance and rerailing teams will arrive at the scene and their specialized knowledge of railway equipment and additional cutting equipment will be invaluable to the regular rescue services.

HAZARDS ON THE RAILWAYS

Although accidents like Quintinshill and Harrow hopefully should never be repeated, there are still many potential hazards on the railways and trains still collide for many and varied reasons. For example a free-running locomotive ran into the back of a stationary train of freight wagons. The result shown in *Fig.* 24.7 clearly illustrates the force of impact and the obvious hazards to the rescue services in extricating the train crew, one of whom was killed.

Hazardous loads, ranging from fuel oils to nuclear waste, are carried by rail and the modern risks were highlighted in December 1984 when a collision occurred in Greater Manchester where a passenger train ran into the back of a train of fuel tankers. On this occasion gas oil from ruptured derailed tankers sprayed over the locomotive of the passenger train and was ignited by its hot exhaust. The conflagration that followed engulfed the 3 derailed tank wagons, the locomotive and the leading 2 coaches of the passenger train. Two people died in the accident and 68 were taken to hospital with minor injuries but all were discharged after treatment.[5] The close proximity of the M602 motorway allowed easy access for the emergency services to contain the incident.

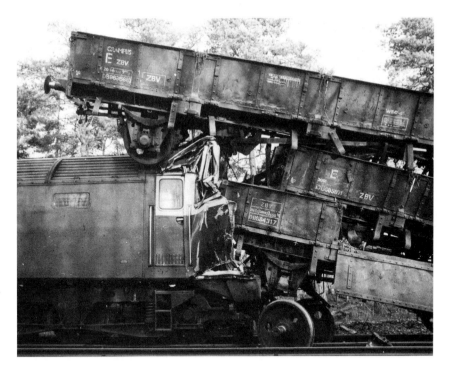

Fig. 24.7. The force of impact when this locomotive ran into the rear of a stationary freight train caused 5 wagons to be lifted off the track and posed a major hazard for the rescue services.
(Reproduced by courtesy of *Basingstoke Gazette.*)

The fire service attending this incident was made aware of the contents of the tank wagons both by the 'HAZCHEM' markings they displayed and by subsequent confirmation from the local British Rail control room. British Rail runs a computer-based system known as the Total Operating Processing System (TOPS) on which every rail locomotive and vehicle is recorded. It produces details of train loads of freight and, therefore, as in the case of this accident, the local control room could question its TOPS terminal and obtain the contents of the tank wagons involved. This information was then transmitted to the fire service control room.

Various specialists may well become involved in railway accidents, depending on the nature of the incident. Contingency plans exist, for example, for accidents to irradiated nuclear fuel rail transport flasks and all emergency service personnel should be aware of them.[6] In any such incident, in addition to all the usual services that would attend a railway accident, a Flask Emergency Team would be mobilized by the Electricity Generating Board. Their role would be to examine the transport flask for damage, carry out radiation monitoring in the immediate area and advise both the railway and the other agencies present on any appropriate action. Similar arrangements exist in other countries.

ACCIDENTS AT LEVEL CROSSINGS

Accidents occurring at level crossings can create a major challenge to the rescue services in that they combine features of both road and rail accidents, often with high speed impact, particulaly on main railway lines. There are over 10000 level crossings on British Rail. They come in 11 varieties ranging from manually operated gates or barriers controlled by closed circuit television to open crossings with no warning devices. Although the numbers are being reduced, there are still over 2000 footpath crossings on the railway network. Some 15 per cent of all fatalities related to railway operation in 1984 occurred at level crossings.

The worst level crossing accident in the UK occurred at Hixton, Staffordshire on 6 January, 1968. Here a train travelling at 70 mph (110 kmph) collided with a transporter carrying a 120 ton transformer. This transporter was only travelling at 2 mph (3 kmph) and had failed to clear the crossing before the automatic barriers closed. The accident resulted in 11 deaths and 45 serious injuries.[7] There were many difficult rescue problems here as a result of the concertina effect of the passenger coaches of the train.

Two cases illustrate the medical problems that can present in level crossing accidents. The first occurred at an automatic open crossing where the train was travelling at a slow speed of only some 10 mph (16 kmph) and was in collision with a car (*Fig.* 24.8). Witnesses stated that they had seen the crossing warning lights flashing prior to the accident. Despite the comparatively slow speed of impact considerable damage was done to the car, which resulted in problems of access to the female driver. She was unconscious and trapped in the upright

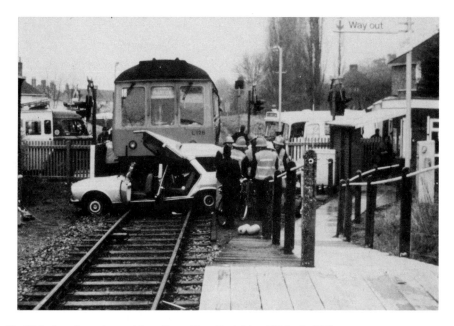

Fig. 24.8. Level crossing accident, Furze Platt, Berkshire, 30 March, 1981.
(Reproduced by courtesy of Transport and Road Research Laboratory.)

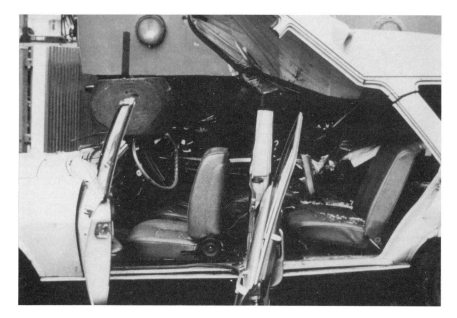

Fig. 24.9. Relative positions of the buffer of the train and the steering wheel of the car.
(Reproduced by courtesy of Transport and Road Research Laboratory.)

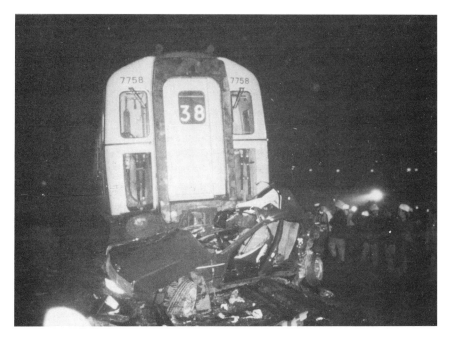

Fig. 24.10. The scene of a level crossing accident at Pooley Green, Egham, Surrey, in which the car
was propelled along the track for some 250 m.
(Reproduced by courtesy of Dr C. Carney.)

position with a poor airway. Clinically she had a fractured base of skull and therefore maintenance of the airway was paramount. It is not difficult to see why she had a severe head injury when one looks at the relative positions of the buffer and the steering wheel of the car (*Fig.* 24.9). Her airway having been safeguarded, an intravenous infusion was commenced because of the likelihood of other injuries resulting from the impact. She was eventually extricated after the fire brigade cut off part of the roof of the car, and she was taken to the local hospital, ultimately to be transferred to the regional neurosurgical centre where she underwent craniotomy to control her intracranial haemorrhage. She made a satisfactory recovery, thus illustrating the importance of aggressive on-site resuscitation prior to extrication.

The second example is of a much higher speed impact at an automatic half barrier crossing. Here a car with 5 occupants zig-zagged around the lowered half barriers and was hit by a train travelling at approximately 40 mph (65 kmph). The train propelled the car along the track, eventually coming to rest some 250 m from the crossing (*Fig.* 24.10). Two occupants of the car were killed outright and a third died from asphyxiation still trapped in the wreckage, despite intubation and ventilation by the ambulance and medical personnel present. The driver of the car was trapped for over 2 hours as a result of the impact and deformation of the vehicle. She had a closed head injury with skull fracture and arterial haemorrhage from an injury to her right arm. Airway control and oxygenation were instituted for her head injury and two intravenous infusions, using Haemaccel and dextrose saline, were required to stabilize her condition during extrication, and thus to ensure her survival.

TUNNEL AND UNDERGROUND ACCIDENTS

Tunnels have claimed lives on the railways both in their construction, as a result of accidents within them, or following environmental problems such as landslips, causing tunnels to collapse.

When complete, the longest railway tunnel in the world will be between the islands of Honshu and Hokkaido in Japan. This will be 53·8 km long and during its construction at least 20 lives have so far been lost. By contrast the longest tunnels in the UK are on the London Underground between East Finchley and Morden, 27·5 km and the Severn Tunnel, 6·6 km, on the London to South Wales route.

The worst underground railway accident in the UK happened at Moorgate on the London Underground on 28 February, 1975, when a train ran into the end of a blind tunnel. This resulted in 2 coaches being compressed into the space of one and impacted within the single tube tunnel. This led to one of the most difficult and protracted rescues ever undertaken on a UK railway and resulted in 43 deaths and 72 people being treated in hospital. The detailed reports of this incident should be read by all medical personnel who are likely to be involved in any railway situation.[8-12] However, it must not be forgotten that Moorgate was unique and one cannot really relate the detail of what happened then to other incidents although the many difficulties of tunnel rescue including poor ventilation, low oxygen levels and high temperatures were all too clearly demonstrated.

What must be remembered about incidents, particularly on any underground railway system, is the effect on other trains in the system. Panic can easily ensue in other trains stopped in tunnels as a result of the accident, particularly if the main lighting goes out. Those medical and rescue personnel controlling the response to such an accident must divert adequate resources to evacuate these trapped trains under safe and controlled conditions. This situation can also occur above ground where there is high density rail traffic.

An example of this occurred on the London Underground system where one train ran into the rear of another at Leyton in East London. The driver was killed and 35 injured. Although this accident occurred above ground there were problems of access to the scene and, in addition, some 2000 people were trapped in several other trains stopped as a result of this accident.

CONCLUSION

The scene of a railway accident can be a frightening place. It will be hostile and unfamiliar ground for many medical personnel. It is therefore of great importance that all who could find themselves involved in a railway incident of whatever type or size should be aware of the kinds of problems they could encounter. No two incidents are ever the same but by sticking firmly to the rules of safety first, then the medical presence at a railway incident can be both rewarding and beneficial. As in all rescue situations the immediate care doctor is part of a team in which all have their specific roles to play. This is nowhere more evident than at the scene of a serious railway accident where so many different agencies can be involved.

REFERENCES

1. Department of Transport (1985) *Railway Safety 1984*. London, HMSO.
2. Marshall J. (1985) *Guinness Rail: the Records,* Enfield, Guinness Superlatives, p. 180.
3. Department of Transport (1985) ibid., p. 38.
4. Hamilton J. A. B. (1969) *Britain's Greatest Rail Disaster*. London, Allen and Unwin.
5. Department of Transport (1985) *Railway Accident. Report on the Collision that Occurred on 7th December 1984 at Eccles*. London, HMSO.
6. Central Electricity Generating Board (1983) *Transport of CEGB Irradiated Nuclear Fuel.*
7. Marshall J. (1985) ibid., p. 182.
8. Department of the Environment (1976)*Railway Accident. Report on the Accident that Occurred on 28th February 1975 at Moorgate Station*. London, HMSO.
9. Medical Staff of Three London Hospitals (1975) The Moorgate train crash. *Br. Med. J.* **3**, 727–31.
10. Winch R. D., Hines K. C., Booker H. T. et al. (1976) The Moorgate train crash. *Injury* **7**, 288–91.
11. *Fire* (1975) 68, Special Supplement.
12. Howard J. (ed.) (1976) *Developments in Disaster Management*. Glasgow: Action for Disaster, pp. 43–66.

Airport and Aircraft Accidents

INTRODUCTION

Since man first learned to fly, the dangers of this unnatural activity have been increasingly recognized and recorded. While man-made disasters involving aircraft attract the widest media interest and coverage, the relative safety of air travel is given little attention. The comparative risks of flying are demonstrated by the fact that 250000 die on the world's roads each year compared with less than 2000 in airliners; the risk of being killed in a car is between 10 and 15 times greater than in an aeroplane.

The risk per hour from all forms of transport has been listed as follows:

Bus	0·03 deaths per million hours
Rail	0·05 deaths per million hours
Private car (UK)	0·6 deaths per million hours
Airline flying	1·0 deaths per million hours
Motor cycling (UK)	9·0 deaths per million hours
Private and sports flying	27·0 deaths per million hours
Mountaineering	27·0 deaths per million hours
Motor cycle racing	35·0 deaths per million hours
Rock climbing	40·0 deaths per million hours

The death rate per million hours from all causes is below 1 until the age of 35 or 40 years when it starts to rise, reaching 5 by the age of 70 and more than 10 by the age of 80.

In a further statistical analysis, it was concluded that flying as a passenger today is no more risky than being 55 years old. While these figures are some answer to the false picture of the danger of flight created by the media, the challenge remains to improve the standards of airport safety and crash management on a worldwide basis.

There are, on average, about 60 fatal air accidents involving airliners every year, of which 35 are non-survivable. However, the fate of many passengers who initially survive an aircraft crash and who later die, could have been prevented by better crash planning and medical response. Air safety requires close co-operation between airline companies, civil aviation authorities and local rescue and medical systems. Survival in air transportation requires acceptable standards of emergency care delivery both on the ground and in the air. All passengers and crew are at risk from any emergency situation including an aircraft crash, hijacking and terrorism, and on-board medical problems.

THE AIRCRAFT CRASH

An analysis of aviation accidents worldwide shows that in general terms the chances of surviving an aircraft crash are greater in wide-bodied jets compared with smaller aircraft, and greater in those accidents occurring on an airport, compared with off an airport, where chances of survival are usually minimal. Much of the original research in this area was done by Bergot[1] from Orly Airport, Paris, who also showed that if there are any survivors on board, there will usually be more survivors than non-survivors. Depending on the forces of impact, seat stability, effectiveness of restraint systems, and whether or not fire has resulted following a crash, injuries will vary from mild neurogenic shock to severe multiple trauma. For the survivors, common injuries include crush trauma to the pelvis, abdomen and thorax, head and cervical injuries, burns, fractures (particularly of the lower limbs) and asphyxia due to hydrogen cyanide inhalation from burning plastic materials in the cabin. It has been estimated that fully one third of all survivors will have long-term disability, including psychological trauma, resulting from the horrific experience. This emotional disturbance may not develop for months or even years later and also may be experienced by rescuers and others, including airline management, who had to cope with the disaster from some distance (*see* Chapter 16).

The Planning

Disaster preparedness for an airport emergency requires an integrated and co-ordinated involvement by the rescue and support services listed in *Table* 25.1 under the headings of those delivering immediate aid, those providing necessary support for the front line services and those who will be involved in the long-term, post-disaster management. All of these groups will of necessity work together to a greater or lesser degree depending on the size of the disaster.

Table 25.1. Airport rescue and support services

Immediate aid (on site)	Secondary aid (peripheral)	Long-term aid (supportive)
Fire services	Traffic control	Psychological services
Medical services	Hospital services	Welfare and community services
Paramedical services	Welfare services	services
Police services	Airline services	Rehabilitation services
Airport management	Community services	
Transportation services		

The Airport Disaster Plan

While all airports should have a contingency plan to cope with an aircraft crash, the degree of response must relate to the relative risks, including size of aircraft using the airport, known hazards such as traffic density, proximity of water and particularly weather dangers, including wind shear.

All airports used for commercial and military purposes should have appropriate fire and rescue services trained in patient handling and first aid, and medical and paramedical responders trained in specific aspects of emergency medicine immediately available. These skills should include triage, airway control, analgesia, extrication, mass casualty management, field hospital or casualty clearing station control, communications systems, toxic gas treatment and immediate care for thermal injuries.

The disaster plan for an airport emergency should clearly answer the following questions:

1. The definition of the emergency—the response necessary and from which services?
2. Communications—how are the services called? What is the form of emergency message?
3. Response—the actions taken by each service?
4. Control of emergency—on site control? Overall control?
5. The specific function, control and communication within each service including fire and rescue, police, medical, paramedical, airport management and security, and the airline.

Each emergency service should in addition have their own in-house disaster plan dealing with call-out, communications, responsibilities, control and equipment.

Regular upgrading of the plan is essential (preferably annually) adding separate sections as necessary to deal with specific emergency procedures such as a bomb alert, hijacking incident or terrorist action within the airport terminal building.

The International Civil Aviation Organization has produced a standardized manual, *Airport Emergency Planning*,[2] which gives guidance for a broad spectrum of disaster management problems. It is a document which can be adapted to suit the needs of both large and small airports.

The Hospital Disaster Plan

Savage,[3] in a number of publications, and this book (Chapter 5), has outlined the requirements for an efficient hospital disaster plan.

The Non-survivable Crash

Crashes away from airports, in the majority of cases, have very few or no survivors, and their recovery needs are often made more difficult because of difficult terrain. Examples include the Potomac River crash in Washington in sub-zero temperatures with a few survivors, the Turkish Airline DC10 crash near Paris in a dense forest, and the DC10 crash on Mount Erebus in Antarctica. The latter was a most difficult recovery under conditions totally alien to human survival. The lesson learned from this disaster was that recovery teams had to be especially selected to cope with such a tragedy and that despite their training, strength and stability they could well need long-term psychological counselling to cope with the aftermath.

Following the Turkish Airline crash out of Paris the relatives of the victims were assembled in a church for a mass burial which resulted in a wave of hysteria and grief sweeping through the assembly, which was soon out of control. It was subsequently realized that it was unwise to allow a large number of mourners to assemble under one roof, as it is inevitable that their grief will soon develop into a situation which goes beyond the powers of existing support services to provide assistance.

Counsellors skilled in grief management, and the aftermaths of disasters, should be available to assist all who are at risk because of their involvement. The need for their services should be recognized at the time of the disaster and not later, when for many it may be too late to heal the psychological injury.

The Response

Communication and Alert

History records numerous examples of disaster mismanagement due to failure to deliver effective emergency care because of a breakdown in communications within a specialized emergency service or between the emergency services. Effective communications require:

a. A fool-proof system of alert: airport to a communications control and thence to medical and paramedical services. Pocket-held 'Bleepers' have improved standards of alerting and communicating but the devices need to be checked regularly and the call-out systems tested to avoid problems. It is now possible to alert a number of emergency services and individuals within each service with one coded signal from a central communications service. The message which is given in response to the alert must be clear, identifying the type of emergency, site and assembly point for the rescue services.

b. A reliable communication link at the scenes between medical and para-medical personnel and three main areas—the crash co-ordination control, the casualty clearing station and the receiving hospital.

The Assembly Point

An assembly point should be designated close to the crash site and all the rescue services except the fire services should gather here prior to being escorted to the crash site. This is necessary, in the interest of safety, in an airport which may still be operating with incoming flights. Important information relative to the details of the emergency can be given to all emergency services as they arrive at the assembly point.

Crash Management

It is expected that the emergency medical services and paramedical services have previously planned a recognized chain of command for all groups. The group leaders will include the following:

a. An on-site medical controller responsible for all medical aspects of triage and emergency care who will liaise with the medical co-ordinator, the chief crash co-ordinator and the paramedical controllers including ambulance and Red Cross. Although the precise designation of these individuals may vary from country to country, the general chain of command is similar at most airports.

b. A medical co-ordinator in charge of all aspects of medical care delivery and evaluation and who will liaise with the medical controllers on site, at the casualty clearing station with the receiving hospital and with the police, fire, rescue and transportation services.

c. An ambulance controller responsible for the provision and movement of ambulances at the crash scene, the casualty clearing station and the hospitals.

d. A casualty clearing station controller. The value of establishing a casualty clearing station close to an airport crash site is being increasingly recognized. While some airports have available large, readily erected tents for casualty clearance and immediate care, others rely on the use of airport hangars which have the advantage of good lighting, warmth and established communications systems. The controller of this station supervises further triage, documentation, and casualty evacuation to hospitals. Other controllers from Red Cross and welfare support services play a most vital role in those countries where their groups are established. The effectiveness of aircraft crash management is easily reduced when, through inadequate or inappropriate uniform and leader identification, rescue workers are confused as to who is in charge and of what service.

There is no place for doctors in white coats at a disaster site, or for nurses in light uniforms. Colour-coded rescue service workers, all with hard hats, are mandatory. Although it is difficult to standardize colours from one country to another, green has become the popular choice for medical personnel. The designation of controllers should be clearly identified with suitable lettering on both the front and back of protective uniforms.

Equipment

Every airport, large or small, should have access to:

1. First aid equipment stored at the airport, to be available within minutes at the crash scene.
2. Specialized equipment to be brought from outside areas such as a hospital or ambulance station.

Airport First Aid Supplies

The type and amount of equipment will depend on the size of aircraft using the airport. Smaller airports servicing light aircraft with few passengers at risk will need minimal supplies of dressings, stretchers, oxygen and blankets. The equipment required to assist a small aircraft accident would usually be carried in the ambulances in most countries.

Bergot[1] has shown that when wide-bodied jet aircraft accidents with survivors are analysed it is generally found that about 20 per cent of passengers and crew will have life-threatening injuries, 30 per cent will have serious but not life-threatening injuries, and 50 per cent will have minor injuries.

The amount of equipment stored at the airport should reflect these findings.

What is of greater importance is that the equipment should be readily available, clean and transportable (preferably on a trailer or in a specially designed vehicle).

A reasonable complement of first aid equipment to be stored on a medicine trailer at an airport servicing large jet aircraft is listed below:

Stretchers—100–150
Large burn dressings—50
Back or spinal boards—10
Splints—50 (wooden box, wire or inflatable)
Blankets—100 (with more in a storage depot)
Triage labels—500 (all passengers and crew should be labelled)
Large plastic bags of clean water—6
Haemostatic dressing pads—50
Portable oxygen and suction units—2

Additional first aid kits containing dressings, large bandages and triage labels should be readily available from an airport depot for the use of first aiders.

Specialized Medical Supplies

These should be available within a few minutes of a crash, even though (except for the larger airports) these are stored away from the airport. Colour-coded containers, each holding identical emergency equipment which is regularly checked, should be light enough to be carried by one or two rescuers. Each case should hold a variety of contents including: intravenous cannulation and infusion equipment (4), airways (6), haemostatic forceps (6), drugs including analgesics, cardiac stimulants, dextrose, bronchodilators, local anaesthetics, tranquillizers, triage labels and dressings. Other cases should house portable oxygen and suction endotracheal intubation equipment, suturing equipment, Entonox, torches and large sterile wound dressings.

Back-up supplies of medical equipment should be readily available from storage depots in the ambulance station or hospital.

Triage

The sorting or triage of passengers and crew is a process which starts with the first contact between rescuers and victims and continues until the final assessments have been done in hospital. The fire and rescue services, the first to make contact with the injured, can initiate triage by quickly deciding which of the victims require the most urgent assistance. Triage labels should be attached by those with some experience in emergency care diagnosis, rechecked by doctors and upgraded or downgraded according to changing circumstances. Most countries now adopt a standard method of injury classification (*see* Chapters 2, 5 and 9).

  a. Priority I colour-coded RED   —those with serious and life-threatening injuries
  b. Priority II colour-coded YELLOW—those with serious but not life-threatening injuries
  c. Priority III colour-coded GREEN —those with minor injuries—including the walking wounded
  d. Priority IV colour-coded BLACK —the dead or unsalvageable

Triage Labels

The most widely used form of labelling internationally is the Mettag system (*see* first endpaper) using a readily identifiable colour-coded, tear-off tag identifying priorities of transportation. It is a strong card with a good numbering system but has the disadvantage that if a patient's category of injury improves (changing from a Priority I to a Priority II or III) a new triage label has to be attached to the patient. The reverse side of the label (*see* second endpaper) is well designed with the body profile available for additional medical information.

The Perth label (*see* third endpaper) is gaining increasing acceptance because it enables the triage category to be upgraded or downgraded by folding the colour-coded cards in any order required. With any one designated colour on the front, the reverse will always show the body profile.

(**N.B.** Further information on the Mettag label can be obtained from Mettag, P.O. Box 910, Starke, Florida 32091, USA and on the Perth label from Dr T. Hamilton, Sir Charles Gardiner Hospital, Nedlands, Perth, Western Australia 6009.)

On-Site Medical Management

The simplest but most workable plan for a disaster site should identify three main areas (*see* fourth endpaper):

    a. A collecting area where the patients are picked up, labelled and given what immediate aid is necessary.

    b. A casualty clearing station to receive Priority I and Priority II patients.

    c. An evacuation and transport area.

This system enables the walking wounded or those with minor injuries to be isolated from those requiring intensive care. Red Cross tents or a sealed-off section of the airport terminal building have been used to accommodate Priority III passengers or crew.

The Casualty Clearing Station

There is increasing international interest in the value of using an airport building as a casualty clearing area where the seriously injured can be stabilized prior to transport by ambulance or helicopter to hospitals. Although some victims of an aircraft crash should be transported directly to hospital, if conditions are favourable, many will benefit from skilled care, with treatment of shock and stabilization in a clean, warm atmosphere, where both doctors, nurses and paramedics have room to work and attend to the injuries.

An aircraft hangar will often provide the needs for a casualty clearing station—heating, lighting, communications, water supply and space. In the hangar, stretchers, trestle tables and colour-coded cones for identifying triage bays may be stored.

Patient documentation is made relatively easier in a hangar, where there can be a designated entrance and exit for ambulances with a tight control over passenger and crew movements following the crash. For those victims who have been certified dead, a temporary mortuary can be established in an isolated room in the hangar away from those receiving treatment. Counselling facilities may also be set up in a hangar as there is usually ample office space and a room such as a cafeteria where welfare services can be housed. Telephone and radio services within the casualty clearing station can be established with other support services such as hospitals, police, airlines and welfare.

THE POST-CRASH PERIOD

In the days, weeks and even months following an aircraft crash, much remains to be done—to record the events, the successes and failures, to recheck and replenish equipment, and to ensure that adequate support and psychological assistance is available for the survivors and the rescuers. A debriefing meeting should be held within a few days, attended by representatives from all emergency services, to upgrade the disaster contingency plans and to identify the weak spots in the response to the disaster.

TRAINING

Disaster preparedness requires 3 types of training:
1. Exercise at a simulated crash attended by all emergency services.
2. Table top exercises where the planning and response is acted out on a scale model of a crash site.
3. In-house training within each emergency service.

Disaster exercises should ideally be held annually and should have a different scenario each year to deal with such problems as a bomb on board, an aircraft crash into water, a crash into buildings or a paddock, a crash at night, etc.

The value of a large field exercise is in testing the effectiveness of communications, site control, casualty clearing station control, documentation and personnel identification. There is little value in testing the standards of emergency care, for this is difficult under simulated conditions; however, triage can be well tested in the field and in the casualty clearing station. One of the problems seen at disaster exercises is that too often time is wasted in simulating injuries when a simple label identifying injuries would be adequate. An umpire with a loudspeaker can help control the teams and identify weaknesses, and a film recording the actions can be of value for the debriefing.

Table top exercises have an advantage over mass exercises in that they can be less stressful, held in an atmosphere more conducive to learning, and they can be stopped and started to clarify any point. They too, require a competent umpire or commentator who can control proceedings.

Training of medical and paramedical responders should also meet in small groups to discuss particular problems relating to triage and emergency care, such as terrorism, explosive injuries, toxic gas inhalation and radioactive contamination. Medical students should be adequately trained in all aspects of disaster medicine in their clinical years with assistance particularly from anaesthetists, surgeons and intensive care physicians. They should participate in regular hospital disaster exercises.

Doctors in the community who are increasingly becoming involved in routine pre-hospital emergency care will require postgraduate training in emergency medicine, triage and mass casualty management. Those who are available to attend airport emergencies should be properly equipped and have effective communications, and suitable protective clothing which identifies them as doctors.

The regular involvement of doctors, nurses and ambulance crews working as a team in airport emergency exercises is excellent training to assist in any other community disaster. Communications have been established, equipment is available and procedures have been rehearsed. A city without an effective disaster plan for its airport has little chance of providing competent disaster management and response for any other major emergency.

MAJOR HIJACKING AND TERRORISM

Terrorism may be defined as the systematic use of extreme fear to coerce a government or community to effect a desired change. Predictions are difficult because terrorism involves small groups of fanatical people. Any country is vulnerable to terrorism, but the strength of the state and its political stability will often determine the degree of success of a terrorist act (see Chapter 28).

Airports, like other special targets such as power plants, petroleum and natural gas industries, are particularly vulnerable both from hijacking and from terrorist activity within the terminal building. Attacks have been particularly common in recent years with indiscriminate slaying of innocent passengers and airport workers. They will only be controlled with increased aviation and airport security to detect terrorist infiltration and concealment of weapons of destruction. The history of hijacking and terrorist incidents over the past decade records common factors in their management and mismanagement.

Describing the Mogadischu-Somalia hijacking in 1977, Renemann[4] showed that the problems of the hijacked are similar to the problems of the hijackers. Both are frightened of the unknown, and both become resigned to death. Both suffer the physical discomfort of confinement for long periods in an unhealthy atmosphere. These are known as the injuries of captivity and are exacerbated by decreased mobility and more evident in the frail or elderly who are, of course, also more vulnerable to cardiovascular and metabolic disturbances. Those who have experienced prolonged hijacking incidents have found that there is usually a need within a day or so for particular medications to help combat the effects of confinement, especially anti-diarrhoea and anti-nausea agents, analgesics and tranquillizers.

An analysis of terrorist incidents shows that the consequences of major acts of terrorism are no different from those of major natural or other man-made disasters. The essentials of management involve skilled triage, medical care of immediate and subsequent injuries, and intelligent contingency planning to cope with specific physiological and psychological derangements including the effects of chemical and toxic agents, general trauma, blast injuries, burns, smoke inhalation, gun shot wounds and dehydration and diarrhoea resulting from confinement for prolonged periods without access to normal food or hydration in an unsanitary environment. Silverstein, through the Washington Center for Strategic and International Studies, has recommended that all commercial aircraft should have special medical kits on board in addition to the standard first aid supplies to cope with the extra medical hazards of hijacking, especially in those areas where hijacking risks are greater.

A terrorist act within the airport terminal building requires an immediate response from trained first aiders who work within the building. Contingency plans should contain a list of all airport workers with good first aid knowledge and a list of readily available equipment to be used before the arrival of the city emergency services.

MEDICAL EMERGENCIES DURING FLIGHT

The lack of emergency equipment and drugs carried by many international airlines shows neglect of an area of emergency care. It has been estimated that less than one third of international carriers provide any form of medical supplies on board other than basic supplies of bandages, aspirin and nasal decongestants.

With increasing numbers of elderly passengers travelling great distances and separated from medical attention for many hours, more problems are being reported by cabin crew which require the services of a doctor and the provision of specific drugs. It is well recognized that air travel exacerbates tension, and medical problems such as asthma and cardiovascular disorders, which may have been stable on the ground. Relative hypoxia occurs because pressurization does not fully compensate for the altitude experienced and may be sufficient to initiate severe cardiac or respiratory malfunction. The effects of alcohol combined with altitude may potentiate some of the problems and hypoglycaemia is another well recognized medical emergency in flight.

As well as basic first aid equipment and additional oxygen, many commercial airlines are now carrying medical cases for the use of a physician on board. The following is a list of drugs and equipment most favoured by airlines for such a purpose.

Pharmaceuticals

4 × adrenaline	1 : 10000 solution	10 ml ampoule	⎫
2 × aminophylline	0·5 g	10 ml ampoule	available
2 × atropine	1·0 mg	10 ml ampoule	in
2 × lignocaine	100 mg	10 ml ampoule	preloaded
2 × calcium gluconate	10%	10 ml ampoule	syringes
2 × dextrose	50%	50 ml ampoule	⎭
2 × diazepam	10 mg	2 ml ampoule	
2 × diphenhydramine	50 mg	1 ml ampoule	
2 × distilled water for injection		10 ml ampoule	
2 × frusemide	40 mg	4 ml ampoule	
2 × morphine	15 mg	1 ml ampoule *or*	
2 × pentozocine	20 mg	2 ml ampoule	
5 × glycerol trinitrate	0–3 mg tablet		
1 × salbutamol inhaler			
2 × sodium chloride injection	0·9%	500 ml bag	
2 × dextrose	5%	500 ml bag	
2 × Haemaccel solutions		500 ml bag	

4 × sodium bicarbonate	8·4%	50 ml ampoule
2 × methylprednisolone	125 mg	1 vial
2 × lignocaine	2%	5 ml ampoule

Equipment

2 × intravenous sets (each containing one intravenous cannula, one tourniquet, 2 alcohol prep swabs, 2 gauze swabs and 1 roll adhesive tape and intravenous giving set.

1 × oropharyngeal airway
1 × emergency tracheal catheter
1 × gauze bandage
1 × sphygmomanometer
1 × disposable syringe   1 ml
2 × disposable syringes 2 ml
2 × disposable syringes 5 ml
2 × disposable syringes 10 ml
1 × disposable syringe   20 ml
1 × laceration pack (needle holder, scissors and sutures)
4 × skin closures
1 × pair of surgical gloves
1 × towel clip
1 × flashlight
1 × stethoscope
1 × suction apparatus

Automatic defibrillators are recommended by a few airlines

It is recommended that all drugs should be listed by both generic and trade names, and that instructions for the use of equipment for emergency states such as hypoglycaemia or acute left ventricular failure be given in at least two languages.

Airports and aircraft are particularly vulnerable to a wide variety of emergency problems requiring competent emergency care. The delivery of this care requires first class training of all emergency services in disaster medicine and emergency care, and a high degree of team co-operation in reducing mortality and morbidity.

'Aviation is not inherently dangerous but the air, to an even greater extent than the sea, is terribly unforgiving of incapability, carelessness or neglect.'[5]

REFERENCES

1. Bergot G. P. (1985) Medical equipment for disasters at airports. *J. World Assoc. Emerg. Disaster Med.* **1**(2), 124–5.
2. *Airport Emergency Planning—Part 7*. 1st edition (1980) International Civil Aviation Organization Doc. 9137–AN/898.
3. Savage P. E. A. (1979) *Disasters—Hospital Planning*. Oxford, Pergamon Press.
4. Renemann H. (1985) Rescue missions following the hijacking of the Lufthansa 737 'Landsheet'. *J. World Assoc. Emerg. Disaster Med.* **1**(2), 199–200.
5. Boom J. (1981) *Head Flight Safety KLM*. Address to 34th Annual International Air Safety Seminar, Mexico.

F. Golden

26

Shipwreck and Exposure

INTRODUCTION

Millions of people throughout the world travel in ships or are engaged in occupations which take them to sea. Occasionally a disaster occurs which attracts the attention of the local or national media, depending on the magnitude of the problem, the prominence of the individuals involved, or some particular mystery surrounding the incident. Infrequently a major disaster occurs which gains worldwide publicity, and comparisons are inevitably made with previous similar incidents such as the sinking of the *Titanic*. The most recent to attain such notoriety was the capsize of the British cross-channel ferry *Herald of Free Enterprise* within 5 minutes of leaving Zeebrugge in Belgium in March 1987. Nearly 200 of the 500 people on board died. Prior to that was the sinking of the Russian passenger liner *Admiral Nakhimov* in the Black Sea in September 1986 with the loss of 400 of the 1234 people on board.

On statistical analysis, however, travel by ship is one of the safest forms of transport; nevertheless, worldwide, thousands of lives are lost annually. The great majority of such deaths occur in capsizings or sinkings of passenger ferries in Third World countries where levels of overcrowding occur which would not be permitted in many more developed countries. International legislation, formulated by the UN International Maritime Organization, demands a minimum standard of safety for ocean-going vessels. Nevertheless, disasters can befall even the most modern ships or oil exploration platforms with all the latest technology in survival aids on board. Examples are the *Berg Istra* in 1975, when 30 lives were lost from a crew of 32; *Alexander Keiland* in 1980, when 123 lives were lost from a crew of 225. The possibility of a collision involving a crowded cross-channel ferry in the busy Straits of Dover has been a perpetual nightmare to all concerned for many years and not without justification as evidenced by the results of the recent incident involving the *Herald of Free Enterprise* in the relatively calm waters of Zeebrugge harbour. Had that incident occurred at sea, the death toll would have been very much higher.

Medical interest in maritime disasters may be a result of one's occupation, e.g. a government agency involved in legislation on maritime safety; a shipping company medical adviser; a ship's doctor; an adviser or active member of a maritime rescue agency; the recipient of casualties from a local disaster, or simply a passenger in a stricken ship. Medical interest thus varies between preventive medicine and the acute management of survivors of such incidents. Accordingly, planning for such possible disasters must be comprehensive, as the permutations of problems which may cause or arise from such disasters are quite wide-ranging. An awareness of the nature of the problems likely to be encountered will assist in the formulation of such plans.

CAUSES OF MARITIME DISASTERS

The principal causes of incidents which may lead to a maritime disaster include:

Unseaworthy vessel.

Environmental conditions, e.g. storm damage resulting in capsize or shipwreck, electrical storm causing fire or explosion.

Collision, caused by human error, poor visibility, or mechanical failure.

Fire, caused by spontaneous combustion of cargo (e.g. grain), or for other reasons in petrochemical bulk carriers. Also, sabotage.

Explosion, in petrochemical tankers with inadequately ventilated tanks or resulting from terrorist attack.

Chemical leakage.

War.

On occasions, the incident leading to the eventual disaster is in itself relatively innocuous with little immediate danger to the crew or passengers. But problems may subsequently arise through fire or loss of containment of the cargo, due to rupture of tanks or breakages of smaller individual containers in a general cargo hold. The picture that springs most readily to mind is the resulting ecological damage from a massive oil spillage. A far more serious threat to human life, however, is the potential for disaster from a chemical leakage, or even worse, a noxious cocktail from the mixing of different chemicals from adjacent ruptured containers. Such an incident, in an inland waterway, e.g. the Mississippi, could cause a major disaster. In many cross-channel ferries, vehicles containing chemicals may be ruptured in collisions, or damaged by fire, creating an unexpected hazard to personnel on board as well as to the rescuers. The antidote to specific chemicals may be known but the possible permutations of cocktails could defy even the most dedicated toxicologist.

In chemical tankers, ships' crews may be well protected individually with specialized clothing and respirators readily available to cater for the occasional accidental spillage, but what about those who come to their assistance in an emergency, or those in an adjacent vessel? Clearly, in incidents involving chemical tankers there are enormous problems. (More specific advice relating to ships may be obtained from *The Chemical Supplement to the International Medical Guide for Ships (IMGS),* International Maritime Organization, London, 1982.)

From the above scenarios it is obvious that the permutations of medical problems which possibly could be encountered in maritime disasters are wide-ranging.

INJURY TYPES

Injury types likely to be encountered in maritime disasters may be of the acute or chronic variety. The acute are those received at the time of the incident which may require immediate attention and include trauma; pulmonary problems due to smoke inhalation, blast injury, chemical inhalation and near drowning; burns, both thermal and chemical, and hypothermia. Chronic ones include the long-term effects of the acute injuries together with chronic hypothermia, cold injury, dehydration, starvation, radioactive contamination and psychological stress.

This particular chapter will concentrate on those injuries peculiar to the maritime environment. Many of the other injuries encountered are common to other areas and have already been extensively covered in previous chapters.

THE INCIDENT LEADING TO SHIP ABANDONMENT

In some instances little can be done to prevent a disaster ensuing from the original incident which led to the ship being abandoned, such as an explosion or a sudden capsize. More usually, the disaster results from lack of forethought, inadequate planning and poor training. The *Titanic* is probably the classic example, although there have been many others before and since, even if not of quite the same magnitude.

In the case of the *Titanic*, few of the 2201 passengers and crew on board were killed or injured when the liner hit an iceberg in the North Atlantic in May, 1912. The subsequent disaster resulted from the ship having insufficient lifeboat capacity for both passengers and crew, leading to the loss of 1489 lives. Most of those who died abandoned ship successfully, all wearing lifejackets, into the calm, near freezing water, only to die within an hour or so, presumably from the effects of the cold. International legislation has since been introduced to ensure that adequate lifeboats and liferafts ('lifecraft') are carried in such ships to prevent a similar recurrence. However, disasters will continue to occur because it cannot be guaranteed that all the lifecraft can always be launched. Severe listing or capsize, heavy weather or damage from fire or explosion, may make some or all of the lifecraft inaccessible or unusable.

Personnel below decks may not be familiar with alternative routes to the upper deck and become trapped if their usual route of access is blocked by fire or smoke or otherwise obstructed. Should there be a power failure, the total darkness between decks can be extremely disorientating.

The ship's doctor should plan and exercise procedures to be adopted for patients under his care, who may be unable to help themselves, to ensure their escape in such a situation. Such plans should include alternative escape routes from the sick bay to the upper deck.

Having reached the upper deck, the preferred means of evacuating ships in such circumstances is by helicopter. Before approaching the helicopter it is important to secure all loose clothing, especially blankets or other loose coverings of patients on stretchers, lest the downdraught from the rotor blades dislodges them and causes an additional incident. In cold, ambient conditions, the downdraught from the rotor blades will be extremely chilling, while in subzero temperatures the wind chill can produce a freezing cold injury of skin in a matter of seconds; therefore, in such environments, all bare skin should be covered before approaching the helicopter.

Should helicopter rescue not be possible then, in larger ships, it will be necessary to abandon ship by boarding a lifecraft prior to its being lowered over the side; in smaller ships, the lifecraft requires to be launched before boarding. This will obviously create problems for injured personnel and plans should also be extant to cater for such an eventuality, making best use of available facilities. Some of the more modern cross-channel passenger ferries, operating between England and France, have escape chutes similar to those used by commercial airliners, but such devices are of little practical value in the event of a capsize.

From the description above, it may appear that abandoning ship is a reasonably safe procedure, but in open seas it is a daunting prospect even in daylight, and frequently associated with tragedy on a smaller or larger scale depending on a variety of circumstances such as weather conditions, sea state, stability of the ship, time available for abandonment, competence of crew, etc. Clearly the ship or company doctor should give careful consideration to methods to be adopted to cater for the sick and injured in such circumstances.

Prior to abandonment, there may be insufficient time for the doctor to collect drugs or other items of equipment to supplement the usual meagre first aid stores in lifecraft. It is therefore advisable for him to keep a small emergency pack in a waterproof container in his cabin with his lifejacket or near the exit of the sick bay. The contents of such a supplementary pack should be decided after studying the contents of the first aid pack of the lifecraft, and will doubtless be influenced by personal therapeutic practices. It is suggested that in addition to any drugs this pack should contain:

1 pair blunt-ended scissors
2 curved artery forceps
12 safety pins (at least 2 sizes)
1 waterproof torch and spare batteries
Bandages and dressings (including tins of vaseline-impregnated gauze dressings)
Antibiotics; analgesics; anaesthetic and antibiotic eye drops and ointments; silicone ointment

Ideally, the pack should be placed in a waterproof container with inherent buoyancy; it should be easy to carry and there should be some means of securing it to the lifejacket or person, lest both hands are required to assist a casualty or to scramble down a rope or ladder. Care should be taken to position it where it will not cause injury if one is forced to jump into the sea from a height.

At times, however, the interval between relative normality and disaster may be so brief that little can be done for anyone other than attempt to save one's own life. In the incident involving the *Herald of Free Enterprise*, sudden capsize (<1 min) occurred as she was leaving harbour; there was no warning before the ship began her inevitable heel to 90 degrees. Loose furniture, hand baggage and breaking bottles tumbled across the 'open-plan' lounges to the dependent sides causing injuries to passengers who were attempting to maintain a secure hold in a totally disorientating environment. The subsequent failure of the lighting, accompanied by the inrushing water at 4°C, added to the confusion and panic. As soon as the immediate disorientation was resolved, passengers were faced with the terrible anxiety of how they were going to escape, whether the ship was going to sink, and what had become of their relatives and companions from whom they had been separated in the mêlée? Those who were partially or totally immersed were confronted with the added problems associated with immersion in very cold water.

POST-ABANDONMENT

Immersion

Survivors who have been unable to board a lifecraft dry and are obliged to jump into the water face a number of immediate problems. Some may sustain traumatic injury from collision with some portion of the ship's structure whilst jumping into the sea, or sustain severe abrasions from sliding or being washed over a barnacle-encrusted hull. On entering the water they may collide with some partially submerged wreckage or flotsam adjacent to the ship's side. Some types of lifejacket, if not correctly secured, will, on contact with the water, ride up and hyperextend the neck and produce little effective flotation support. Should such an individual be jumping from a height, then a fractured mandible or hyperextension cervical injury may occur.

Regardless of how one comes in contact with the water, if it is cold ($<15°C$), and the individual is unused to such low temperatures, a sympathetic reflex response mediated through the cutaneous thermoreceptors will produce a transient tachycardia, hypertension and hyperventilation, so-called *cold shock*. Under normal circumstances, in fit young adults, the response will be little more than unpleasant, unless they are particularly sensitive to the cold when the hyperventilation may be of sufficient severity to produce tetany. Clearly, the resulting incapacitation is highly undesirable in such circumstances. In some, the hyperventilation, although not quite leading to tetany, disrupts the synchrony of swimming and respiration and leads to drowning within minutes of immersion.

The involuntary, uncontrollable hyperventilation associated with cold shock is undesirable in another sense in that it occurs at a time when there may be a requirement to breath-hold, or at least synchronize breathing with the rebound wave splash off the side of the hull to prevent aspiration of water.

In addition to these reflex responses, a variable degree of cardiac overloading will be present, caused by a generalized peripheral cold vasoconstriction and venous squeeze from the hydrostatic pressure acting on the surface of the immersed body. Both these factors will produce a significant rise in CVP which will vary, depending on water temperature and angle of flotation. The colder the water and the more vertical the angle of flotation, the greater will be the rise in CVP. In a vertical flotation posture in thermoneutral water, the hydrostatic pressure alone will increase venous return such that there will be a 30 per cent increase in cardiac output in a physiologically intact subject.

Clearly, therefore, individuals who have underlying cardiovascular disease may suffer cardiac failure, myocardial ischaemia or a cerebrovascular accident, which if not fatal in themselves, may lead to incapacitation and drowning, or simply be an added complication to manage following rescue.

The transient reflex cold shock response wanes after 2 or 3 minutes, and has usually disappeared completely within 5 minutes. The response is not found in cold-habituated individuals, and being mediated through the peripheral thermoreceptors it is attenuated by protecting the skin from sudden contact with the cold water with, for instance, extra layers of clothing or, ideally, special waterproof suits.

Having survived the initial effects of entry into cold water, the survivor must then swim clear of the side of the ship, not an easy procedure if the hull drift rate is high, or as is frequently the case, the water is covered with fuel oil and littered with flotsam. Once clear of the hull, if it is not possible to get out of the water, then in order to reduce body heat loss the survivor should float passively with legs together, elbows adjacent to the chest wall, hands out of the water holding the collar of the lifejacket, and await rescue.

Survival Times

From the foregoing it is apparent that there are a number of interacting physiological and physical factors which influence the likely survival times of the immersed individual. The most important of these are cardiovascular fitness, degree of cold habituation, body insulation, sea state, effectiveness of lifejacket and any protective clothing. *Fig.* 26.1 shows the average expected survival times for normal adults in conventional clothing in relatively calm water at varying temperatures. Clearly some will die within minutes of immersion for the reasons given above, while others will survive for considerably longer.

A dilemma occurs when advice is sought on the duration of the search for survivors. As a general rule of thumb, the minimum search time should be at

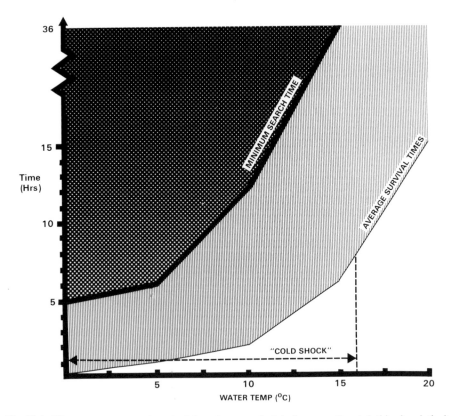

Fig. 26.1. The average expected survival times for normal adults in conventional clothing in relatively calm water at varying temperatures.

least 6 times the average survival time. Thus in water at 5°C the search time should be at least 6 hours and about 12 hours if the sea is calm. When to abandon a search for survivors in a capsized hull is always difficult, as survivors may not be immersed, or only partially so. Other considerations include the volume of available oxygen and the contamination of the atmosphere in a confined space by chemicals or fuel vapour.

Immersion victims who have adequate flotation support will eventually lose consciousness through hypothermia when the core temperature falls to around 30°C, while death from cardiac failure (possibly VF) occurs at a core temperature of about 24°C. More usually, however, as consciousness becomes impaired, at core temperatures in the region of 34°C, immersion victims are no longer able to protect their airway, aspirate water and drown. Even relatively short-term survival, then, frequently depends on being able to board a lifecraft, although this does not in itself guarantee survival.

Lifecraft Survivors

The problems confronting survivors in lifecraft may be conveniently divided into short-term and long-term. Short-term hazards refer to those specific problems confronting the survivor during the first 24 hours. They are largely related to maintaining the seaworthiness of the craft and thus are outside the scope of this text. From a medical viewpoint the most important is ensuring adequate protection against environmental conditions, particularly low ambient temperatures. Many deaths from hypothermia have occurred within 24 hours of boarding liferafts even in the 'temperate' waters of the English Channel.

Long-term problems again are predominantly governed by environmental conditions. It is significant that all lifecraft voyages of epic duration have occurred in tropical waters. The longest to date lasted 117 days in the Pacific, undertaken by the Bailey husband and wife team following the sinking of their yacht. In general, shortage of drinkable water, although responsible for many dramatic stories, is less important than thermal problems for survivors adrift in temperate waters. By comparison, nutritional difficulties fade into insignificance. Inadequate ventilation in enclosed survival craft may lead to CO_2 intoxication if some air flow is not maintained.

Thermal problems will include acute and chronic hypothermia, depending on ambient conditions, available insulation, duration of exposure, nutrition and other factors. In subarctic and arctic environments, local cold injury, freezing (frostbite) and non-freezing (trench/immersion foot), will also be a problem.

Fluid Balance

Most survival craft carry sufficient potable water to provide each occupant with about 600 ml per day for 3 days. As no water should be consumed during the first 24 hours, except by casualties who have burn injuries, there should be sufficient water for all occupants for 4 days. Except in the tropics, this quantity of water should ensure that the occupants should survive for at least 7 to 10 days before suffering serious ill effects, provided all possible behavioural techniques are adopted to ensure maximum physiological water conservation. About 450 ml/ day appears to be the minimum requirement to keep an inactive individual fit for about 6 days in a temperate climate. However, 1·0 to 1·5 litres per day are required for indefinite periods. In the Second World War, the critical amount of water for survivors adrift for 6 days was about 150 ml/day but this was associated with a 22 per cent mortality rate; with between 150 and 450 ml/day, the mortality rate was reduced to 0·6 per cent.

In survival situations associated with starvation, there will be increased catabolism of tissue protein with a resultant increase in urea production. Excretion of this urea will require additional fluid intake to prevent body fluid loss. The temptation to eat fish and sea birds must be avoided, therefore, unless there is a plentiful supply of drinking water. Ideally, the diet should consist largely of fats and carbohydrate, which have a metabolic end product of CO_2 and water. In healthy young men, a diet of 100 g of carbohydrate per day, ingested without water, reduces protein catabolism from 78 to 43 g, resulting in a reduction in urinary output from 680 ml to 360 ml/day. Thus 100 g of carbohydrate will conserve more than its own weight in water.

In warm climates, sweating can be reduced by optimum use of shade, breezes and the wetting of clothing with sea water. Sea water or urine should never be drunk; both contain salt—and urine, urea—in concentrations in excess of tissue fluid, even when the body is severely dehydrated, and thus will require to be excreted in turn involving a loss of body water in excess of the volume consumed.

Food

Modern communications, satellite location devices and search and rescue techniques make it unlikely that survivors from large ships will spend sufficient time adrift to suffer any serious nutritional deficiency. However, yachts may be weeks or even months overdue before anyone is even aware that they are missing and then there may be little to indicate where to commence searching for survivors. In such survivors, starvation may well prove to be a serious problem, but only if they have had adequate drinking water available.

RESCUE

While in transit to the stricken ship, or awaiting receipt of casualties, try to ascertain the nature of the problem which caused the incident, the number of personnel on board and thus the possible number of casualties, and the nature of any cargo carried. If chemicals or other toxic materials are likely to be present then it is advisable to have closed-circuit breathing apparatus and specialized protective clothing at hand. In addition, specialist advice should be sought from a toxicological centre.

Plans should be made, if contingency ones are not already extant, regarding the techniques to be used to rescue survivors; the identification of a suitable triage site adjacent to the rescue area; preparing stores likely to be required (e.g. drugs, fluids, oxygen, splints, blankets, etc.). Personnel should be delegated and briefed for specific tasks such as the rescue party, first aid, and the recording of survivors as they come onboard. Ideally, waterproof numbered labels should be at hand to attach to survivors, preferably to their wrists.

Survivors may be rescued direct from the stricken ship, the water, lifecraft or delivered by helicopter without necessarily having received any treatment but the most rudimentary first aid. Those rescued from the sea are frequently too weak to assist in their own recovery, or may have injuries which prevent them from doing so; in either event, arrangements must be made in advance to devise a means of lifting such survivors inboard. In the *Herald of Free Enterprise* incident, difficulties were encountered in rescuing survivors from inside the capsized hull. Some passengers were able to hold on to ropes lowered through 'windows'. For many of those immersed, however, the loss of tactile discrimination, manual dexterity and muscle power made any attempt at holding a rope impossible. After 10 minutes' immersion in water at that temperature (4°C), hands are virtually useless. Therefore, in most circumstances some form of lifting net or basket is ideal. Manhandling is usually difficult as survivors are frequently covered in fuel oil. In heavy weather it may also put the rescuers' lives at risk.

The dangers of the rescue period are apparent from the following extract from the writings of Sir Salisbury MacNalty, the official historian of the British Medical Services at War:

> '. . . commonly many survivors, who had managed to get themselves to the point of being helped from the sea, collapsed when safety was within reach and required to be handled in the same manner as those who had been helpless while still in the water.'

There are numerous anecdotal stories of survivors attempting to climb up the sides of the rescue ships, only to fall back into the sea and be lost. Whatever the precise physiological mechanism of the collapse of such survivors during rescue (possibly due to the sudden reduction in cardiac output associated with the removal of the supporting hydrostatic squeeze), it is tragic to come through such an ordeal only to be lost when salvation is at hand.

Every effort should therefore be made in advance to prevent such a tragic outcome. If lifting nets or baskets are not available, then, weather permitting, the rescue ship's boat or lifecraft may be used as a suitable platform onto which the survivors may be rescued before being recovered inboard. This avoids a vertical lift by rope or harness which is not advisable for hypothermic survivors—victims who have been immersed for 30 minutes or more in cold water. However, despite advance planning, there will be occasions when it is necessary to recover survivors by any means practicable in the conditions.

TRIAGE OF SURVIVORS

An easily accessible sheltered compartment on the upper deck, adjacent to the rescue area, should be chosen in which to make a cursory examination of survivors as they are rescued and decide on disposal and priorities for treatment.

It is important to remember that many hypothermic casualties collapse and sometimes die on or shortly after rescue (*see below*). For this reason survivors should not be required to climb down ladders to treatment centres; the nearest easily accessible sheltered area should be used for triage. It is also important to remember that immersion victims rescued from cold water, particularly the young, may appear to be dead but respond to resuscitation efforts.

The Immersion Victim

For the purposes of initial management, no attempt will be made to differentiate between survivors suffering from hypothermia or drowning. Such distinctions are artificial and unnecessary at this stage. It is advisable to assume that all survivors are suffering from hypothermia and drowning to a varying degree until proven otherwise. Initial treatment is therefore the restoration of adequate ventilation and circulation, with prevention of further heat loss.

All personnel involved in the rescue should be aware of the necessity to maintain an adequate airway, prevent postural hypotension and provide adequate insulation. The importance of speedy and persistent resuscitative efforts should also be emphasized to first aid parties. First aid team members should be warned that about 60 per cent of near-drowning victims vomit or regurgitate during resuscitation. Conscious patients should be encouraged to cough and take deep breaths. One hundred per cent oxygen should be administered initially as a significant degree of hypoxaemia may be present even in an alert patient when other obvious signs of hypoxia are absent. The possibility of there being an internal traumatic injury (e.g. ruptured spleen) should be borne in mind.

Acute Hypothermia

Survivors who do not show overt signs of ventilatory problems but appear to be only mildly hypothermic—shivering but rational—and have been immersed for less than 30 minutes may be rapidly rewarmed in a hot bath (41°C, hand-hot), if facilities are available. They should be undressed in the bath. Care should be exercised when removing and disposing of clothing to avoid loss of vital documentary evidence. It is best to put all the clothing in a polythene bag labelled with a number corresponding to the casualty's number.

The patient should remain in the bath until he subjectively feels warm. He should not be permitted to remain in the hot water until he starts to sweat. After leaving the hot bath, he should be placed in a warmed bunk and insulated with blankets. During rewarming he should be given warmed sweet drinks, but no alcohol.

Should a hot bath not be available, conscious, shivering survivors may be placed in warm showers, but attendants must be watchful for postural hypotension. If there are a large number of cold survivors, a lifecraft from one's own ship—placed in a sheltered position on deck—could be used as a receptacle for hot water, but careful supervision will be required.

Cold lifecraft survivors or those who have been immersed for long periods and are severely hypothermic, showing signs of unconsciousness or confusion, should be gently undressed, dried and placed in a horizontal position, or slightly head down, in a sleeping bag or in blankets insulated from the deck. They should then be permitted to rewarm spontaneously at a rate not exceeding about 1°C per hour. Oxygen via an oronasal mask will be of help if shivering is severe. Hotwater bottles or other techniques for skin rewarming should be avoided.

There is no specific treatment for acute hypothermia other than rewarming. Cardiac arrhythmias frequently seen at temperatures below 33°C usually revert to normal on restoration of normal core temperature.

Complications to be safeguarded against include postural hypotension, hypovolaemia and airway obstruction. Appropriate monitoring of such casualties is therefore called for. Intravenous fluids are not advised unless absolutely essential; physiological, autoregulatory control will usually cope satisfactorily and keep pace with the changing metabolic and cardiovascular adjustments unless artificial heat is supplied to the surface of the body.

Drowning

Cardiopulmonary resuscitation for drowning victims will be limited by available resources, equipment and manpower. If there are many near drowning victims it will be necessary to apportion treatment priorities to optimize the use of precious resources. Hopefully a number will be successfully resuscitated. What must be safeguarded against, however, is the death of survivors who may have aspirated water, are conscious at the time of rescue but subsequently develop pulmonary complications. Such patients should not be placed in ships' cabins without adequate supervision.

As a general rule, all immersion cases who have aspirated water, experienced chest pain, or have physical signs in the chest, should, where possible, be admitted to hospital for chest X-ray, blood gas analysis and general assessment.

Oil Contamination

Shipwreck survivors are frequently covered in oil and many may have swallowed or inhaled some. Oil has a negligible systemic toxicity although, if swallowed, it may cause vomiting, or if inhaled, may produce an aspiration pneumonia. In the eyes it will produce a conjunctivitis which may last for several days.

Initial cleaning of oil from around the mouth, nose and eyes is all that is required. The remainder of the body can be cleaned later when time permits. This is best achieved by standing the victim under a hot shower, removing all clothing and gently wiping with cloths or paper towels to remove excess oil from the skin. Hair shampoo and toilet soap may then be used and specialized non-toxic skin cleaners (e.g. 'Swarfega') will deal with any obstinate patches, but solvents and scouring compounds not specifically designed for use on the skin should be avoided. The eyes may be cleaned with liquid paraffin followed by a topical steroid to relieve the conjunctivitis.

The Survival Craft Survivor

Dehydration and malnutrition are only likely to be problems for survivors adrift in tropical waters. In temperate and subarctic waters castaways will probably succumb to the effects of cold long before dehydration and malnutrition become manifest.

Chronic Hypothermia

The difference between acute and chronic hypothermia, apart from the rate of onset, is principally one of variation in retained body fluid. The intense peripheral cold vasoconstriction in both acute and chronic hypothermia, is physiologically compensated for by a cold diuresis and an intravascular/interstitial fluid shift. In chronic hypothermia there is in addition a significant interstitial/intracellular fluid shift while the cold diuresis is considerably protracted. Furthermore, if renal temperatures are low, renal tubular function is impaired and the diuresis becomes massive. Overall circulating blood volume is usually adequate to meet the metabolic demands and the reduced circulatory capacity. However, a sudden restoration of body temperature without a concomitant increase in circulating fluid volume will result in rewarming collapse and frequently cardiac arrest. Slow (internal) spontaneous rewarming, as described above, with careful fluid replenishment (warmed dextrose 5 per cent) will help a redistribution of body fluids without collapse. Overzealous intravenous transfusion may, on the other hand, overload the central circulation; ideally, therefore, CVP monitoring is called for.

Associated peripheral cold injuries to the hands and feet should be managed as outlined in Chapter 17.

Dehydration and Malnutrition

In cases of long-term lifecraft survival, the survivors are likely to be suffering from starvation and dehydration. Caution should be exercised in attempting to reverse either condition rapidly. Intravenous feeding may be necessary but usually the survivor will be able to take fluids orally. A light diet with minimal roughage, containing sugar, essential proteins and small amounts of fat is recommended for a day or two until the gastrointestinal tract has recovered sufficiently to cope with normal food. A diet of beaten eggs containing sugar mixed with milk or water should satisfy the initial requirements. Although survivors do not usually display overt signs of vitamin deficiency, it is essential to supplement their diet during treatment to prevent avitaminosis.

Psychological Effects

Many shipwreck survivors are subsequently haunted by the memory of sights and sounds of loved ones or acquaintances in agonal throes. Many will feel an overwhelming sense of guilt that they could have done more to help others; most will harbour a sense of deep shame that they have themselves survived. Forgotten will be the extreme difficulties encountered in endeavouring to save their own lives under the circumstances and the fact that there was little or no spare capacity remaining to save others. If relatives have also been lost in the disaster then the survivors are deprived of traditional sources of support and conciliation. Sedation is therefore important in immediate care; in the long term, psychiatric care and group therapy with fellow survivors, with whom they can more readily identify, is advised (see Chapter 16).

CONCLUSIONS

Disasters at sea are rare. Casualties may suffer a variety of injuries similar to those encountered in most disasters on land in addition to those peculiar to a maritime environment. As in all disaster planning, careful forethought and preparation is necessary to ensure the optimal use of facilities and labour to relieve suffering, prevent unnecessary loss of life, record accurate identification where possible and maintain adequate communications. The rescue and management of shipwreck survivors is no exception to this policy.

Chemical Accidents

On 7 December, 1917 the French freighter *Mont Blanc* sailed into the harbour in Halifax, Nova Scotia, Canada to meet up with the British cruiser *HMS High Flyer*. The former vessel was loaded with TNT, picric acid, gun cotton and barrels of benzene. These supplies were urgently required for the war in Europe. The *Mont Blanc* collided in the harbour with a Belgian ship *Imo*. An enormous explosion followed. Damage to life and property was immense. The explosion blast was felt 96 km away. The total number of fatalities was never established but was between 2000 and 4000. Of 550 children at school that morning in Halifax, only 7 survived. Some 8000 people were injured; 25000 were made homeless. Four square kilometres of the city centre were flattened. The severity of the disaster was reduced by the courageous action of the marine superintendent who went aboard the British ammunition ship, *Pictou,* anchored in the harbour and opened the sea valves. He set the vessel adrift and within minutes the ship and cargo sank. Thus a second massive explosion was avoided.

The rescue effort was hampered by appalling weather with fog, driving snow and freezing temperatures. Trains were used to bring medical supplies and doctors from Boston and New York. The military barracks were used to house women and children whilst 500 tents were used for the troops. The Academy of Music and other public buildings were used for the injured.

In December, 1984, 45 metric tons of methyl isocyanate escaped from a pesticide plant in Bhopal, India. The highly toxic gas spread rapidly over the local residential area killing many inhabitants immediately and creating considerable panic as people started to flee the area. An estimated 2500 died, with up to 100000 others affected. Many bodies were buried en masse to avoid risk of epidemics. Medical aid was rapidly forthcoming from all over the world.

In November, 1984, a liquefied gas explosion in Mexico City claimed the lives of 450 people and 4250 were seriously injured, many badly burnt. A similar incident involving a tanker containing LPG which crashed on a camping site in Spain also claimed many lives.

In the United Kingdom the worst industrial explosion devastated the Nypro plant at Flixborough, near Scunthorpe, on 1 June, 1974. Twenty-nine people died and over 100 were injured. Many homes in the adjacent village were destroyed and the blast was felt 30 miles away. Three thousand people were evacuated for fear of a further explosion. It took over 24 hours to bring the fire under control.

Another major evacuation was organized in Barking, East London, following a fire and explosion at the Walmsly Chemical Plant. It was feared that a toxic

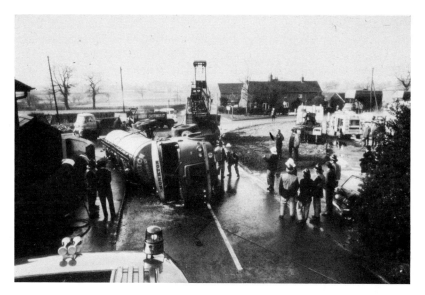

Fig. 27.1. Consequences of a chemical accident.

cloud from the fire could contain significant levels of cyanates. A housing estate of about 8000 residents was evacuated, in an orderly manner, to local rest centres set up by the local authority. These were in schools and halls, according to a pre-arranged plan.

It is accidents like these, and many others that have occurred throughout the world, that have led planners to be particularly concerned about chemical accidents and our preparedness to deal with them. The consequences of some chemical accidents for a community can be devastating for many years to come (*Fig.* 27.1).

PREVENTION

In an ideal world, planning to prevent accidents is all that would be needed. However, it is unfortunately also necessary to plan to treat casualties. Accidents do happen! Stringent efforts have been made in many countries to control and regulate the production, storage, transport and use of toxic or otherwise hazardous materials. In Great Britain the Control of Industrial Major Accident Hazards Regulations 1984 (CIMAH Regs.) require the operator and the local authority to prepare both on-site and off-site plans to deal with an emergency situation. The health authorities should also be consulted in the planning process. Many of these sites present a fire and explosion risk. Some could require wide evacuation in areas downwind of a leak of a toxic substance such as, for example, chlorine.

HAZARD WARNINGS

In order to provide swift, safe and effective response to an incident involving chemicals that may be toxic or explosive, it is essential that the precise nature of the substances involved is accurately identified as quickly as possible. Laws now require tank vehicles or tank containers carrying prescribed dangerous substances to display the name and address of the manufacturer, importer, wholesaler or supplier and a hazard information panel (*see Fig.* 27.2). The following information is given:

1. The United Nations Diamond-Shaped Hazard Warning Label

This shows the primary hazard—such as inflammability, corrosivity, toxicity or liability to spontaneous combustion. In cases of mixed loads with no general hazard there is an exclamation mark within the diamond.

2. The HAZCHEM Code

This gives information about suitable fire-fighting methods, types of personal protection required, whether the substance is likely to react violently, whether it may be safely washed into drains and whether the danger is such that local evacuation of the public from surrounding areas should be considered. The HAZCHEM code is available on all fire appliances. It should be available also in all ambulances, police and immediate care doctor vehicles (*Figs.* 27.3 and 27.4).

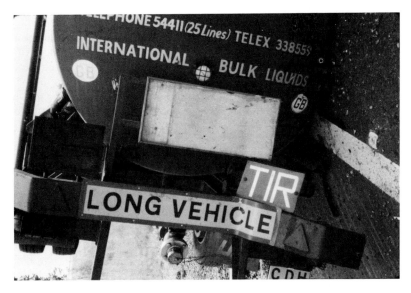

Fig. 27.2. Information displayed on a vehicle.

Front

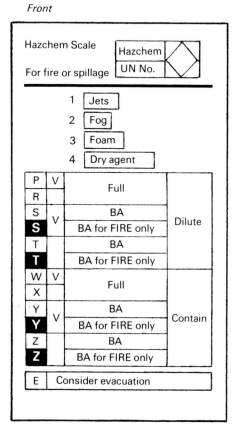

Fig. 27.3. The HAZCHEM code (front).

Back

Notes for Guidance

Fog
In the absence of fog equipment a
fine spray may be used.

Dry agent
Water must not be allowed to come
into contact with the substance at risk.

V
Can be violently or even explosively
reactive.

Full
Full body protective clothing with BA.

BA
Breathing apparatus plus protective
gloves.

Dilute
May be washed to drain with large
quantities of water.

Contain
Prevent by any means available, spillage
from entering drains or water course.

Fig. 27.4. The HAZCHEM code (back).

'UKHIS' BOARD

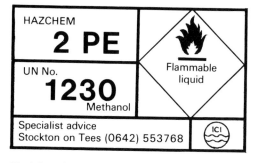

Black lettering on orange background.
Black symbol and letters in red diamond on
white square background.

Fig. 27.5. Example of signs displayed on vehicles carrying hazardous chemicals.

ECE-ADR 'KEMLER' BOARD

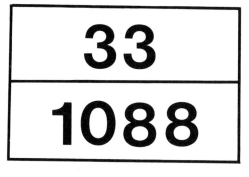

Black figures and border on reflective
orange background.

Fig. 27.6. Example of signs displayed on vehicles carrying hazardous chemicals.

ECE-ADR 'KEMLER' SCALE

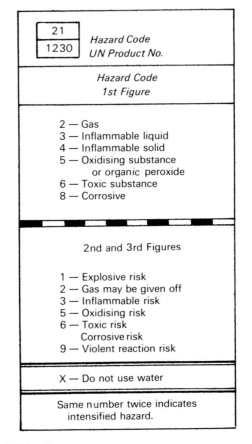

| 21 | Hazard Code |
| 1230 | UN Product No. |

Hazard Code
1st Figure

2 — Gas
3 — Inflammable liquid
4 — Inflammable solid
5 — Oxidising substance
      or organic peroxide
6 — Toxic substance
8 — Corrosive

2nd and 3rd Figures

1 — Explosive risk
2 — Gas may be given off
3 — Inflammable risk
5 — Oxidising risk
6 — Toxic risk
    Corrosive risk
9 — Violent reaction risk

X — Do not use water

Same number twice indicates
intensified hazard.

Fig. 27.7. The CHEMLAR scale.

3. The United Nations Number

This is specific to the substance and allows for its rapid identification by name.

4. Specialist Advice Telephone Number

Composite labels giving all of the above information have been devised for the UK (*Fig.* 27.5) and European Community (*Figs.* 27.6 and 27.7).

Transport Emergency Cards (TREM cards or CEFIC cards) should be carried by the drivers of tankers. The cards give written instructions about first aid, fire-fighting methods and the management of spillage. Similar cards are produced by some industrial waste disposal firms. Copies of these cards should be held in all accident and emergency departments and emergency service controls.

Toxic substances transported by rail carry the composite labels and a two-letter identification code for the use of the railway control office.

RESPONSIBILITIES AT A CHEMICAL INCIDENT

The *police* and *fire services* have a duty to ensure the safety and protection of the public in general terms after incidents involving toxic or corrosive substances and the health authorities have a responsibility to recover and care for any casualty—however caused. Fire brigades have equipment to protect brigade personnel from the effects of smoke and other toxic vapours. These will include full enveloping gas-tight suits which, when worn with breathing apparatus, will give almost complete protection from a hostile environment. The fire service, therefore, takes a leading role in incidents involving toxic substances. The police will set up a cordon around the affected area. They will be responsible for traffic diversions and evacuation of any area at risk. The police would normally make contact with the owners or carriers of the substance involved so that they can assist in removing or containing the hazard. The role of the ambulance service is to provide aid to any casualties, to transport casualties from the site to suitable medical facilities, either an established emergency department or, in an incident of disaster proportions, to an improvised field hospital. From time to time transport, direct to specialist hospitals, may be appropriate. Examples would be burns units, plastic surgery units or hospitals equipped to deal with radiation contaminated casualties.

Doctors or *nurses* may, from time to time, be called upon to assist at emergencies where toxic or corrosive substances are involved. It is vital that such staff are given adequate training and preparation for such incidents. They can then make a safe and effective response to alleviate distress and treat injuries to casualties without putting themselves at unnecessary risk. If not, they become a liability and are better withdrawn from the scene to their more familiar hospital environment.

The nature of the hazard will differ from incident to incident. Local liaison and planning is essential and local arrangements must be clearly understood by all involved. They should be familiar with the language, radio procedures and rank structure of the other rescue services. As part of their preparation they should be familiar with the HAZCHEM coding system and the steps involved in decontamination procedures. Where possible they should have visited local chemical works, power stations and other local establishments with disaster potential.

Other agencies and organizations may also be involved and their responsibilities, depth of involvement and arrangements for attendance will be different in each local authority area. Local or regional emergency planning officers, highways departments, water authorities, environmental health departments and specialist industrial chemical accident teams may also become involved. In certain situations the Armed Forces may also become involved.

REPORTING OF INCIDENTS

It is essential that the first emergency service officer or immediate care doctor at the scene of the accident communicates full and accurate details for chemical identification to the authorities. This enables all the other services to be fully alerted and acquainted with the situation at the scene of the incident to which they are going. All chemical names should be carefully spelt out, using the international phonetic alphabet. Any available information from drivers, chemical plant workers and others involved should also be obtained and passed to Control. Early consideration of the direction of the prevailing wind and the direction of flow of liquids is important and, where possible, other services arriving should approach from uphill and upwind of the incident.

COMMUNICATION AND CALL-OUT PROCEDURES

The police are normally responsible for the overall control and co-ordination of all services and agents during a chemical incident. The fire service are normally responsible for the collection and dissemination to the other services of any scientific advice about the nature of the chemical hazards, first aid requirements and any other data of relevance to the chemical hazard, such as the risk of explosion, volatility and solubility in water. Normally the ambulance control have the responsibility to enlist medical advice and assistance wherever necessary. Any further additional medical aid would be requested by the medical or ambulance incident officers. Where possible it is appropriate to send a doctor to chemical accidents whenever an ambulance is also despatched, even if there is little to do. This attendance is most useful as practice for the really big incident. The ambulance control should also alert appropriate hospitals, informing them of the nature of the hazard, if known. Neighbouring hospitals should also be informed as patients who have been involved may take themselves to any hospital by private means. The senior doctor called to the scene should play the role of Medical Incident Officer. His function is purely administrative, rather than clinical. In conjunction with the Ambulance Incident Officer he should liaise with the receiving hospitals.

Remember, when dealing with a hazardous substance:
  Do not touch it
  Try to identify it
  Inform Control
  Seek expert advice

PROTECTION OF RESCUE AND MEDICAL STAFF

Any personnel with pre-existing skin conditions, including wounds involving breaches of the skin, should avoid attending chemical incidents if at all possible. Utmost care should be taken to avoid personal contamination. Protective clothing should be worn at all times and, as a minimum, should include eye protection, impervious gloves, boots and overalls. There should be no smoking, drinking or eating at the scene, although early provision of food and rest away from the scene is much appreciated. All personnel who are exposed to the risk of contamination should wash under a shower as soon as practicable. Any wounds sustained during the incident should be flooded with water before being dressed. Any contaminated clothes or dressings should be sealed in a plastic bag until disposal is arranged (*Fig.* 27.8).

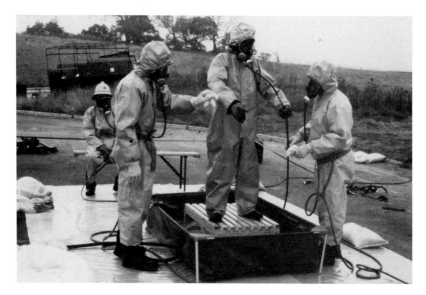

Fig. 27.8. Security of contaminated material.

PROCEDURES AT THE INCIDENT

Although there is considerable variation between authorities as to details, generally speaking the arrangements should be as detailed below. Most fire services have access to CHEMDATA, a computerized record of some 30 000 or more chemicals and there is generally a national centre ready to provide assistance in identifying chemicals not on local computer records. There is enormous value in having chemical experts on scene in difficult cases. Barriers should be set up to indicate a hazardous area. Only persons properly equipped with protective clothing appropriate to the nature of the hazard should be permitted to enter the contaminated zone. All persons and equipment coming out of the contaminated zone should follow a predetermined path under the direction of decontamination officers. If casualties are involved they would normally be removed from the hazardous area by fire brigade personnel as quickly as possible. The way in which this is done would be entirely dependent on the nature of the chemical hazard or contamination. In the case of toxic vapour, smoke or gas, removal to fresh air may be all that is necessary. For a few highly toxic and persistent substances it may be necessary to decontaminate casualties at the scene.

DECONTAMINATION

Decontamination would normally be effected by stripping and washing down thoroughly. Water alone, or water and detergent, are the most suitable agents for decontamination in almost all cases. On rare occasions, dry methods of cleaning, using intrinsically safe vacuum cleaners for dry powder contamination, and scraping, when tarry or viscous substances are involved, are employed.

Emergency life-saving procedures take precedence over any other decontamination. It is extremely rare that a victim will be so heavily contaminated with so toxic a chemical that the rescuer's own life is put at risk—assuming that the victim has been removed from the source of the contamination. Many authorities now have especially equipped decontamination vehicles which will provide the necessary equipment for decontamination, protection and shelter for contaminated casualties. When such facilities exist it is most important to exercise the equipment regularly with the other emergency services and medical teams. In other authorities, equipment only exists for the decontamination of firemen in protective clothing. Any other decontamination facility has to be improvised. The actual decontamination process basically consists of stripping and washing down the injured or contaminated casualties. If patients require stretchers then the easiest type to decontaminate casualties on is the scoop stretcher, but it should not be used to carry them any distance. In the case of females, reluctance to strip and wash them down must be balanced against the hazard involved. Contaminated property and clothing should be kept together and labelled. Polythene bags are useful for clothes and personal effects. It is most important that any contamination is contained and confined as closely as possible to its site of origin. To do this it must be ensured that as far as possible no persons, equipment or vehicles are allowed to leave the site until 'clean'. There may be occasions, however, when it is necessary for casualties to be removed from the scene to hospital for treatment whilst still contaminated to a greater or lesser degree. In such situations, especially if the contaminant is a volatile liquid, every precaution must be taken to avoid increasing the concentration of toxic fumes in the relatively confined space of the ambulance. This can be achieved by closing the door between cab and rear of the ambulance, opening all windows and wrapping the casualty in a polythene bag leaving his head uncovered. The practice of driving an ambulance with its rear doors open is probably unsafe.

It is also necessary for emergency departments to be prepared to receive injured contaminated casualties. Suitable rooms with adequate ventilation, extraction systems, showers and trolley baths are important. It is equally important that other casualties are kept away from contamination and that further spread is kept to a minimum.

Any ambulance that is used to convey contaminated casualties should not be used again until expert advice has been obtained about monitoring levels of contamination and cleaning.

Some patients who are contaminated may well take themselves to any hospital they consider appropriate for treatment and it is important that any such patients are identified and recorded as being from the incident.

Facilities at hospitals vary greatly from area to area and the on-site medical and ambulance staff should make themselves aware of local resources.

FATALITIES

Once a body has been certified dead by a doctor, it becomes the responsibility of the coroner or his equivalent. The police will normally take responsibility for decisions about further management but may well take professional advice from an on-site doctor. Depending on the nature of the incident and any possible criminal proceedings, corpses can either be decontaminated at the scene by hosing them down or they can be bagged at the scene and removed to the local mortuary. The former may destroy some forensic evidences; the latter spreads the risk of contamination considerably. All personnel handling corpses should be adequately protected. Much commonsense and initiative should be used, depending on the nature and degree of contamination. In incidents of disaster proportions temporary mortuaries may need to be established. Mass graves should be considered and, wherever possible, full documentation and, if possible, photography should be arranged before disposal.

EVACUATION

In an incident where toxic chemicals are liberated into the atmosphere in the form of smoke, powder, fumes or gases, it may become necessary to consider the possible need to evacuate the area at risk. The extent of such an area is dependent on many factors, such as wind velocity and direction, weather conditions and local topography. Clearly the decision to evacuate is one of urgent priority, if necessary. Evacuation of an area at risk would normally be undertaken by the police but, clearly, as they are not trained and equipped with breathing apparatus and protective clothing, it is usual for fire brigade members to deal with evacuation of the immediate area of contamination. Cordons around the area and security of evacuated property is the responsibility of the police. The local authorities are required to make contingency plans for mass evacuation in such instances and may plan to open rest centres. These rest centres are often in schools or halls and arrangements can be made for food, drinks, blankets and other requirements. Often the voluntary aid societies and other bodies can be mobilized to assist in them. The local authorities should also have plans for emergency transport. For the walking wounded and the uninjured, this may include local bus companies. Ambulance transport should only be used for those too ill, infirm or handicapped to use other transport. Evacuation from toxic vapour clouds can generate a great deal of panic and the whole operation needs firm and tactful policing. Public address systems and loud hailers are of considerable use in marshalling the people and offering explanations and reassurance.

A medical or first aid presence at each rest centre should be arranged to provide care for the frightened or distraught and for those who, during the evacuation, forgot important medication or left drugs behind. All those present at each centre should be recorded and their disposal to other places documented. This information should be collated subsequently, possibly by the police casualty bureau, or other responsible authority.

Plans for major chemical incidents need to be prepared in advance, in just the same way as most areas have plans for a train or air crash. Specified hospitals should be equipped and staffed to deal with contaminated casualties and those suffering from the acute effects of poisoning. In Sweden, 4 hospitals in the Stockholm area are included in a toxic chemicals plan. Two mobile units are equipped so that they can be taken to the scene of the incident. A series of suitable antidotes is stored at each hospital, and on the mobile units, to deal with the most common cases of chemical poisoning. The emergency store of antidotes is intended to supply the requirements of 10 severely poisoned persons for 3 days. A special routine is required to sort out expiry dates and the exchange of drugs within the store. In cases of severe emergency, one hospital will back up the other. It is clear that anyone poisoned or affected by toxic chemicals in the Stockholm area must be conveyed to one of the 4 participating hospitals and not taken to one that is nearer, just because it is nearer.

PRINCIPLES OF FIRST AID

Always use personal safety and protection equipment relevant to the known hazard. Unconscious patients should be cared for in the normal way using the recovery or semiprone position. Controlled or assisted ventilation and external chest compressions may be necessary. Inhalation casualties should be removed to fresh air and given absolute rest where possible. Oxygen should be administered in high concentrations and at an appropriate flow rate for as long as is necessary. With smoke inhalation, there may also be burns to the respiratory tract which may not be immediately apparent until the secondary pulmonary oedema develops. Where there is contamination, all affected clothes should be removed, together with wrist watches and shoes. The victim should be washed copiously with water and soap. If the eyes are affected they should be washed gently with a jet of water or normal saline. A simple arrangement is to use normal saline and a standard giving set to irrigate the eyes continuously, with a tap to control flow. Where irritant gases are involved it is useful to be able to use inhaled or nebulized beclomethasone. For hydrofluoric acid burns, a paste made from calcium gluconate is used to cover the burn area. Organophosphorus compounds often produce symptoms which may require injections of atropine. Phosphorus gel ignites spontaneously in air. If a patient has this adherent to skin or clothes, the affected area needs to be kept under water, or covered in very wet compresses or towels. In hospital the phosphorus can be removed under water by scraping with a spatula. Phosphorus is luminous in the dark.

CHEMICAL ACCIDENT FIRST AID SUMMARY

Skin Contact
1. Remove all contaminated clothing, including shoes, watch and jewellery, unless stuck to skin.
2. Drench affected area with running water using soap as well, if appropriate.
3. Check for burns and systemic signs of poisoning.
4. Set up intravenous infusion.
5. Refer to hospital, if required.

Eye Contact

1. Wash eye thoroughly using normal saline for at least 10 minutes.
2. Refer for specialist eye examination.

Ingestion

1. Do not make casualty vomit.
2. If unconscious, do not give anything by mouth.
3. Check breathing and pulse. Give artificial ventilation, if necessary, using a self-inflating bag (not mouth-to-mouth in cases of cyanide or hydrogen sulphide ingestion) or automatic resuscitator. Give external chest compressions, if necessary. Set up i.v. infusion.
4. If unconscious, but with pulse and breathing normally, place in the recovery position. Set up i.v. infusion.
5. If conscious, give a pint of water to drink immediately. If the chemical is corrosive, give 1 pint of milk unless the chemical contains phosphorus, chlorinated hydrocarbons or degreasing solvents, in which case continue giving water.
6. Transfer to hospital.

Inhalation

1. Remove from exposure, wearing appropriate protective clothing and breathing apparatus.
2. Check breathing and pulse, as above. Commence treatment with artificial ventilation and external chest compressions, if required. Set up i.v. infusion.
3. If appropriate, use the recovery position for unconscious patients who are breathing spontaneously.
4. Give oxygen.
5. Remove to hospital.

Advanced resuscitative measures should be provided to supplement first aid as soon as possible and follow the principles of dealing with the seriously ill, as indicated in Chapter 3.

REFERENCES

In this general review of procedures at chemical accidents, it is impossible to cover the individual effects of thousands of different chemicals. This detail is covered in three companion volumes which are essential reference sources for anyone involved in the medical response to a chemical incident:

Dangerous Chemicals Emergency Spillage Guide
Dangerous Chemicals Emergency First Aid Guide
Substances Hazardous to Health

All of these publications are available from The Administrator, Croner House, 173 Kingston Road, New Malden, Surrey KT3 3SS.

FURTHER READING

A Guide to the Control of Industrial Major Accident Hazards Regulations 1984. (CIMAH): Further Guidance on Emergency Plans. (1985) Health and Safety Executive, UK (Ref: HS/G25).

Approved Substance Identification Numbers, Emergency Action Codes and Classification for Dangerous Substances Conveyed by Road Tankers and Tank Containers. (The approved list) (1984) Health and Safety Executive, UK.

Chemical Industry Scheme for Assistance in Freight Emergencies (CHEMSAFE) (1976) Chemical Industries Association.

HAZCHEM Codes—Joint Committee on Fire Brigde Operations and Health and Safety Executive, UK. (1977) HN(77)167. London, DHSS.

National Arrangements for Incidents Involving Radio-Activity (NAIR) (1976) HC(76)52. London, DHSS.

28

Terrorism – General Aspects, Aetiology and Pathophysiology

INTRODUCTION

Terrorism may be defined as acts of violence carried out in peace time with the object of invoking fear and panic in the population. Nearly always these acts involve a threat to a life and/or the injury or death of innocent citizens. The infinite variety of methods by which they are committed, together with the total unpredictability of time and place make medical planning almost impossible. Justifiably therefore, in medical terms, terrorism may be classified as a disaster.

Terrorism is probably as old as the communal life of man. Historical purists, however, believe it should be dated from 'the Reign of Terror', synonymous with the French Revolution, since it was then that certain ideologists first stated that 'violence is necessary for the good of the people'. The second half of the 19th century saw the development of the modern concept where small groups of individuals carried out violent acts for political ends which in themselves were often of an anarchistic nature. In the last few decades the advent of the mass media has provided a launching pad for the image we know today.

The terrorist seeks to further his aims by causing fear and panic. This he hopes will stimulate the population to bring pressure to bear upon the authorities upon whom demands are being made. Apart from the actual demands being made, the aim is often to produce a disruption of the organization and daily running of society which often deliberately entails the humiliation of authority by demonstrating the inability of a government to protect its citizens. Profound emotions are stimulated and may result in strengthening the resolve of parts of the target population and their government, but paradoxically this may increase divisions within such society.

Three facets of man's modern social evolution encourage terrorism and will ensure its place in society for the foreseeable future:

Development of the Mass Media

This may now, for example, allow live coverage of a terrorist incident to be seen by millions around the world. The terrorist cause is advertised by such publicity and effectively increases the humiliation of authority.

Weapons of Mass Destruction

The incredible sophistication of man's ability to destroy his fellow man has now reached the stage where superpowers have the ability to produce total mutual destruction. The threat of total war may well have become outdated as an option by which one nation can express pressure on another. From this, therefore, terrorism might be considered as 'the new warfare'.

Modern Technology Aids the Terrorist

Technological developments in weaponry, coupled with the complexity of modern installations which make them more attractive targets, allow small, relatively impecunious groups to carry out acts of major destruction, which in turn encourage the humiliation effect since they allow 'the greater roar from smaller mice'.

Not only is terrorism, therefore, here to stay but undoubtedly its incidence will increase over the next few decades. Over the last few years the incidence of such acts has increased in frequency, in severity as judged by potential danger, and in diversity of location in all countries in the Western and Third World. Even the 'Utopian Societies' of Scandinavia have recently had their delusions of relative immunity shattered by the assassination of a Swedish prime minister. Figures for countries in the Eastern Bloc are not available.

Incidents may involve all three groups of the medical profession, namely general practitioners, hospital clinicians, and community medicine specialists.

General Practitioners

General practitioners may find themselves providing attention to the victims of an incident, either directly by being close to the scene or indirectly in the follow-up and rehabilitation of victims and their relatives.

Hospital Specialists

Those normally involved in the front line management of trauma, such as anaesthetists and surgeons, have an obvious role. Later, comparisons will be made between injury to those sustained in war where the injured are often fit young soldiers, and the victims of terrorist violence who are often those least able to withstand major trauma, such as the very young, the old and the pregnant. Therefore, various specialists not usually associated with violence, such as paediatricians, geriatricians, and obstetricians, may become involved. In psychopathological language the terrorist's aim could be said to be deliberately to produce a mass acute anxiety state within the population. Hence psychiatrists, again not usually associated with the management of trauma, may also become involved.

Community Medicine Specialists

The authorities have a duty to provide medical facilities which will support the population at these times and community physicians are required to co-ordinate the clinical services as well as plan and prepare the emergency services to deal with incidents should they arise.

Victims of terrorism frequently involve a large cross-section of the population, often previously unconnected with each other; for example, the passengers of a large civil airliner. In these circumstances it is by no means unlikely that one or more of the victims may be a doctor. Apart from the obvious role of tending any sick and injured, by virtue of his position in society many of the group may look to him for leadership and advice.

The types of injury that may be sustained by victims of terrorism are varied. Many sustain conventional trauma injuries, the pathology and management of which are described elsewhere. Terrorist violence, however, often brings into the area of the general practitioners' civilian practice or the catchment area of any district hospital injuries of the type usually seen only in war. Military medical specialists may, therefore, be required to assist in the planning and management of such incidents. This chapter, and the next, will deal with the preparation for, and the pathology and management of these injuries and also cover two fields of which they may have no knowledge, namely forensic psychology and pathology.

Before considering these matters, however, comment on ethical dilemmas is required.

ETHICAL CONSIDERATIONS

Codes of medical ethics require physicians to care for the sick and injured with compassion and skill, treating all equally without emotional involvement and without allowing their own moral or religious judgement to temper opinions and actions.

Management of the vast majority of the victims of terrorist violence will give rise to few problems but occasionally some may arise in respect of management and confidentiality. In addition to the 'innocent' members of the population, casualties may include members of the terrorist organizations involved and/or the forces of authority, i.e. the anti-terrorists.

For some centuries it has been normal in war-like conflicts for physicians to treat the wounded and sick of both sides, although this was not always the case. Enemy wounded receive the same skill and compassion on the battlefield, priority of treatment being based upon the patient's individual clinical needs. Even in the heat of battle, the medical services feel little rancour towards enemy wounded in their care. In fact, there may be a positive trade-off in that treating enemy wounded may help to secure similar management for those captured by the enemy. Professional soldiers have a respect for the enemy which involves providing protection and succour for him when he surrenders and a lack of bitterness, based on the fact that a soldier was doing his duty for his country. In the terrorist situation, however, a doctor may find that he has to go from the bedside of the mutilated victim of what may appear to be senseless violence, and who may be perhaps a child, a colleague or even a relative, to the bedside of the perpetrator of this act who has been injured during his capture. Despite emotion, which may run high, the physician must treat both the same. Like the anti-terrorist who is required to act, and be seen to act, within the laws of his country, so must the physician act and be seen to do so within codes of international medical ethics. Should he fail he will subsequently be subjected to censure which may, in the long term, aid and abet the terrorist.

On the battlefield a wounded prisoner, once assured that he will receive humanitarian care by his captors, will normally readily submit to appropriate medical and surgical management. In contrast, however, the captured terrorist may regard health care services as part of the hated target against which he has been directing his violence and will often act in an uncooperative manner, hurling both physical and verbal abuse at those attending him. When terrorists themselves are patients, problems of confidentiality and other ethical dilemmas may bring the physician into conflict with established authority which may be making demands upon him. It is necessary to draw a distinction between those demands made upon him by an authority which are required by law and those which are not. Only national law may override ethical conduct under these circumstances. When in doubt the doctor is best advised to take the advice of his senior professional colleagues whenever possible.

AETIOLOGY

Discussion of the causes of terrorism is beyond the scope of this book. However, since doctors may find themselves having to care clinically for terrorists, it may be helpful in their management to have some concept of motivation. Motivation is of three types:

Political or Religious

Here the stated aims and demands may in fact hide the true aim, which often is designed to destroy society itself.

Criminal

Here the aim is usually to achieve some form of personal gain, usually financial. There may, however, be other aims, such as freedom for colleagues or safe conduct to a place of sanctuary.

Delusionary

Superficially this may appear to be one of the groups above but the aims may, in fact, be the delusions of a mentally disturbed mind.

Distinction between these groups may often not be clear-cut. For example, criminals may claim political motivation in an excuse to seek asylum or avoid prosecution. Likewise, what may appear to be a criminal act, such as robbery, may be committed under the umbrella of a politically motivated underground organization. Distinction between a normal and abnormal state of mind in terrorists may be even more difficult to define. In practical terms, most governments regard all terrorist activity as criminal, irrespective of the motivation. Nevertheless, an understanding of the motivation is important for the doctor who may occasionally find himself involved with the forensic psychology of such conduct.

THE PATHOLOGY OF TERRORISM

The mechanism of violence inflicted upon victims of terrorism depends upon the nature of the incident. Sometimes the harm is potential rather than real, as may occur with kidnapping and hijacking.

The method chosen by the terrorist depends not only upon his aims but also upon his own abilities in terms of training, resources and access to facilities. Certain acts require far more sophistication and preparation than others. The main types can be considered in descending order of sophistication:

Kidnapping
Hijacking
Assassination
Mass hostage-taking with barricades and sieges
Bombing
Riot stimulation

Some hostage and/or hijack situations, however, may be unplanned. This is usually when more sophisticated plans have gone wrong in the criminal type of incident.

Over the last few decades the most common type of incident has involved explosive devices. These are responsible for at least 80 per cent of all incidents, and approximately 62 per cent of incidents in the European theatre. Bombs have been responsible for 95 per cent of the casualties inflicted by terrorists. Other causes of injury are gunshot wounds and stabbings. Rarely victims may be involved in fires, usually secondary to an explosion, or blunt trauma sustained from body blows or blunt missiles. The latter are common in riots.

In contrast to the rural scene where explosive devices may be used to ambush small parties of personnel, usually belonging to military or police forces, explosive devices in the urban situation cause anywhere between 20 and 200 casualties.

Types of injuries resulting from terrorism tend to differ from those sustained in other disasters described in this book in the following ways:

1. The frequency of selection by the terrorist of targets involving a density of population.
2. The vast majority of injuries are of a type seen only in war.
3. Fear and panic among the population, which although common to many disasters, have been deliberately invoked by the aetiological agent and lead to an increased element of psychiatric problems. Acute physical crises brought on by this fear, such as cardiac arrhythmias, especially amongst those susceptible, can also occur.

APPLIED FORENSIC PSYCHOLOGY

In certain terrorist scenarios, such as a siege or when hostages are held, doctors may be required to advise and help the anti-terrorist forces to bring the incident to a 'successful conclusion'. From the physicians' viewpoint the definition of a 'successful conclusion' must be to end the incident by a course of action which results in minimal loss of life or injury to all concerned. Rarely will non-specialists be required to advise in this manner and in some countries there are now specifically trained specialists for this purpose. However, for the non-specialist doctor who might occasionally find himself in this position it is necessary to understand the problems since, at a later date, they may often have to care for victims or terrorists.

The Terrorist

Doctors may be asked to advise on the state of mind of terrorists and for this they are referred to standard textbooks on forensic psychiatry. To produce a 'successful conclusion' experience shows that once the law enforcement or anti-terrorist forces have constrained the incident, a forced conclusion should be delayed for as long as possible. As time proceeds, sleep deprivation and other factors depress the terrorist's psychological 'high' from its peak at the onset and often the futility of his situation gradually becomes apparent. American experience suggests that the main exception to this rule is the prison revolt where hardened criminals, often serving genuine life sentences and, therefore, with little to lose, tend to become more hardened, more resolute and more dangerous as time passes. Early resolution by force is, therefore, often advocated in such circumstances.

The Hostage

From the moment of capture hostages are in a state of existential fear. This is a mixture of fear for life or limb coupled with the psychological stresses which threaten the image of the individual, resulting from his helpless detention against his will. Such a threat to self-esteem can be almost as significant as the reaction to physical threats and, as will be seen later, may be more important in producing the long-term after-effects.

During their period of detention hostages find that there are recurrent episodes of sheer terror usually associated with feelings of complete helplessness. The fear produced by this sensation is one over which the victim finds he can exert little control. A similar example is the fear which grips the passengers of a crashing aircraft, contrasted, for example, with that of the flight deck crew who are attempting to resolve the situation. It may be contrasted also with the feelings of a soldier on a battlefield, who is still fighting and can still fire his weapon.

This fear is further exacerbated by gross distortions of sensory input. On one hand there may be a total overload caused, for example, by the noises of conflict, both deliberate noises by the rescuing authorities intended either to stun or to prevent sleep amongst terrorists and prolonged harangues by fanatical ones. At the other extreme there may be sensory deprivation by isolation in a dark, unknown, locked room. Total disorientation in time and space is thus produced.

The most common response of hostages to these problems is the syndrome of 'frozen fright'. Here there is a paralysis of affect and logical thought. Outwardly, however, the victims often appear calm and seem to obey their captor passively and co-operatively. Emotions expressed, if any, are often inappropriate, illogical and may appear to be sympathetic towards their captors. Sometimes there is definite resentment against the authorities attempting to rescue them.

Psychologists explain some of this emotional response as 'traumatic infantilism' in which conditions of extreme fear cause the psyche to resort to a child-like state where there is a total dependence upon 'the hand that feeds', irrespective of the treatment received from that individual. Battered children often demonstrate considerable affection for the parents upon whom they are totally dependent. They may be quite defensive of their violent parents and will seem to resent intervention by the public authorities. The same tends to be true in the hostage situation with the hostages developing positive feelings for their captor upon whom they are dependent for their lives. These syndromes of 'frozen fright' and 'traumatic infantilism' are of considerable practical importance to authorities planning hostage rescue. The authorities must appreciate that they can expect little co-operation from the hostages. Hostages may behave in an illogical or irrational manner which may hamper their rescue. Rescuing authorities must not expect hostages to assist them in either a practical or theoretical way, since they may not even support their rescuers' ideological point of view, irrespective of the view held by them prior to being captured.

An extreme variant of this has been described as the Stockholm Syndrome, named after an incident in 1974 in that city. Here a bank robber, who had taken a female employee of the bank hostage, was besieged in a vault. During the siege, a positive relationship developed between the two such that not only did marriage subsequently occur but on release the hostage roundly complained to the authorities about the treatment of her captor. A similar case occurred when Patti Hearst, an American newspaper heiress, was kidnapped by the anarchistic Symbianese Liberation Army and next heard of actively fighting for them in an armed raid.

In order for the syndrome to be complete, it is necessary not only for the hostages to have developed positive feelings for their captor and negative feelings for authority but also for the captor, secondarily, to develop positive protective feelings for the hostages. Many besieging authorities deliberately attempt to foster the development of this syndrome in the hope that it will help to ensure the safety of the hostages. However, the syndrome will usually only develop under certain circumstances, which usually require that the hostages have a relatively immature personality and that the captors themselves are exposed to a degree of psychological stress or danger. Such a syndrome, for example, did not develop during the New Mexico State Penitentiary riots in 1980, where the hardened criminals had no wish to develop such relationships and their hostages were mature prison officers. In the American Embassy siege in Teheran there was likewise no such development, and this was due, possibly, to the fact that the guards were at no time in any danger.

Immediate management of hostages upon release is one of considerable practical importance. At the moment of release, victims are still in a state of frozen fright and possibly traumatic infantilism and if allowed immediately to be reunited with friends and relatives will often break down into a submissive infantile type of behaviour. The knowledge that they have done so, in retrospect, will be detrimental to their ultimate recovery and humiliating to all concerned. It is, therefore, recommended that victims are permitted an hour or two, usually in isolation and in privacy, before reunion and before facing the outside world again.

THE PATHOPHYSIOLOGY OF TERRORIST VIOLENCE

Explosions may injure many people indirectly as a result of being thrown through the air, violence from striking blunt objects or the ground, or injury from falling masonry, sometimes resulting in being crushed and/or trapped beneath collapsed buildings. Occasionally a fire may cause burns. All these forms of injury are dealt with elsewhere and remarks will be confined to the injuries caused by explosives and the effects of missiles set in motion by them.

Injuries from Explosives

Ever since man invented explosives, he became aware that injury could occur as a result of the explosion alone without any penetration. It was observed that many die with no external evidence of violence. Until the earlier part of this century it was commonly believed that this was the result of either toxic inhalation of chemicals produced or possibly anoxia due to rapid consumption of oxygen by the chemical reaction of the explosion. As early as 1758, however, Jars had suggested that these injuries were a result of the acute expansion of gases, as described in his paper *Dilatation d'Air*. Many victims of blast injury do, however, have elevated blood levels of toxic substances, including carbon monoxide and other substances released from modern explosives, which in themselves are potentially lethal and so may have contributed towards the pathology. The theory of acute hypoxia, however, probably cannot be substantiated as being of any significance, since within a few seconds there is an inrush of air from the surrounding atmosphere. However, explosions may cause massive fire storms which consume all available oxygen as was seen following bombing raids in World War II.

The explosive blast in a conventional explosion is caused by the very rapid expansion of a mass of hot gas, which apart from setting in motion missiles which are discussed below, has 3 primary physical effects:

1. The formation of a blast shock wave.
2. The release of radiant heat to cause burns.
3. The production of rapidly moving columns of gas in the surrounding air, called the blast wind.

The Shock Wave

This is a front of overpressure expanding rapidly away from the centre of the explosion. Initially it travels very fast but rapidly settles down to the speed of sound which is approximately 300 m/s in air. The extent of the overpressure falls off rapidly according to the inverse cube law. The effects of such a pressure wave obviously depend upon the size and duration of the overpressure produced. Since the wave is passing rapidly through the air the duration may be described as a 'thickness' of the pressure front. This thickness depends upon the type of explosive material. A standard high explosive, such as TNT, will produce a shock wave with the duration of a milli-second whilst at the other end of the scale a thermonuclear device, which will not be further discussed, may produce a shock wave with a duration in the vicinity of a complete second.

The peak and/or thickness of the shock wave may also depend upon other physical phenomena; for example, reflection from a nearby solid surface effectively doubles the pressure peak.

Armament manufacturers have attempted to overcome the effect of the very rapid fall-off of overpressure from the centre of the explosion by developing weapons in which the explosive material covers a large volume. Such weapons, known as fuel air weapons, consist of a cloud of potentially explosive material several metres across, which may be either a true gas, droplets or solids absorbed onto particles, which are subsequently ignited. Blast overpressure remains high throughout the cloud and, therefore, a much larger area is subjected to overpressure than from a point explosion. Such a weapon is difficult to use and requires sophisticated equipment, probably beyond the ability of the majority of terrorists. From the traumatologist's point of view, however, the effects produced will also be seen when any cloud of potentially explosive material is ignited, possibly accidentally, in industrial accidents or in domestic coal gas explosions.

Two hundred years after Jars originally propounded the concept of blast injury, the exact mechanism by which it produces damage to the body is still not completely understood. For a time it was thought likely that the wave of high pressure passed through the upper air passages into the trachea and lungs, directly injuring the bronchial tract. In World War II, after animal experiments, it was concluded that most of the damage resulted from a compression effect on the body as a whole.

On striking a mammalian target, some of the pressure wave is reflected, some is deflected and some is absorbed by the tissues. The latter may be increased by a phenomenon of damming up before penetration. Once absorbed, the pressure wave passes through the various tissues at different speeds in proportion to their density, but in all cases this is much greater than that of its speed in air. It has long been observed that the majority of the damage is inflicted at tissue/air interfaces. In terms of physics 4 different phenomena occur, almost certainly simultaneously:

a. There is a general compression of the body as the pressure wave strikes the presenting surface first, which may be likened to the body being thrown against a solid brick wall, and generalized contusion of organs occurs in proportion to the duration of the wave of overpressure.

b. A shock wave passing through a dense medium reaching an interface with a less dense medium, for example a gas, throws off small particles of the former into the latter. Such a phenomenon is seen following an underwater explosion in which quantities of water will be thrown into the air from the surface, and is also seen when small particles from the inner surface of protective armour plates and/or bunkers are thrown off injuring personnel. This phenomenon is known as 'spalling' and is presumed to occur in the body when the shock wave reaches the tissue/air interface, such as the lining of upper and lower respiratory tracts and the bowel. Cellular disruption is caused on the surface of these membranes. This is in complete contrast to the original concept of the pressure wave travelling down the trachea and damaging the lungs from within. This is probably the method of damage to the olfactory end organs overlying the ethmoid plate, the shock wave reaching the plate via the bones of the skull before it reaches it through the air passages.

c. Minor variations in density between different tissue planes will also cause differential speeds of the shock wave and, likewise, the degree to which these tissues will be set in motion relative to each other will differ since they have different constants of inertia. Sheer effects may, therefore, occur and this is probably the mechanism by which submucosal and subserosal haemorrhages are produced, which in turn result in ischaemic changes in the devitalized surface lining.

d. Gas trapped within the organs, such as the alveoli or gut lining, will be compressed or displaced when surrounded by the shock wave producing the phenomenon of inplosion. During the re-expansion phase, perforation may occur and gas may enter the circulation through ruptures of vessel walls.

Since all 4 mechanisms occur simultaneously, both in experimental and real conditions, it is academic to apportion responsibility. Of greater import are the clinical syndromes produced from studies of human victims and animal experiments. Two groups may be considered, those who die a sudden death and those who survive the initial insult.

Sudden Death

Many mammals subjected to a particularly high incident pressure wave may die instantly with no external evidence of injury. Animal experimentation, however, suggests that many cases die from air embolism. Air is believed to be forced directly through breaches of the alveolar membrane or ruptures of arteriovenous shunts in the lung parenchyma as a result of the physical phenomena described above. Air emboli can be tolerated by many tissues which can withstand end artery ischaemia for the time taken to absorb the gas. Brain and myocardium, however, are exceptions and it is believed that sudden death is the result of fatal coronary air embolism. Direct cardiac contusion, due to sudden thoracic compression, is another possible aetiology, although animal experimentation does not support this. Cardiac arrest in humans, however, following severe thoracic compression or a blow over the myocardium, is not unknown and it may well be that the human myocardium is more susceptible to injury than those of experimental mammals due to anatomical differences.

Survivors

Tympanic membrane. First to be damaged is the tympanic membrane which will rupture when there is an overpressure of 30 kPa. Fortunately the majority of such perforations heal spontaneously. The most significant clinical point is that intact tympanic membranes make it unlikely, but not impossible, that the patient has been subjected to a serious blast overpressure. Further rise in overpressure may produce direct sensoneural damage to the cochlea producing clinical signs of deafness similar to those seen in severe acoustic barotrauma.

Lungs. Once overpressure starts to reach the vicinity of 70 kPa, evidence of lung damage begins to appear, being almost certainly present with an overpressure of 200 kPa. A 50 per cent mortality occurs once the overpressure reaches 300 kPa. The amount of damage is, of course, also determined by duration of overpressure in addition to its degree. Lesions produced include rupture of the alveoli, their lining membrane, and also damage to arteriovenous shunts. A common result is intra-alveolar haemorrhage which in survivors may produce an increasing degree of diffusion block with concomitant increasing respiratory failure over a period of time. The subsequent course of this condition is very similar to that seen in adult respiratory distress syndromes, with an increasing diffusion effect. The syndrome of blast lung, however, differs from other cases of ARDS in the early phases in that air may enter the circulation.

Cardiac effects. Animal experimentation shows an intense bradycardia occurs after subjection to high overpressure. This effect is abolished by denervation, and is probably explained by direct pressure on the carotid sinus. Primary cardiac contusion can also be seen, but rupture is said to be rare.

Abdominal viscera. Overpressure sufficient to produce pulmonary damage is also likely to produce effects below the diaphragm, mainly affecting the hollow viscera, although retroperitoneal and subserosal haemorrhage of the solid viscera, such as liver and spleen, are commonly recorded. Thirty-four per cent of fatal cases have lacerations of the liver. In the gastrointestinal tract, haemorrhage may occur in the submucosal or subserosal planes and occasionally into the lumen of the bowel itself. Perforation, due to shearing effects in an area of ischaemic bowel, may occur at the time of injury or after an interval. In man the ileocaecal region, for reasons unknown, is the area most commonly affected.

Cerebral effects. Assessment of the effect of blast alone on man is difficult since concomitant blunt head injury is very common. A study of blast fatalities in Northern Ireland showed 66 per cent to have suffered severe brain injury and 51 per cent to have skull fracture. Air embolism certainly occurs and may progress some time after exposure producing a clinical picture of increasing loss of cerebral function, possibly over a period of several hours, sometimes proceeding to fatal massive cerebral softening. Dissection of the carotid artery in its intraosseous course has also been considered a possible cause. There are many well known clinical syndromes in which victims appear to be in a totally dazed or confused state and have been described with labels such as 'shellshock'. It is by no means clear to what extent physical stresses, as distinct from psychological stresses, are responsible for these syndromes. Animal experimentation shows that there are alterations in EEG patterns following blast which are quite dissimilar to those following blunt trauma, in which there is a cessation of all electrical activity. Electron microscopy shows evidence in animals of diffuse intraneural damage following such a shock wave. The clinical significance of these factors, even if they occur in man, is unknown.

On occasions the shock wave may be transmitted to the body through a solid or liquid medium. In the case of solids this may, for example, be the deck of a ship, and the net result tends to be a contusion to the part of the body in contact with the solid. Clinical syndromes describing this in war have been known as 'deck slap' and 'destroyer heel'.

Explosion shock waves transmitted through the water have specific characteristics. The incompressability of water means that there is far less absorption of the shock wave, causing it to be propagated over a much wider area. Its fall-off tends to follow the inverse square rather than the inverse cube law, as seen in air. The velocity of the shock wave in water is approximately 4 to 5 times that in air and, therefore, it will surround a body in the water much more quickly than in air, and the 'squeeze effect' will occur with a wave of much shorter duration. The maximum point of overpressure tends to be at a distance of approximately 1 m below the surface of water. Casualties floating horizontally on the surface tend, therefore, to be relatively protected in contrast to those who are perhaps treading water in the vertical position. This may also account for the observation that underwater blast tends to increase the preponderance of intra-abdominal injuries (rectal perforation is common) in contrast to injuries to the chest. There is also some protection given to vertically floating victims since the upper part of the chest may well be protruding from the surface. Even in patients whose head is protruding from the water cerebral manifestations appear which are probably secondary to arterial air embolism.

Other Primary Effects of Explosions

Flash Burns

Depending on the type of explosive, the sudden release of energy may give off a short burst of thermal radiation sufficient to produce flash burns in those in relatively close proximity. These burns are usually of a superficial type and tend only to affect exposed skin, normally the face and hands. It is worth noting that hair tends to protect the scalp even if there is a temporary ignition of the hair. The bald scalp is, by contrast, extremely vulnerable to a flash burn.

Blast Wind

This is a column of gas generated initially from the explosion, and later air displaced by the explosion, which moves outwards at high speed, many times that encountered in hurricanes. The injuries produced by such winds are often bizarre and may be severe. Close to the explosion, total destruction and atomization occurs, the victims literally being torn apart. However, on the outer limits of the area of lethality there will be some survivors and traumatic limb amputations occur. In this type of traumatic amputation, structures will be avulsed at different levels. The nerves may often be torn off at a far more proximal level than the other tissues. In the upper limb this may well be at the level of the brachial plexus. Blast winds are often channelled by surrounding features, such as furniture, producing bizarre pictures. For example, a victim sitting at a table may have severe damage to the lower limbs while the trunk, upper limbs and head remain unscathed. Likewise one body may protect another; for example, a person suffering a traumatic amputation will shield the person sitting next to him so that he remains relatively unscathed.

Penetrating Missile Injury

The vast majority of injuries are produced by missiles set in motion by the explosion. These may be considered as primary or secondary missiles.

Primary Missiles

Primary missiles are those integral to the bomb itself being packed around the explosive. In military devices they may form part of the casing of the weapon, being prestressed to fragment at particular points. The Mills 36 grenade was so designated since its casing was designed to fragment into approximately 3 dozen pieces of metal, each about an inch square, which gave it the chocolate bar appearance. In more modern devices the explosive is surrounded by a material, often wire, intended to fragment into many thousands of pieces, each only a few grains in size, but having a kinetic energy of up to 200 J. Bullets may technically be considered to be solitary primary missiles from an explosion which differ from bomb fragments because they are aerodynamically stable, may be directed and are much heavier, with a kinetic energy of as much as 2500 J. Non-military explosive devices, as commonly used by terrorists, are usually 'home-made'. Here the missiles may be an assortment of articles around the explosive, including stones, nuts, bolts, nails, etc. The outer casing which may fragment unpredictably can be any form of bag, case, box, filing cabinet and, particularly popular in rural districts, a milk churn. The unpredictable nature of such a device on detonation is responsible for bizarre effects, seen in some explosions, where people in close proximity may escape relatively unharmed, whilst a solitary individual has been killed some distance away by one missile from such a device.

Secondary Missiles

Secondary missiles are objects set in motion in the vicinity of the explosion that are not part of the bomb itself. Some may achieve velocities similar to those of the primary missile. The number and nature of such missiles depend not only upon the quantity of material around but also its tendency to fragment. Obvious examples of easily fragmented material are wood and glass. Any materials found in the construction of modern buildings, or their contents, may be involved and can include at one end of the spectrum modern plastics, formica and laminates, and at the other, major heavy construction materials such as concrete. Bizarre injuries have been reported, varying from serious injury produced by almost microscopic particles, to complete through-and-through penetration by missiles as large as a piece of 4 × 2 inch (10 × 5 cm) timber. Injury from fragmentation of other individuals may occur.

Missiles produce damage by several pathological mechanisms. These are:
1. Momentum effect
2. Laceration and penetration
3. High energy transfer

Momentum

An individual struck by several fragments suffers multiple contusion from the change of momentum. In some cases, this may be sufficient to produce a major traumatic amputation. This should be contrasted with the avulsion type of amputation due to blast winds. Here the structures will tend to be amputated at a similar level but the wound, which will often be jagged and irregular, will be complicated by retention within the tissues of fragments and possibly gas from the explosion. Such a situation is extremely common in lower limb injuries sustained by treading on anti-personnel mines.

Laceration and Penetration

Any tissue in the track of a missile may suffer such an injury. The missile will often carry into its track secondary missiles from the outside, such as protective clothing, or any tissues through which they have passed such as skin and bone fragments. Some missile fragments may be fairly clean, such as the smooth surface of glass or inorganic material, and others e.g. wood splinters may be extremely 'dirty' and contain millions of micro-organisms within their structure. Horrendous infective inflammatory reactions were well described by naval surgeons in the era of wooden battleships.

High Energy Transfer

A missile, during its retardation after striking a target, gives up some (or in the event of it stopping, all) of its kinetic energy. Initially the kinetic energy released is used to form the track through the target and some will be given off as heat, but this is of little clinical significance. Should a missile have a level of kinetic energy higher than that required to form the track, then the excess energy will be transferred to the tissues to cause a so-called 'high energy transfer wound'. For a missile to have the potential to produce high energy transfer it normally requires a velocity greater than that of the speed of sound in air and the energy available is proportional to the square of such velocity. Some, but probably not the majority, of bomb fragments found in survivors have such a capacity. Bullets from most rifles and machine guns do, but those from hand guns do not normally come into this category. The transfer of these high levels of energy to the tissues (a rifle bullet transversing a human thigh will release approximately 400 horse power), produces the phenomenon known as cavitation. Here a temporary cavity many times the size of the bullet track is formed in tissues, all tissue being forced out of position for a few thousandths of a second. Two secondary physical phenomena then occur. Apart from the obvious tearing of structures as they are forced out of the way by the cavity, tissues in the surrounding area will be subjected to an overpressure of up to 400 kPa. Tissues tolerate such an overpressure but as the cavity collapses the same tissues are then subjected to an underpressure of as much as 200 kPa which produces severe disruption at cellular level. The tissues will, therefore, in a wide area surrounding the track, contain a large number of dead cells and an even greater number of cells whose viability might be described as critical. Massive tissue swelling occurs, due to cloudy swelling, oedema arising from capillary leakage by compromised cells, as well as haemorrhage. If restricted, this swelling initiates a vicious cycle of reduced tissue perfusion, producing further hypoxia, oedema and cell death. As the temporary cavity collapses, the negative pressure also causes a mass of debris to be sucked into the wound through both exit and entry wounds. Such contamination is in addition to the particles that are carried in by the penetrating missile, and includes skin contaminated with invisible faecal dirt that covers the majority of human skin from the waist to the knees. Following such an injury, therefore, there will be 100 per cent bacterial contamination of an area of widespread tissue damage.

Relative Significance of Blast and Fragment Injury

Injury by missile fragments is of far greater clinical significance than that due to primary blast effect. Estimates show that in terrorist bomb incidents, between only 2 and 4·5 per cent of patients subsequently treated in hospital sustain significant blast injury. When military devices are used this figure is probably even lower, since the more efficient fragmentation design of such weapons tends to insure that the area of lethality due to fragment injury is far greater than the area of lethality due to blast.

29

Terrorism – Management and Forensic Aspects

This chapter will consider planning, the management of blast and penetrating missile injury and the simple psychiatry of terrorist victims. It ends with a brief discussion of the forensic aspects of terrorism which may involve medical practitioners.

PLANNING

Prevention of these disasters is in the province of politicians, security officers and law enforcement agencies. Many incidents are prevented by intense security precautions, but some, like assassination, occur just outside the security screen. For example, it is the public bar in which soldiers drink rather than their heavily defended military headquarters that is blown up and the late Lord Mountbatten and Mr Airey Neave are examples of individuals assassinated in this manner.

Medical authorities have a duty to make appropriate preparations and contingency plans for terrorist incidents. The existence and rehearsal of such plans may lessen considerably the ensuing chaos of such an incident and so reduce the impact which the terrorist is attempting to achieve. Two scenarios should be planned for:

1. Mass casualties, such as caused by a bomb.
2. Incidents where a small number of casualties, real or potential, may occur.

1. Mass Casualties

When planning for these incidents they should be considered in the same way as any other mass casualty situation. For practical purposes it should be noted that the majority of bomb incidents in an urban setting produce between 20 and 200 victims. In the face of an increased security threat, the authorities must strike a fine balance between making adequate preparations and increasing the public awareness to a point where their apprehension will so increase that the terrorist is assisted in achieving his aim.

2. Small Group Incidents

These include situations where harm, potential or real, may occur to a small number of individuals. This includes assassination of specific persons, hijacking and sieges. Sometimes there is merely a threat and sometimes incidents have occurred where there is the potential for considerable injury and possibly death caused either by terrorists or security forces operating against them. In the latter case, even if no physical harm results, there will always be some psychological damage. Planning should involve the availability, at short notice, of teams with specialized expertise in life support together with the appropriate equipment and facilities to transport such patients to a surgical centre as rapidly as possible. The surgical centres which could be involved should also be involved in the planning and should have appropriate communications and warning to prepare to receive any such casualties. Staff in such a centre should, if possible, be personally acquainted with members of the specialized teams on sight to reduce any confusion and improve team work should they arrive in the hospital with their patients.

Predetermined concepts of triage, along with pre-arranged documentation, such as labels, should form part of the plan as for all other major disasters (*see* Chapter 2). Administrative back-up and casualty evacuation should follow standard mass casualty procedures, although the following special problems which occur in relation to bomb incidents, etc. should be noted:

a. The security problem continues after the incident and may hamper treatment and evacuation. Likewise medical services may, in themselves, hamper security operations. Collaboration between security and medical services in both the planning and at the time is essential.

b. There is a large element of panic at the scene involving a number of dazed, bewildered and mildly injured casualties. This is complicated by the well-known 'spectator' syndrome seen at other disasters. The panic induced is, of course, part of the result required by the perpetrators of the act and may serve to confuse the rescue of casualties. The acute fear may in itself precipitate a large number of 'collapses' some of which may be a sheer fright response, whilst others may be genuine.

c. A very real fear which may hamper rescue arrangements and must always be remembered is the possibility of a second explosion, sometimes deliberately engineered by the terrorists.

d. Unlike other disasters described in this book, once the victims are clear of the scene of the incident and admitted to hospital they are not necessarily safe. Security may entail a protective screen at the hospital. Attacks on hospitals, specifically aimed at assassination of certain patients, are by no means unknown. Patients have been shot whilst lying in an intensive care unit.

e. In riot situations where tensions between different factions have been running high it may be necessary to arrange for victims of different sides to be treated in separate hospitals, otherwise the conflict will continue.

f. There may be particular problems with members of hospital staff in that they may receive direct, or indirect, threats from terrorist organizations should they attempt to treat the victims. In some countries, where terrorist acts are committed by a party with considerable popular following, it may also have sympathizers within the hospital staff.

MANAGEMENT OF BLAST INJURY

Resuscitation both on site and in hospital should follow standard lines. The following specific points should, however, be noted. Diagnosis, especially on site, can be very difficult. Initially a blast injured patient may have no signs of external damage and appear unhurt but may suddenly deteriorate either in the next few minutes, or a few hours later. Associated injuries, such as inhalation burns or penetration by small fragments, which may initially appear to be of minor import, may in fact be severe. A very conservative approach, therefore, should be taken.

Whenever there is a possibility of significant blast damage, positive pressure ventilation should, if possible, be avoided for at least the first hour after the exposure to blast in order to reduce the risk of air embolism. There is possibly a case, if positive pressure must be used, for performing prophylactic pleural drainage because of the high risk of pneumothorax. Fluid overload should be avoided in view of pulmonary and possibly cardiac lesions produced by blast. Likewise positive end expiratory pressure should be avoided whenever possible for several days, and there is some experimental evidence in animals to suggest that even an increased inspired oxygen level can be detrimental, by producing an increase in intra-alveolar haemorrhage. Some advocate the immediate prophylactic administration of corticosteroids but their value has never been cofirmed. There is perhaps some justification for their use where smoke inhalation has occurred in conjunction with major burns.

On arrival at hospital, once resuscitation has been commenced, a thorough top-to-toe examination of the patient is necessary. In bomb victims an early examination should include examination of the tympanic membranes. Management of a perforation itself is minimal, and healing is usually spontaneous. However, the presence of an intact tympanic membrane may well indicate that the patient has not received significant blast injury. Early general neurological examination for base line purposes should be performed, and olfactory sensation recorded, since anosmia is not uncommon.

Immediate and repeated assessments for signs of respiratory or cardiac failure should be performed, and these may include base line blood gas estimations. Chest X-ray is mandatory and frequent examinations of the fundi for air embolism in the retinal vessels advocated. Should respiratory failure begin to appear, aggressive management is required, but a fine balance must be made to avoid the complications described above. Central venous pressure should be kept either below, or in the lower range of normal.

Where there is no evidence of missile penetration, careful assessment of the abdomen, including erect X-ray, is mandatory. Generalized abdominal tenderness is common due to multiple small internal haemorrhages and, since such patients do not fare well with general anaesthesia because of the accompanying pulmonary injury, a conservative line should be taken whenever possible. Nasogastric suction, with carefully monitored intravenous therapy, is required. Only if signs of local peritoneal irritation, massive intraperitoneal haemorrhage or radiological evidence of free gas in the peritoneum appear, should laparotomy be performed.

Traumatic amputations caused by the blast winds will require aggressive life-saving first aid measures and immediate care personnel should not be afraid to use a tourniquet. There can be few greater tragedies than death due to exsanguination in such a case when a tourniquet has not been used because the 'first aider' has been overcautioned about the dangers of its application. These amputations are avulsive in nature, the internal structures, especially the nerves, often being avulsed at more proximal levels. Therefore, even if the limb is available, re-implantation is not a practical proposition.

Acute neurological deterioration may occur in cases of closed blast injury. As described above the pathology is not clearly understood, although on occasion it obviously may be the result of massive air embolism, and sometimes the services of a specialized neurological centre are required. In most cases it is doubtful whether any therapeutic intervention will affect the prognosis.

PENETRATING MISSILE TRAUMA

The most common injuries caused by bombs are due to penetrating missiles. Such patients may also have blast injury. Victims may have been hit by one or two missiles or even several hundred. Gunshot wounds may be considered under this heading as 'small number' missile injuries. Sometimes it is possible to determine the potential of the injuring missile to have caused a high energy transfer wound, and this may influence the management. For example, if the sole injury is known to be a through and through injury of soft tissue by a bullet from a hand gun, with relatively low velocity, then the injury may be treated as one of low energy transfer.

Diagnosis

Two questions must be asked when examining a patient who has been injured under these circumstances. Has the patient been injured by a penetrating missile? What is the possible track through which the fragment, or bullet, may have passed?

Diagnosis of Penetration

Any patient injured under circumstances where there has been an explosion or gun fire, who has any form of wound at all, must potentially be considered to have sustained an injury by a penetrating missile. A suspicion that a penetrating missile has been responsible must be maintained until proved otherwise. Many wounds may appear to be small abrasions or cuts and may even be considered by the patient to have been sustained in this manner.

'A patient reported to his doctor some 4 hours after being involved in a riot, saying he had received a small cut above the lateral malleolus from a piece of flying glass. The small wound appeared perfectly clean and was sutured. Only 3 days later, after the patient complained of persistent pain in the leg, was an X-ray arranged which showed a low velocity bullet lodged at mid-calf.'

Where there could be any suspicion of missile penetration X-ray is mandatory.

Possible Track

This may be difficult to determine since fragments may be deflected en route through the body, and often it is impossible to determine the posture in which the patient was at the time of impact. This is of particular importance when studying penetrating wounds of the trunk. Wounds of the thoracic cavity, in patients who survive to reach hospital, often carry a good prognosis and require little treatment, other than perhaps chest drainage. The converse, however, applies to the abdomen where penetrating missile injuries almost always require surgery and postoperative morbidity and mortality is high. There is a tendency to think of the abdomen as being represented by the hexagonal drawing usually placed in the clinical notes to represent the anterior abdominal wall when recording physical signs. However, this only indicates the region between the costal margin and the inguinal ligaments. Remember that the abdominal cavity extends for a further third of its distance above the costal margin and also down into the true pelvis. Not only does the abdomen have a front, but sides and a back and, especially important to remember, a top and a bottom represented by the diaphragm above and the pelvis and its outlet below. Missiles may, therefore, enter the abdomen through the chest, or through thighs, buttocks or perineum. Suspicion of abdominal involvement in all such injuries must be borne in mind. Such injuries, especially those where the missile has passed through the back, thighs, buttocks or perineum, are especially dangerous because of the risk of contamination of large muscle masses with faecal material.

Principles of Management

It should be remembered that all penetrating injuries are contaminated and, whenever there has been high energy transfer, contamination will be mixed with necrotic tissue which provides an ideal tissue medium. The principles of treatment of such a wound are:

    a. Removal, as far as possible, of any non-viable tissue.
    b. Removal of foreign contaminants wherever possible.
    c. Allow the wound to heal without an increase in wound tension.

The practical details of achieving this are as follows:

a. Removal of Non-Viable Tissue

The wound must first be explored through wide surgical incisions. In the limbs these should be in the longitudinal axis, and the practice of joining entry and exit wounds should be avoided. Excision of devitalized skin should be kept to an absolute minimum, except that the contused area around the edge of entry and exit wounds should be excised. Subcutaneous fat whose vitality is in doubt should be ruthlessly removed. Non-functioning or devitalized voluntary muscle should be removed and its viability should be judged by the physical signs of capillary bleeding when cut, contraction when squeezed by forceps, colour and consistency. The latter two features require a degree of clinical experience. Bone fragments, unless totally devitalized and detached from their periosteum, should not be removed. Major nerves and blood vessels should not be removed unless irreparably damaged. Under some circumstances, with distal limb wounds, the surgeon will find it useful to apply an exsanguinating tourniquet prior to exploration. This will enable the major anatomical structures to be defined amid the oedema and disruption that present. However, once he has identified these structures, the tourniquet should be removed in order to assess viability of tissue. The inevitability that there is bacterial contamination present is an absolute bar to the use of any prosthetic material within the wound at initial surgery. Internal fixation for fractures or prosthetic vascular repair is not, therefore, possible. Major arteries must either be repaired by direct suture whenever possible or by autogenous vein graft. Tendon and nerve injuries should be identified by a non-absorbable suture in their ends and left for secondary repair.

b. Removal of Contaminant

Much of this is done as wound excision proceeds above. (For care in fragment removal *see* comments in forensic section.) As far as possible all foreign material likely to be contaminated, for example wood splinters, cloth, gravel and dirt, should be removed. Small metallic or glass fragments, and these may include bullets, should not be deliberately sought after since during the last few centimetres of their trajectory through tissue there will have been minimal energy transfer, and the surrounding tissues may be relatively undamaged. The main exception to this rule is lead fragments lying within a synovial joint, since synovial fluid has a particular affinity to dissolve lead rapidly, producing a very active chemical synovitis, and similarly with fragments within the spinal canal where an arachnoiditis may be caused. Bomb explosions in modern buildings often fragment modern materials, such as formica and plastic, but fortunately these are often brightly coloured and hence may be easily seen. Their smooth surface also prevents them adhering to the tissues, making removal easier. Once wound excision and mechanical removal of fragments is complete, thorough irrigation of the tissues must be performed. Suitable agents for this purpose depend upon availability and personal preference of surgeons concerned. In most cases large quantities of a sterile crystalloid are sufficient, but many advocate the use of hydrogen peroxide since the foaming action on contact with the tissues produces a mechanical cleansing effect. Some advocate the use of an antiseptic at this stage and the most effective known is a mixture of hydrogen peroxide and povidone-iodine in equal proportions. However, the bactericidal value of this procedure is doubtful.

c. Allowing the Wound to Heal Without an Increase in Wound Tension

Wound tension rises primarily when swelling is not permitted to occur. Secondarily, it is caused by movement of the tissue. The principles, therefore, of preventing this happening and so permitting the tissues the maximum chance to defeat infection is, firstly, to allow for massive swelling and, secondly, to prevent unnecessary movement. The first is achieved by wide fasciotomies of the deep fascia, and closing wounds initially only where there is sufficient elasticity of the tissues to allow gross distension. In practice this refers to the face, the male genitalia and possibly the dorsum of the hand. All other wounds should be left open and closure performed only once such swelling has subsided. Details of the dressing are important. Regrettably there is a great tendency by both doctors and nurses to insert a pack into a large wound. Such a device has the same effect as closure, i.e. it does not prevent a rise of wound tension. The wound should be dressed with a large soft dressing of fluffed dry gauze laid on, rather than in, the wound. The over-dressings must be large enough to soak up the exudate which will be produced over several days without its reaching the surface dressing, thus providing a route for infection. A large dressing will also provide a degree of support and splintage for the tissues. Delayed closure of the wound can usually be performed between the 4th and 6th day after wound excision. In all but the smallest wounds this should preferably be performed under a general anaesthetic. Dressings which may have become adherent can therefore be removed without causing distress, so it is not necessary to apply a non-stick dressing. Excessive anti-stick substances, such as paraffin, are not beneficial to the wound. Closure at this stage does not depend upon the development of granulation tissue, so even if early granulations are removed when taking off adherent dressings, no harm has been done. The wound edges do not require freshening and the skin alone should be closed by delayed primary suture without tension. If there has been loss of skin substance such as to make closure impossible, split skin grafts should be used. Unnecessary active movement at this stage can be prevented by large dressings, possibly supported by a plaster cast over the top, which should, of course, be split.

d. Antibiotics and Antiseptics

It is doubtful if the incidence of infection in such wounds has been reduced by the advent of either antiseptics, used liberally in World War I, or antibiotics, first introduced in World War II. The value of antiseptics under these circumstances is extremely doubtful. Antibiotics do possibly reduce mortality due to early septicaemia, and may buy some time when surgery has been delayed. Penicillin is specifically useful to prevent infection by streptococcal and clostridial organisms. However, neither are any substitute for adequate surgical wound excision. Which antibiotic should be used, and it is normal practice to arrange for them to be administered as soon after wounding as possible, is a matter of choice. All wounds should receive a penicillin unless the patient is sensitive, and in some cases of gross contamination, a penicillinase-resistant penicillin combined with antibiotics active against gram-negative strains. Wounds involving the central nervous system should, in addition, receive a sulphonamide and those in which the oral and/or abdominal cavity are involved should receive a suitable antibiotic active against anaerobic organisms.

Wounds in Special Sites

a. Soft Tissue Injuries

Management along the above lines for pure soft tissue wounds will be the most common operative procedures performed, these being between 34–40 per cent overall. Some trunk wounds will be shown on exploration to involve body wall structures alone. One study showed that 20 per cent of clinically apparent penetrating wounds of the thorax had not breached the pleura.

b. Fractures

Fifty per cent of all wounds will involve the limbs and in 15 per cent there will be unstable fractures, some with bone loss. Early stabilization to prevent movement, thus allowing soft tissues to recover, is important, and whatever method is used, the other target is the maintenance of length. Accurate reduction, initially, is not important. The different methods available will not be discussed but internal fixation is usually contraindicated, and undoubtedly external fixation is becoming increasingly popular.

c. The Head

In penetrating wounds that involve the cranial cavity, except for those where only the most minute fragments are involved, wound track toilet should be performed. The fragments driven into the skull are often contaminated with skin which is more dangerous than the metallic fragments causing the injury. Whenever possible the services of a neurosurgical centre, and preferably one where computerized axial tomography scanning is available, should be used. However, in the absence of such facilities, adequate knowledge can be obtained from straight X-rays taken in two planes. Standard access to the brain should be obtained, either by means of a formal flap or, where there is only a small penetration, by local craniectomy. The wound track should be adequately cleaned of all fragments with removal of any pulped brain. Closure of the dura is a matter for debate, but primary skin closure of the surgical incision should be performed with drainage. Antibiotics and prophylactic anti-convulsant therapy are mandatory. Where the appropriate intensive care facilities are available, elective hyperventilation of the patient for 48 hours may be advocated, but this should only be carried out where there are full facilities. Steroids should not be given. The patient's level of response on admission according to the Glasgow Coma Scale Score provides a relatively accurate guide to prognosis in penetrating missile brain injury. Even in the centres where maximum facilities are available, a survival rate of more than 10–15 per cent cannot be expected in any patients in whom the level of response is less than drowsy. Where the patient is neurologically unresponsive a 100 per cent mortality is likely. Exceptions to this are children who show a greater capacity for recovery. Where a large number of cases are presenting, and facilities are limited, this should be taken into account when assessing priorities.

d. Eyes

Analysis of a large number of terrorist bomb victims accumulated over many years in Northern Ireland show that approximately 40 per cent have significant eye injuries for which expert ophthalmic opinion and treatment are necessary at an early age. Half of these are closed and half penetrating. Since the precise diagnosis of eye injury may often be difficult in the first place it is reasonable for all victims to be reviewed by such a specialist.

e. Otological Damage

The incidence of damage here is likewise high. The vast majority, however, comprise simple rupture of the tympanic membranes, which will normally heal spontaneously. A significant percentage have sensoneural damage which is probably permanent. In a small number there may be middle ear ossicular dislocation and, in patients in which there is profound conductive deafness, audiometry to confirm it is necessary. If found, referral to an appropriate specialist is required. Visualization of the tympanic membrane and simple clinical tests for hearing loss are mandatory in all cases.

f. Maxillofacial Injury

Multiple fragmentation is associated with a high incidence of damage to the facial skeleton, and hence the reason why the injuries are more commonly seen in wartime than peace. In any possible wound around the face, underlying bone damage should be suspected until proved otherwise and facial wounds should not be sutured until underlying bone damage has been excluded. Penetrating wounds should be managed along the general lines for other structures except that the elasticity of facial tissues can allow swelling without a rise of wound tension. Thus primary skin closure, provided there has been no loss, can be obtained. Bone fragments should always be covered by deep tissue and, if this is not possible, they should be removed. It goes without saying that there may be a high incidence of upper airway problems when such injuries occur, and establishment of a secure airway has maximum priority at all times.

g. Chest Injury

Detailed management of penetrating chest injury will not be described other than to stress some important points. Occlusion of open wounds should be performed as an emergency life saving first aid measure, and pleural drainage should be instituted in any case of penetrating injury as soon as possible. This procedure should take priority over intravenous infusion, even on site, and should be second only to securing the patency of the upper airway. Patients with penetrating missile injuries of the chest tend either to succumb rapidly to major intrathoracic damage, often involving the mediastinal structures, or survive, providing adequate simple emergency measures, such as relief of tension pneumothorax and replacement of blood volume, are performed early. The percentage that come to open surgery in the second group may be small. Dramatic urgent thoracotomy in the first group is seldom successful, this being in contrast to penetrating chest injuries caused by stab wounds.

The low density of lung tissue tends to reduce significantly the degree of energy transfer and it is, therefore, quite possible for a through and through high velocity missile wound to occur in the chest with relatively little damage, provided the mediastinal structures are not within the missile track. The thoracic wall is a remarkably good deflector of smooth missiles and it is not unknown for a patient to present with what appear to be entry and exit wounds diametrically opposed, suggesting a through and through wound. Upon exploration, it is found that the thoracic cavity itself has not been breached, the missile passing extra-costally right round the chest wall.

A small percentage of patients may require open operation and the indications for this tend to be persistent blood loss and/or persistent air leak. Usually haemorrhage is from major vessels in the chest wall and, more rarely, from the lung parenchyma. In the latter case, where the haemorrhage is significant, it may be necessary to dissect and occlude the vessels of the lung root rapidly before any further procedure can be performed. Although the pericardium may have been untouched by a missile, in a significant number of cases a sympathetic post-operative pericardial effusion may occur, possibly producing fatal tamponade, so it is always wise to open and leave the pericardium adequately drained.

h. Abdomen

Laparotomy is nearly always required. This is a time-consuming procedure since it is necessary to carry out a thorough search for small areas of bowel perforation amongst oedematous loops of bowel and omentum, in the presence of the inevitable intraperitoneal haemorrhage. When high energy transfer has occurred there may be massive faecal contamination associated with generalized cellular damage and multiple bowel perforation. The risk of septic complications with anastomotic breakdown is extremely high. Therefore, the most conservative approach to bowel anastomosis is necessary. Essentially, no primary anastomosis should be performed when both ends involve colon or rectum, and only limited segments of extensively damaged small bowel should be resected. Debate exists as to whether major injuries of the caecum and right colon should be treated with ileal diversion with or without hemicolectomy or with ileal transverse anastomosis. Available evidence at the moment tends to support the latter. Injuries of the more distal large bowel should always be defunctioned by a double barrel colostomy. Extensive paracolic drainage of the peritoneal cavity is necessary. Standard laparotomy closure should be used but missile entry and exit wounds through the soft tissue of the abdominal wall should each be treated with adequate excision, toilet, irrigation and delayed primary closure.

i. Spinal Injury

Lesions of the spinal cord are regrettably common in penetrating missile injuries. Usually the missile has not damaged the cord or its meninges or even the vertebral column, the effect being produced by high energy transfer. Prognosis for recovery of such cord lesions tends to be poor. Management should be along the lines for spinal injuries in general, and operative intravention is normally only indicated where there is an obvious CSF leak due to direct penetration of the meninges. In practice this will often come to light during wound exploration.

Of far lesser importance in terms of pathology, but a much more common clinical problem, is the high incidence of soft tissue paraspinal injuries described, usually in the cervical region, often as the result of the sudden translocation of the victims. 'Whiplash' injury is notorious for its persistence and slow recovery.

PSYCHIATRIC MANAGEMENT

Specialist management of those terrorist victims who suffer severe psychiatric disorder following their trauma will not be dealt with here. However, recent studies have shown that a high percentage, if not all, of those injured and also those without physical injury, will show evidence of post-traumatic stress reaction. This will require management and support by their medical attendants, be they surgeons, accident and emergency officers or general practitioners. Three groups may be defined: the physically injured, the released hostage (with or without physical injury) and relatives of both.

For most, treatment will be simple psychotherapy. Like so many psychological syndromes which follow physical illness, relief is obtained by forewarning. When symptoms are present explanations as to why, and as to the fact that they are by no means unique to the individual concerned also help. To facilitate this the physician must be aware of the recognized post-traumatic syndromes which may develop. Post-disaster neuroses, and occasionally psychosis, are well recognized and have a definite morbidity and mortality.

The Physically Injured

The sequence of mental events that follows serious physical injury is well recognized and has been compared to that which follows bereavement. Initially there is a state of numbness and reaction almost of disinterest to his injury by the patient. He tends to be submissive to those around him. As days of disability and pain continue, the patient tends to withdraw and become more resentful. Military surgeons recognize well that protracted pain and recurrent surgical procedures do not make men more brave, as the poets suggest. Eventually the most stoical of individuals tend to become almost infantile and their threshold to withstand discomfort and pain decreases daily. This must not be confused with the elective surgical patient who often undergoes a solitary operative procedure, and may be free of pain within a few days, and well on the way to recovery. The multiple injured patient often requires recurrent surgery over many weeks or months. A state of depression develops, associated with self-resentment and constant expressions on the theme of 'Why me?'. At times there may be total non-cooperation with medical attendants, and undoubtedly some of this may be the result of the biochemical changes which follow such injury, related to gross catabolism. This is especially true when there is sepsis involved, and under these circumstances it is sometimes difficult to distinguish between the psychological reaction and a toxic confusional state. It is important to identify the latter. Patients normally have to be permitted to work themselves through this phase and it is extremely difficult to gain satisfactory motivation and co-operation until this phase is over. In the long term patients will often develop recurrent episodes of depression and certain syndromes which are described below. Surprisingly, many bear few feelings of bitterness towards the perpetrators of the acts of violence. Their feelings tend to be either of ambivalence or positive sadness for such people. Strangely it is almost as if the severity of injury is in inverse proportion to the degree of rancour.

Motivation towards recovery is dependent upon the patient's attitude to his injury. There is a distinct difference between those who can possibly rationalize their injuries as having in some way been of benefit to their sense of duty or to society, in contrast to those who see them as a total waste. A significant difference can be demonstrated when comparing the response to rehabilitation of comparable physical injuries sustained under two different circumstances. Traumatic amputations at a fixed level are obviously such comparable injuries, and it has been shown that in battle casualties in whom the injury was the result of enemy action, as contrasted to accidental explosions following the cessation of activities, the rate of recovery is different. As far as victims of terrorism are concerned there may, therefore, be a difference between injured members of security forces and innocent bystanders.

Contrary to popular belief, financial compensation and its receipt under these circumstances seldom seem to affect the rate of recovery.

Psychological support for those with minor injuries in some ways should be stressed more, if only to emphasize the fact that because of the low level of physical injury the psychological problems may well be missed, overlooked or even dismissed. A study with matched controls of comparable levels of minor injury (patients attending a casualty department but not admitted) for victims of terrorist violence have shown the period of disability in the post-injury period to be approximately two and a half times that of the control. Their sickness record, once they have returned to work, does not appear to be affected, but performance at work is and there is also an increased incidence of breakdown of marital and other family relationships. Anxiety symptoms are common and many become dependent on medication in an attempt to control them, while others tend to self-medicate with an increased consumption of tobacco and alcohol, the latter sometimes proceeding to frank alcoholism. Behaviour patterns in the post-disaster victims of terrorism contrast both in the short and long term with those of other types of disaster in this book. Victims of human violence often find themselves rejected by fellow members of society, even by friends and relatives, which is in complete contrast to the attitude of society to those victims of natural disasters. The explanation suggested for this is that the victims of violence are in some way partially responsible for it, and that in the case of terrorism this presumably means that the victim is a member of the society the nature of which itself has provoked the acts. This also applies to members of security forces who although, initially, may have been seen to have been acting as heroes, later may meet rejection. The same is true of casualties from an unpopular war. In the case of natural disaster, society sees this as an act of God for which no human being can be accountable.

Victims of natural disasters often adopt unnatural and excessively heroic profiles, and will tend to work long hours to the point of exhaustion (which makes them totally inefficient), in an attempt to seek some form of glory, whilst helping to alleviate the mess of a disaster. Strangely such individuals can also develop, at the same time, acutely antisocial behaviours, such as looting at the time of disaster. Victims of terrorism contrast on both points. They attempt to take as low a profile as possible, often avoiding social contact to the point where it is deemed antisocial, and antisocial behaviour of the looting type is not seen.

A third contrast in behaviour is that, following natural disasters, many victims suffer from an often irrepressible desire to return to the scene. Terrorist victims do not, and in fact will often go to the stage of deliberately avoiding the locations.

Despite a full recovery from physical damage, which may have been minor, recurrent post-disaster neurosis may be detected months or years after the event. Sleep disturbances, often with nightmares, are common for up to 2½ years and irrational phobias are often reported. There may be episodes of reactive depression manifested by early morning waking, low tear threshold and feelings of worthlessness. There is also an increased incidence of psychosomatic conditions, such as irritable bowel syndrome, various allergies and headaches. There is evidence that some organic conditions often thought to be related to psychological stress will develop more commonly in such victims, including hypertension, duodenal ulcer and cardiac arrhymias.

MANAGEMENT OF THE RELEASED HOSTAGE

Much has been written in the past about the effects of long-term detention producing such problems as prisoner-of-war or concentration camp syndromes. These studies have emphasized the permanent residual effects, such as premature ageing, reduced life expectancy and varied behaviour patterns. Recently it has become appreciated that detained hostages, perhaps detained for even as short a time as a few hours, may have suffered severe psychological damage from which it takes a considerable time, if ever, to recover. Released hostages can be considered in 3 groups. Approximately one third, and this will obviously depend upon the cultural background of the particular hostages, appear very often to take the whole matter in a stoical fashion. These are often described as stoical, rural people who appear to suffer few problems. A smaller sub-division of this group is an odd collection of people who actually describe it as a life-enhancing experience. However, two-thirds overall of released hostages develop significant post-traumatic problems which require help.

Immediate management has been covered previously. The problems from which the hostages suffer can nearly all be related to the extreme existential fear to which they have been subjected, also described earlier. For a considerable period of time after release feelings of this existential fear and the acute anxiety may suddenly return, precipitated by minor stimuli, such as a noise or sight of something which can be associated with the terrifying experience. The degree to which certain individuals suffer depends not only upon the experience which they have been through but also upon their underlying personality. Young, immature adults tend to do less well, as do those with a history of previous psychiatric disorder and/or repeated exposure to similar traumatic experiences. In contrast, those who during their period of captivity were able to render active aid, for example to the sick or injured amongst their fellow hostages, or were able to keep themselves occupied in a more useful way, tend to suffer less. This can, of course, be related back to the situation of utter helplessness described earlier.

The threat to self-esteem and self-image is regarded by the psyche in a similar manner to that to life and limb and, not surprisingly, therefore, many released hostages will undergo a great number of the syndromes and behaviour patterns described above for those injured physically as a result of human violence. Again there is the increased incidence of marital and family breakdown, and also the presence of psychosomatic disorder.

Particularly marked are sleep disturbances which may persist for a considerable time, often with many nightmares and sudden awakening with night fears.

It has been claimed by some that pharmacological support with sedatives and tranquillizers does not help the post-traumatic anxiety of these patients and in some has been known to make them much worse.

Those hostages who developed a degree of transference of affect towards their captors, with negative feelings towards authority, continue to persist with these upon release. Sometimes they are able to see the illogicality of this but the feelings still remain, and this is thought to be due to a persisting fear of retaliation which may have little logical basis. For many, however, there is the realization that during their captivity they may, as a result of their frozen fright, have behaved in a manner which they may even now consider reprehensible and there could well be guilt complexes concerning this. It is, therefore, extremely important to emphasize that there was nothing wrong in anything that they did to survive, in as much as they did it by animal instinct.

Relatives

The management and support of relatives of the above groups can be likened to those of any seriously ill patient. During a crisis the situation is similar to that during a very critical illness. Later, support similar to that needed for the seriously physically disabled over a protracted period of time is required. Explanation and constant support may be necessary.

FORENSIC ASPECTS

In most countries, acts of violence committed by terrorists, irrespective of motive, are considered criminal. Doctors concerned in the management of the injured may find, therefore, that they have specific obligations. Examination of the dead is a matter for the forensic specialist and the reader is referred to Chapter 14. However, the majority of victims survive and the clinician then becomes responsible for the recording of the evidence. This also applies to patients who may ultimately come to the pathologist's autopsy, but treatment during a short period of survival may have removed vital evidence, for example by excision of wounds.

Why Record Data?

Doctors must, therefore, be aware of the reasons as to why they must be careful to record data, what data they should record and the form in which they do it. This information may subsequently be required under the following circumstances:

1. In providing information which may assist the investigating authorities.

    A fireman fighting a fire in a bonded warehouse where arson was suspected was seriously injured by an explosion. The emergency services considered the explosion to have been due to the ignition of alcohol. However, during resuscitation the surgeons experienced in this type of injury concluded that the patient had been injured by a bomb deliberately exploded, probably by remote control. This altered the whole significance of the incident.

2. In providing evidence in a Court of Criminal Law.

    The clinician may find he is appearing on behalf of a prosecuting authority in the trial of apprehended terrorists or, on the other hand, may be giving evidence concerning injuries received by terrorists where anti-terrorist forces have not acted within the law. At all times evidence must be impartial. Unlike the evidence that he may give in the situation above, which might be a verbal opinion, his evidence in Court will only be admissable provided it was collected and recorded in a manner which conforms to established rules of evidence.

Doctors also have a duty to the patient because their evidence may enable a Court or Tribunal to award the patient adequate financial compensation for his injury. There is also a general responsibility to record accurately certain information which, at a later date, may be essential in retrospective research into the pathology of injuries sustained.

When to Record Data

Theoretically, detailed notes of the wounds and their progress in all patients should be made from the moment of first medical care, possibly at the scene of an incident, through all stages of treatment until final recovery. At the scene of an incident, and possibly during essential resuscitation in an accident and emergency department, this may prove unpractical. Time spent making such records must be balanced against time required for life-saving procedures either on the patient concerned or on others. Fortunately those for which the most accurate records are required tend to be those who have received gunshot wounds and the total number of these casualties is relatively small.

Provided the injured patient's condition is stable, the best time to pause to make accurate observations is often once the patient has been anaesthetized in an operating theatre and before any preparation of the skin is made prior to surgery. In more minor cases, these observations should be made prior to treating wounds.

What Data to Record

Unless specially experienced, doctors should not necessarily attempt to correlate their findings with an opinion as to the nature of injury but should record accurately observations which can be later interpreted by an expert. An accurate description and measurement of all wounds should be noted with diagrams if possible. Measurements should be recorded in at least two dimensions and the unit of measurement should be millimetres or centimetres. Entry and exit wounds should be identified as such, if possible, but this is not always easy. In general an exit wound caused by penetrating fragments tends to be larger than an entry wound, but in the case of a bullet wound the two may be identical in size, if by chance the bullet leaves the body in a stable phase of its flight. This also may apply when the wound has been supported either by tight clothing or an external object, such as a floor or a wall. Careful examination of entry wounds may show a small ring of abrasion around the wound, but even this may be present in certain exit wounds where there has been support of the skin. Bullet wounds sustained at close range may be contaminated by powder particles fired from the gun which may lie on the surface or be tattooed into the layers of the epidermis. Careful recording of such contamination and measurement of the total area involved should be carried out because forensic experts may be able to calculate the weapon range later. Where a gun muzzle has been held against the skin two other observations may be relevant. In incidents with loose contact gas may have escaped between skin and muzzle, leaving powder tattoo markings which spread away from the point of contact. There may also be an impression on the skin from parts of the muzzle, such as the foresight. If, however, at the moment of firing the muzzle had been pressed firmly into skin then the gas from the discharge will have dissected subcutaneously causing a multi-lacerated entry wound. Occasionally a patient is injured only tangentially by a bullet causing a graze on the surface of the body. This may leave a small furrowed track through the skin with small lacerations on either side. The tips of these lacerations point towards the weapon and it is thus possible to establish the direction of the bullet. When a shot-gun has been used there may be multiple entry wounds, and it is important to record the scatter by measuring the distance between the entry points that are farthest apart.

Care of Forensic Specimens

During surgery fragments of missiles will be removed. Removal should be performed on clinical grounds and only rarely solely to obtain the specimen for forensic purposes. In order to preserve vital evidence, however, fragments must be removed with special care. Preferably the gloved finger, or non-metallic instruments, should be used whenever possible, to prevent any scratches on the fragment surface. Microscopic examination of this surface may prove of considerable forensic importance and help to identify the origin of the missile. Individual firearms, for example, leave their own specific scratch pattern on a bullet and may subsequently be identified. If entry and exit skin wounds are excised as part of the operative procedure they should be placed on card or X-ray film and then placed in formal saline, using a marker stitch to orientate them. All fragments and tissue thus removed should be placed in a rigid plastic container and sealed and labelled. The container should not leave the operating room until the end of the case and should then be kept under lock and key until it can be handed directly to a member of the investigating authority either by the surgeon or the nurse in charge. Rules regarding the continuity of evidence mean essentially that the fewer the people that handle the evidence the better. The prosecution at trial may be required to prove, and this may require evidence from many people, that any such exhibit could not have been tampered with in any way since removal from the patient. After surrendering these exhibits to the investigating authority a receipt should be obtained and a note made in the patient's record to this effect. Should the doctor be asked to give evidence at a subsequent trial, and have to identify these fragments, he is advised to see the exhibits immediately beforehand.

If photographs are to be taken, before or during surgery, they are best done by an official police photographer if they are likely to be used as evidence. Otherwise they are unlikely to be admissible as evidence unless carefully corroborated. Any other photographs or X-rays taken should be signed immediately, preferably by a doctor.

All of these facts should be meticulously recorded in the patient's case notes and very often the operating note may be the best place. The doctor is advised, if time is available, to retain a personal copy. Should he subsequently be required to give evidence in Court only that evidence written at the time may be used to refresh his memory whilst he is in the witness box.

'A young man was shot in a public house by a terrorist. The surgeon who treated him was required to give evidence in Court 8 years later concerning the incident, and his original statement to the investigating authority had been destroyed as 'time expired'. Fortunately the operating notes containing the essential measurements were still available.'

Medical Reports on Injuries

After the incident patients may claim financial compensation for injuries sustained. The quantity of such compensation depends entirely on medical evidence, usually in the form of a written report, but sometimes, especially if the claim is contested, involves the doctor giving evidence in Court. An unbiased, honest, factual account is essential in the interests of justice. Referral to notes made at the time, as in the criminal evidence, will be useful. However, in the event of serious injury, or where there is likely to be a residual disability, the doctor preparing the report should arrange to examine the patient once a static level of recovery has been achieved. Sometimes, if recovery is still proceeding, an interim report will be required. Such a report should contain a description from the patient of exactly what happened, how he was injured and what he noticed at the time. This should be corroborated whenever possible with evidence from the case notes, witnesses and possibly relatives. The degree of pain and suffering undergone should be recorded but, since these are essentially subjective, Courts prefer an attempt to make an objective assessment if possible. The time spent in hospital and observations made from the case notes may be obvious in this respect. Once the patient has returned home useful guidelines, which should be recorded, include the time the patient was confined to bed and to the house, and the total duration of time off work. Some objective indicators of pain and suffering can be estimated from the amount of analgesia and/or hypnotic drugs that the patient required and the duration for which they were prescribed. The date that he first achieved a normal night's sleep without pharmacological support is a useful point to note. Preparation of reports and the re-examination of a patient may prove a very salutary lesson to hospital clinicians who are often unaware of the time that patients take to recover from such injuries after discharge from hospital. Once the history has been recorded, and notes made of all residual disabilities and/or symptoms, a careful general clinical examination must be performed. Any residual scars should be noted and measured accurately, along with any limitations of joint movement. X-rays taken previously and at the time of examination should be reviewed and interpreted for the purposes of the report in lay terms. Opinion should be given as to prognosis and as to whether or not all the patient's symptoms are compatible with the findings. The language in which the report is written should be in simple lay terms since it will be interpreted by legal rather than medical officials.

Finally, comment should be made as to how the disabilities of which the patient complains have affected his life style and their authenticity. This will be an appropriate part of the report in which to include what may be considered psychiatric morbidity. Specific comment should be made about nightmares and phobias which have developed and as to whether or not this has influenced the patient's habits. Problems described in the previous section should be specifically looked for since some patients may associate them with a feeling of guilt and are reluctant to admit them until asked. In contrast other patients will attempt to overemphasize their symptoms and tend to volunteer the importance of their psychological symptoms from the outset.

Some degree of psychiatric morbidity is nearly always present and it has been noted by many observers that, contrary to popular medical opinion, many of the symptoms are not relieved by financial compensation.

30

Nuclear Accidents

INTRODUCTION

The hazards of radiation have been known since the discovery of X-rays. With the discovery of nuclear fission and fusion, and the use of the energy they generate, as both a power source and weapon, there is now a potential hazard that involves every soul on this planet. There are currently tens of thousands of nuclear warheads in existence, and hundreds of nuclear power stations, built, building or planned.

In a brief chapter, it is possible to draw little more than a sketch of the field. It is hoped this is adequate for the doctor involved with an accident or disaster involving radiation injury. Far fuller accounts can be found in the sources listed in the bibliography.

Since it is not relevant in the short term, the long-term effects of radiation have been ignored. These are, of course, of great importance. The fact that 20, 30 or 40 men died as a result of burns and radiation after the Chernobyl disaster pales into insignificance if many thousands die years later from leukaemia or other malignant conditions.

NUCLEAR WAR

The disasters covered in the previous chapters in this book cover a whole range of circumstances and affect from one or two in a road accident to hundreds of thousands in earthquakes, or even millions in famines. None, however, have the potential for the obliteration of the human race. The worst conceivable disaster of all is man-made, and does. It is nuclear war.

It is not the intention of this chapter to consider war as an accident. Nevertheless, a vast literature exists on the effects, both social and medical, of nuclear war. It all comes to the same conclusion. It is impossible to plan a rational, workable medical response to an all-out nuclear exchange between the two superpowers that involves their NATO and Warsaw pact allies. Indeed, 'civilised life as we know it, and the human value and ethical standards on which the practice of medicine is based, would cease to exist in vast areas . . . It would be impossible to run even a basic medical care service without minimal standards of law and order. Survivors would be preoccupied exclusively with the search for food and shelter. They would be unlikely to devote attention to the care of the sick and dying'.[1] And further, 'We do not doubt that doctors would wish to give help, even in the midst of such devastation . . . but their impact on the situation would be minimal".[1]

Discussion has also considered the effect of one demonstration nuclear explosion over a populated area. Remembering that the bomb at Hiroshima was equivalent to 12·5 kilotons and the one at Nagasaki was 22 kilotons, most are now in the 150 to 200 kiloton range, but many are up to or over 1 megaton. The explosion of just one of these weapons in the UK would surely produce so many patients as a result of trauma and burns, that the rest of the National Health Service would be completely overwhelmed. For instance, how could 50000 burned patients be treated in 100 or so specialized beds? 'Even the death and disability that could result from an accidental explosion of one bomb from among the enormous stockpile of weapons could overwhelm national medical resources'.[2]

If nuclear war and weapons, therefore, can be excluded from the consideration of nuclear accidents, then attention can be directed solely to accidents involving the civilian, peaceful use of nuclear energy. This is particularly relevant when the number of nuclear power stations in existence and in planning are remembered, but particularly so after the events at Three Mile Island, Pennsylvania in 1979, and at Chernobyl in 1986.

UNITS OF MEASUREMENT

The absorbed dose of radiation is measured in grays (Gy) and is a measurement of the energy imparted to matter by ionizing radiation. One gray is equal to 100 rads, a unit which it has now replaced. One centigray is, therefore, equivalent to 1 rad.

The damage done by different forms of radiation differs. To take this factor into account the dose equivalent, measured in sieverts (Sv) is used. This is equal to the absorbed dose times a factor that allows for the action of each particular form of radiation. For alpha particles, the factor is 20; so, 1 Gy of alpha radiation will provide a dose equivalent to 20 Sv. For beta particles, gamma rays and X-rays, the factor is 1. Thus, 1 Gy of, say, beta irradiation, is equal to 1 Sv. Like the gray, the sievert is often considered in fractions. So, just as 1 rad (the older unit) equals 0·01 Gy, so 1 rem (older unit) is equal to 0·01 Sv.

MEDICAL EFFECTS OF RADIATION

Four main groups of radiation injury can be described. These are:
1. External whole body radiation.
2. External contamination with radioactive material.
3. Internal contamination from inhalation or ingestion of radioactive material.
4. Local burns from high dosage beta or gamma radiation.

External Whole Body Radiation

The effects of increasing the radiation dosage are shown in *Table* 30.1. The effects, particularly the death rate, will depend to a great extent on the avail-

Table 30.1. The effects of increasing the radiation dosage

Dose Gy	Symptoms	Survival with treatment %
0–1	Asymptomatic	—
1–2	Nausea, vomiting, bone marrow suppression	100
2–6	Nausea, vomiting, severe leucopenia, loss of hair	2–100
6–10	As above, plus severe gastrointestinal syndrome	0–10
10+	As above, plus acute encephalopathy and cardiovascular collapse	0

ability of treatment. They will be modified by the age, general fitness of the patient, and any other injuries that have been received.

The elderly and very young have a worse prognosis than those in the prime of life. Burns will have a synergistic effect, the result being a higher mortality than expected from either the degree of exposure to radiation or the percentage area burned, on their own.

The period over which radiation is taken up is also of importance. The longer the period over which a particular dose is received, the better the chance of survival of the patient. A large dose in a short time has a more lethal effect than the same dose over a much longer time.

The vast range in the salvageable group, those receiving between 2 and 6 Gy, is the result of comparing fit and sick patients, and those where the whole range of modern medical technology has recently become available.

There has been much debate in recent years as to the LD_{50} (lethal dose for 50 per cent mortality) in humans. It had been thought to be in the 4 to 4·5 Gy range, with survival being unlikely above 6 Gy. However, after the Chernobyl accident, some patients have survived doses of 8 Gy, and one is reported to have survived 11 Gy, despite the failure of marrow transplantation.[3]

At the lower end of the scale, around 2 Gy, Rotblat has presented data suggesting that there may be far more severe effects in the elderly and sick especially, as it is already known that this is so in children.[4]

Clearly, there are considerable differences of opinion about the amount of radiation that is survivable. However, few would disagree that most patients will survive 2 Gy and below, but few above 6 Gy. Medical skills, the fitness of the patients and, no doubt, a degree of luck, will affect the survival of those in between.

Syndromes

Neurovascular Syndrome
This arises with massive exposure to 20 or 30 Gy. It occurs within the first hour or by 2 days. It presents with confusion, delirium, fits, stupor and shock. It is

universally fatal within 4 days. It would be important to differentiate it, if possible, from other causes of encephalopathy.

Gastrointestinal Syndrome

This syndrome will appear with increasing severity from exposure to 6 Gy and upwards. It is characterized by nausea, vomiting, bloody diarrhoea and haemorrhage from other mucosal surfaces. The electrolyte and fluid balances of the patient are grossly deranged. There is also a severe leucopenia. Death is inevitable within 2 weeks, provided initial resuscitation is successful, unless haemorrhage and infection can be controlled in the longer term.

Haematological Syndromes [5]

Lymphocyte numbers fall immediately. The degree of fall provides an excellent indicator of the severity of injury. Levels of around 100 will prove lethal.

The neutrophils may show a small rise for up to 48 hours, and then fall progressively to reach their lowest level around 30 days. There may be a brief, spurious rise around the 15th day. If the patient survives, spontaneous recovery may start around the beginning of the 5th week. If the brief rise is absent the prognosis is likely to be worse.

Platelets, also after a brief rise, will fall steadily towards that lowest level around the 30th day. During recovery they may be present in well above normal levels.

So the early fall in lymphocytes may act as a useful prognostic sign, but the period of greatest danger may not be reached until a month after exposure to the high doses of radiation which cause haematological syndromes.

Triage

The level of exposure needs to be known to determine appropriate treatment. If thousands of victims were involved, it would be impossible to treat those who had received massive doses of radiation. A form of triage would be needed. Even when only small numbers needed to be treated, triage would help. The following factors should be considered:

1. Nausea, vomiting and diarrhoea within minutes, or ataxia, coma and shock within hours—a fatal dose will have been received.
2. Diarrhoea, with blood, within 4 days, lymphocytes around 100 within 3 days, and severe platelet changes within a week—a fatal dose, again, may have been received. The fatality rate would certainly be around 80 per cent.
3. Extent and intensity of skin burns due not to heat but to intense beta and gamma irradiation. These can involve 90 per cent of the body surface and will affect the mortality rates adversely.

Treatment

Treatment of anything more than a minor exposure to radiation will require the full range, extent and skills of modern medicine and intensive care. This is possible in peacetime but, clearly, is totally unrealistic under wartime conditions.

Generally, with awareness of the pathological changes induced by radiation, the treatment is exactly what would be expected. It involves fluid replacement, transfusion with white cells and platelets, plus red cells if haemorrhage has occurred. Parenteral nutrition will be necessary while gastrointestinal symptoms remain. Infection will need to be combated with appropriate antibiotics, and the patients need to be nursed in a sterile environment. They will need single rooms with laminar air flow and possibly full isolation in plastic-lined 'life islands'. Burns will need to be treated appropriately. Bone marrow transplantation may be attempted, though there is some doubt about its efficacy.[6]

Milder cases, presenting with nausea, vomiting and anorexia, may only need intravenous fluids, including electrolytes, antiemetics and antibiotics.

External and Internal Contamination with Radioactive Material

Material produced as the direct result of a nuclear explosion, or radioactive material deposited on exposed skin or clothing after spillage or splashing, will cause further radiation injury.

Inhaled and ingested material will have the same effect, but will have become inaccessible to the decontamination processes described below.

Decontamination

The military forces of most states are regularly drilled in decontamination procedures. There is no point in decontaminating the surface of a patient if the medical or nursing staff become contaminated in their turn. Therefore, there are essential requirements both for the decontamination site as well as the actual procedures themselves.

The site requires a plentiful clean water supply so that patients can be washed repeatedly on drained sluicing tables. It needs to be away from other buildings, separate from the rest of a hospital, with its own entrance and clean air supply. Personnel need to be dressed in fully protective garments, including masks with respiratory filters, and gloves. Radiation monitoring equipment will be required and personal dosimeters should be worn at all times.

The patient, having been removed from the contaminated area, will need to be undressed completely. The mouth and nose will need to be rinsed with water. Then the whole body must be washed with soap and water, paying particular attention to the hair and body orifices. This may need repeating several times. Great care must be taken to avoid abrading the skin, as this is likely to increase absorption of radioactive material. Hair may, in fact, need to be shaved.

Repeated surveys with monitoring equipment will tell when decontamination is complete.

Prophylaxis

Radioactive fallout, from a leak or explosion, contains many radioisotopes. The most important is iodine-131. To prevent, or reduce, its uptake into the thyroid, potassium iodate can be given. 100 mg need to be given before, or immediately after, exposure. Any delay will reduce its value. If a delay of 1 hour occurs, it will provide protection of only 80 per cent. After 3 hours it will be only 50 per cent effective.[7] It should then be repeated daily for 10 days as I^{131} has a half-life of 8 days.

Other radioisotopes with a longer half-life that may affect long-term survivors of a major disaster and the environment for years to come include strontium-90 and caesium-137. The worst, of course, is plutonium which has a half-life of around 25 000 years. As an alpha emitter it is also an internal hazard, but of course will only be produced by accidents involving weapons.

NUCLEAR ACCIDENTS

A nuclear accident can be defined as an unexpected event in a nuclear weapon, fuel transporter or reactor which leads to a radiological hazard external to the facility, the building or the equipment in which it should have been contained. Thus, the release of appreciable amounts of nuclear radiation may occur from nuclear power stations, nuclear fuel or weapons in transit, or nuclear reactors in some ships and submarines. The last group will not be considered as they only exist in a military context and a few ice-breaking ships. However, Public Safety Schemes do exist at all naval berths.

Transport of Fuel

Authorities responsible for the movement of nuclear material by road and rail take extensive precautions to prevent an accident. These extend to the use of damage-proof transport flasks, carefully designed, manufactured and tested. Nevertheless, should an accident occur on the road, the transporter crew will notify the power station concerned and then remain with the vehicle. A Flask Emergency Team will be sent for. The police will keep the public out of the area. The fire brigade may be needed. The same authorities will need to be involved in the event of a railway disaster. Contingency plans exist to cover all areas, and specially trained and equipped teams exist so that they can be called out promptly.

In the event of an accident involving a nuclear weapon in a convoy, and in the extremely unlikely event of fire breaking out and radiation escaping, the dominant isotope released would be plutonium. This could result in contamination of a wide area. Most fuel accidents would cause no radiological problem, as the decay heat of the fuel is so low that even a loss of coolant in the flask is most unlikely to lead to any release of fission products.

Power Stations

If the cooling system in a nuclear power station fails for any reason, and the safety processes do not function, the core will overheat, rising from normal operating levels of around 315°C to over 1815°C. At this point the core will melt its cladding and fission products will be released into the atmosphere as a plume of radioactive material. Fires and explosions may also be added to the problem, releasing further radioactive material, and indeed radioactivity could enter the groundwater if the containment pressure vessel is damaged.

The plume of radioactive material may or may not be visible. It may be of quite short duration but can last much longer, 10 days for instance at Chernobyl. It travels in the atmosphere, depending on the wind and atmospheric conditions.

Injuries will be caused by the initial event to those in close proximity to the power station. As already discussed, these will include burns, trauma and high dose radiation injury. As the distance from the source increases, radiation becomes the sole source of injury. Locally, direct gamma radiation will emanate from the radioactive cloud. Deposited particulate matter will coat all surfaces. This will cause most local and early deaths. Long-term effects are more likely to be caused by inhalation and ingestion of radioactive particles.

At Chernobyl[6] it was calculated that between 3·5 and 5 per cent of the core inventory was released into the atmosphere, much as fine particulate debris. One ton was spread over the Chernobyl site and a further 6 tons over the surrounding 20 km. This, it has been calculated, will give a collective dose of 86 000 man-Sv in 1986, and 290 000 man-Sv over the next 50 years. During the same time, natural background radiation will total around 100 000 man-Sv. Because of the enormous explosion, actual reactor debris, in addition to fission products, were deposited all over Europe.

The worst likely scenario in the USA allows for 15 per cent of a core to be released.

RESPONSE TO A NUCLEAR ACCIDENT

Prophylaxis

The use of potassium iodate has already been mentioned. It must be emphasized that treatment must be prompt, within 1 hour of exposure. It would be needed throughout the area over which the radiation might spread, which can be up to 320 km downwind of the power station. The trigger level for the administration of stable iodine is gauged to balance the risk of any allergic reaction.

Shelter

Sheltering protects people from radiation. The protective factor (PF) gives an indication of the degree of protection provided. Thus, a PF of 1 provides no protection, while a PF of 5 lets in one fifth of the radiation that would have been received in the open.

In the event of a radioactive leak, the population in the surrounding area, but again, particularly downwind, should be told to stay indoors with doors and windows kept closed. There they should stay.

Evacuation

Depending on the scale of the leak and the weather conditions, evacuation of the population from the area of risk may be necessary. This, if taken to its limit, should reduce the number of people at risk to zero. It will prove a massive exercise. Again, the trigger level for evacuation is gauged to balance the risks of evacuation itself. Some authorities have suggested everybody within 30 km of a plant should be evacuated; others argue that 55 km downwind is safer. More than 10 million Americans live within 30 km of a nuclear power plant, and 20 million within 50 km. Also, there are at least 9 reactors within 15 km of 100 000 people.[8]

For evacuation to function smoothly, adequate warning, preceded by public awareness and education, is needed. A functioning transportation system must exist with somewhere to take all the population to. These requirements will pose immense social and organizational problems. A sudden change of wind will steer the radioactive plume in a new direction, and cause any plan to be altered at short notice. All the time, there is likely to be a large population, frightened by something they cannot see, smell or measure, which effect will pass unnoticed at the time and may even only appear years later.

Later Actions

Restrictions will be needed for some time as a result of contamination of the environment. The consumption of certain foodstuffs will be limited, though the levels of acceptability vary from country to country. Decontamination of the accident site and surrounding area will be necessary. Levels of radiation may make the surrounding area uninhabitable for several years.

TWO EXAMPLES

Thus far the problems posed by nuclear radiation have been considered largely theoretically. However, two recent events have provided practical experience with leaks from nuclear power stations.

Three Mile Island

On 28 March, 1979, a failure in the cooling system at the Three Mile Island Nuclear Generating Station allowed a leak of radiation into the environment. The leak was, in fact, very small and most of the radiation was contained within the plant itself. It then took 4 days to sort out the serious problems that arose with the reactor's nuclear core.

Although no injuries were caused to workers within the plant or to the surrounding area and its population, it has provided an excellent example of the problems caused in the mass evacuation of a heavily populated area. A particular area of concern was the evacuation of medical facilities within the threatened area, where problems of communications, transportation and manpower arose.[9] One thousand, three hundred and eight short-term patients, 2400 nursing home patients and 30 outpatients on dialysis needed evacuation. By 4 April, the hospital census showed 621 patients only left. This success was fortunate on another count, in that a severe shortage of medical staff had also developed, and the request for help from the military had been denied. Hospital facilities had to be arranged to receive patients, some over 80 km from the site of the incident.

For future plans it was clearly important that evacuation should be in a radial fashion, outwards from the site of the incident, and not in directions that crossed each other. Thus, with the proviso that the area downwind is avoided, people north of the incident go north, south go south, etc. Exit corridors need to be identified and traffic control must be strict.

Chernobyl [3,6,7]

As a result of the explosion and fire in the Number 4 reactor at Chernobyl in the Ukraine, USSR, on 26 April 1986, a plume of radioactive material was released into the atmosphere. It reached Scandinavia, 1500 km away, later next day.

Two men were killed in the initial explosion; 29 more were treated on the site within the next hour; 132 were admitted to hospital within the day, 129 being then transferred to Hospital Number 6 in Moscow for specialist care; 72 with acute symptoms of radiation sickness were admitted to hospital in Kiev. All were plant workers or firemen. No members of the general public were affected by acute radiation sickness.

Iodine was distributed to 45000 people in Pripyat, 3 km from the plant. They were told to stay indoors, and were evacuated next day anyway. Ten days later an area of 30 km was evacuated, affecting a further 90000 people. The average dose of radiation received was estimated at 350–500 mSv (35–55 rem).

Of the patients in Moscow, 21 out of 22 patients who had received more than 6Sv died within 28 days. Of those receiving between 4 and 6Sv, 7 died, but all had severe burns. Only one died who had received under 4Sv. The extent of the burns, in fact, as well as marrow damage, was the chief cause of death.

The major factors affecting survival were good clean nursing, good assessment initially, prophylactic antibiotics, and the replacement of blood and blood products. It is doubtful if the much heralded bone marrow and foetal liver transplants made any difference to survival rates.[6]

The immediate problems being over, the reconstruction and long-term problems stretch out into the foreseeable future. Decontamination of the affected reactor site, so that the other three can be restarted safely, is underway. Normal economic and social life in the neighbourhood is likely to be delayed for several years. Restrictions on foodstuffs will depend on locally acceptable levels of contamination. Estimations of additional deaths from cancer are speculative, and certainly will need many years and much epidemiological study to assess. It will provide the largest study since that of the survivors of Hiroshima and Nagasaki.

SUMMARY

Despite the fact that the word 'nuclear' has worrying, or even frightening, connotations in the minds of many people, and that both nuclear power and weapons have been considered in this chapter, it is vital to remember that they are separated by a huge gulf. Apart from the physics, there is little connection between them. Indeed, they obviously exist for very different reasons. It is important that this vital difference is clearly understood.

Nevertheless, nuclear war is clearly, unavoidably, international. Nuclear disasters, on any but the smallest scale, are international too, as Chernobyl has shown. It is only right that this one, so small in effect when compared with the potential catastrophe of nuclear war, should stimulate international co-operation and the sharing of knowledge and experience.

Awareness of the effects and implications of a civilian disaster only serve to emphasize the unthinkable devastation that would be caused by nuclear war. Since there is no cure, it must be avoided. It is as simple as that.

REFERENCES

1. *The Medical Effects of Nuclear War* (1983) Report of the BMA's Board of Science and Education. Chapter 6, p. 117. Chichester, Wiley.
2. WHO (1984) *Effects of Nuclear War on Health and Health Services.* Geneva, WHO.
3. Geiger H. Jack (1986) The accident at Chernobyl and the medical response. *JAMA* **256**, 609–12.
4. Rotblat J. (1985) Acute accident mortality in nuclear war. Presented at the Symposium on the Medical Aspects of Nuclear War, Washington DC.
5. Andrews G. A. (1980) Medical management of accidental total body irradiation. In: Hubner K. F. and Fry J. A. (eds.) *The Medical Basis for Radiation Accident Preparedness.* Holland, Elsevier.
6. Editorial (1986) Living with radiation after Chernobyl. *Lancet* **ii**, 609–10.
7. Medical News and Perspectives (1986) Physicians' reaction to Chernobyl explosion: lessons in radiation—and co-operation. *JAMA* **256**, 559–68.
8. Leaning-Link J. (1985) Emergency response to nuclear accident and attack. *J. Wld. Assoc. Emerg. Disaster Med.* **1** (Suppl.), 385–95.
9. Stanley Smith J. and Fisher J. H. (1981) Three Mile Island. The silent disaster. *JAMA* **245**, 1656–9.

FURTHER READING

Clarke R. (1986) *London Under Attack.* Report of GLAWARS Commission. Oxford, Blackwell.
Emergency Reference Levels: Criteria for Limiting Doses to the Public in the Event of Accidental Exposure to Radiation. (1981) National Radiological Protection Board. HMSO.
Glasstone S. and Dolan P. J. (eds.) (1977) *The Effects of Nuclear Weapons. US Department of Defense and the US Department of Energy.* 3rd edition. Washington DC, US Government Printing Office. Published in UK by Castle House, Tunbridge Wells.
Greene O., Rubin B., Turok N. et al. (1982) *London After the Bomb.* Oxford, OUP.
Hubner K. F. and Fry J. A. (eds.) (1980) *The Medical Basis for Radiation Accident Preparedness.* Holland, Elsevier.
National Radiological Protection Board (1986) *Living with Radiation.* London, HMSO.
Protection of the Public in the Event of Major Radiation Accidents; Principles for Planning. (1984) ICRP Publication 40. *Annals of the ICRP*, Vol. 14 No. 2. Oxford, Pergamon Press.

A Directory of Organizations Related to Medicine for Disasters

AMBULANCE SERVICE INSTITUTE

The objects of the Institute are to hold examinations from time to time in educational, administrative and technical subjects appertaining to the United Kingdom Ambulance Service. The Institute grants certificates of qualification in four classes—Licentiate. Associate, Graduate and Fellow. The Institute aims to promote, encourage and improve the theory and practice of ambulance service organization and administration in the UK and all operations connected therewith. The Institute exists to enable members to meet and correspond and to facilitate the interchange of ideas on ambulance service subjects. For this purpose branches of the Institute have been formed around the country.

Correspondence should be addressed to:
  The National Secretary,
  The Ambulance Service Institute,
  Ambulance Service Headquarters,
  Elm House,
  Belmont Grove,
  Liverpool L6 4EG,
  UK

ASSOCIATION OF ANAESTHETISTS OF GREAT BRITAIN AND NORTHERN IRELAND

The International Relations Committee of the Association of Anaesthetists of Great Britain and Northern Ireland concentrates much of its activities in promoting improved standards of anaesthesia and resuscitation in the developing countries. It provides aid by the subsidy of visiting teachers and certain publications to assist in the education of local anaesthetists to provide an appropriate anaesthetic service to patients suffering from natural disease and trauma. The expertise of local anaesthetists is of particular value in times of both natural and man-made disasters.

Correspondence should be addressed to:
  Assn. of Anaesthetists of Gt. Britain & Ireland,
  9 Bedford Square,
  London WC1B 3RA,
  UK

ASSOCIATION OF CHIEF AMBULANCE OFFICERS

The Association was formed in 1949 by a group of Chief Ambulance Officers in the UK and amended in 1976, following the National Health Service reorganization of 1974, when ambulance services were transferred from a Local Government function to become completely integrated into the National Health Service. The objectives of the Association are to promote and maintain efficient and economical ambulance services within the National Health Service by fostering mutual help amongst Chief Ambulance Officers throughout the UK and other countries, through the pooling of experience and by providing opportunities for co-operation between chief ambulance officers of Health Authorities. For the same purpose meetings and conferences are held regularly to discuss problems, and exchange information and ideas appertaining to the successful management of ambulance services.

It should also be the focal point for other professions and bodies from which advice or information may be obtained relative to the administration and operation of an ambulance service, and the association should publish such reports, handbooks and literature, as are deemed to be of general importance and interest.

Correspondence should be addressed to:
  The National Secretary,
  Association of Chief Ambulance Officers,
  c/o Dorset Ambulance Service H.Q.,
  Ringwood Road, St. Leonard's,
  BH24 2SP,
  UK

ASSOCIATION OF EMERGENCY MEDICAL TECHNICIANS

The Association of Emergency Medical Technicians (AEMT), formed in February 1978, is a Registered Charity and is affiliated to the British Association for Immediate Care. It is a non-political body primarily formed to raise the standard of immediate care given to the public by members of the Ambulance Service and intimately involved professions, such as Accident and Emergency Nurses, Armed Forces Medical Assistants and doctors in an emergency situation. The Association aims to encourage and promote training of ambulance personnel to an advanced level of knowledge and expertise in line with developments and advances in emergency care. In addition to an Examination Board that holds examinations biannually, the Association publishes a Training Manual to combine with the Training Syllabus. Public Education in cardiopulmonary resuscitation is undertaken by most of the Association's branches throughout the United Kingdom.

The Association publishes a quarterly journal *Emergency Care* and holds an annual conference, 'Medtec'. The Association has five grades of Membership: Medical, Registered (Paramedics), Associate, Student, and Subscribing.

Correspondence should be addressed to:

Dr Stephen Mather,
President, AEMT,
Department of Anaesthesia, Bristol Royal Infirmary,
Bristol BS2 8HW,
UK

AUSTRALIAN RESUSCITATION COUNCIL

The Australian Resuscitation Council was established in February 1976 for the purpose of fostering and co-ordinating the practice and teaching of resuscitation, as defined and set out in its Constitution. The formation of the Council was sponsored by the Royal Australasian College of Surgeons, including its Faculty of Anaesthetists, in response to the need for uniformity and standardization of resuscitation techniques expressed by participants from ambulance and voluntary organizations in several public seminars conducted by the College on topics including resuscitation.

The College invited the Australian Institute of Ambulance Officers, the Australian Red Cross Society, the National Heart Foundation of Australia, the Royal Life Saving Society of Australia, the St John Ambulance Association of Australia, the Surf Life Saving Association of Australia and the Resuscitation Research Council of New South Wales, which were the major bodies responsible for teaching and practising resuscitation, to join a Steering Committee to advise upon the constitution of a voluntary co-ordinating body, to be known as the Australian Resuscitation Council. The College Council then accepted the advice of the Steering Committee that the Australian Resuscitation Council should consist of representatives of the national bodies so convened, together with the Australian Defence Medical Services and the College of Nursing Australia. It was agreed that the Australian Resuscitation Council should be funded principally by application to government sources and to private endowment organizations while only a small membership fee should be levied on member organizations.

For the purpose of the Council, 'resuscitation' is defined as the preservation or restoration of life by the establishment and/or maintenance of airway, breathing and circulation, and related emergency care, and in its discussions the Council gives primary consideration to resuscitation as it applies before definitive hospital care. Among the objectives for which the Council was established are:

1. To provide a forum for discussion of all aspects of resuscitation.
2. To gather and collate scientific information regarding resuscitation techniques.
3. To promote simplicity and uniformity in techniques and terminology.
4. To pursue the development of standards for equipment and training.
5. To foster interest in and promulgate information regarding resuscitation.
6. To provide an advisory and resource service regarding techniques, equipment, teaching methods and teaching aids.
7. To foster research into methods of practice and teaching of resuscitation.
8. To establish regular communication with other bodies, in Australia or overseas, with similar objectives.

Membership of the Council consists of the following organizations:
1. The Royal Australasian College of Surgeons.
2. The following health-professional organizations teaching and practising resuscitation:
    a. The Australian Defence Medical Services
    b. The Institute of Ambulance Officers Australia
    c. The College of Nursing Australia
    d. The Royal Australian College of General Practitioners.
3. The following voluntary organizations teaching and practising resuscitation:
    a. The Australian Red Cross Society
    b. The National Heart Foundation of Australia
    c. The Royal Life Saving Society—Australia
    d. The St. John Ambulance Association of Australia
    e. The Surf Life Saving Association of Australia
    f. The Electricity Supply Association of Australia.

Because Council policy is implemented at State level, branches have been established in six States. The Council publishes a Newsletter and has issued policy statements on many aspects of resuscitation and first aid and published criteria and content for courses in cardiopulmonary resuscitation and a course in instructional techniques.
Correspondence should be addressed to:
Australian Resuscitation Council,
PO Box 369,
Spring Hill,
Queensland 4000,
Australia

BRITISH ASSOCIATION FOR IMMEDIATE CARE

The aims of the British Association for Immediate Care (BASICS) are to foster co-operation between existing immediate care schemes and to encourage and aid the formation and extension of schemes in the United Kingdom; to develop and strengthen co-operation between all services in dealing with emergencies; to encourage and assist research into all aspects of immediate care and accident prevention; to raise the standard of immediate care and training; to produce publications for the dissemination of information; and to evaluate specialist emergency equipment. The Association now has some 1500 members dispersed throughout the UK, most of whom are family practitioners, but there is also considerable participation by consultants in accident and emergency medicine, anaesthesia, cardiology, surgery and military medicine.

The Association publishes the *Journal of the British Association for Immediate Care* three times per year and subscriptions can be taken out by arrangement with the Administrator at the address below. Other publications are planned including a series of *Monographs on Immediate Care*. This series aims to provide up-to-date and practical advice for the immediate care doctor and the series includes topics such as *Chest Injuries, Pain Relief, Major Disaster* and *Entrapment in Road Traffic Accidents.* More titles are planned on both clinical and administrative aspects of immediate care.

The Association has developed close links with its counterparts in other countries and with international organizations involved in immediate and emergency care.

Correspondence should be addressed to:
Mr R. Bailey,
The Administrator, BASICS,
31c Lower Brook Street,
Ipswich,
Suffolk IP4 1AQ,
UK

BRITISH RED CROSS SOCIETY

The British Red Cross is an independent voluntary organization which, in the terms of the Geneva Convention, maintains a membership trained principally in first aid and nursing to act as an auxiliary to the public services in time of emergency. In addition to training its own members it also gives training to the public. The Society's voluntary members work to alleviate suffering among the injured, the sick, disabled and frail elderly people. To train its members and maintain its services it relies on donations from the public.

The Society operates through local offices in England, Wales, Scotland, Northern Ireland, the Channel Islands, the Isle of Man and Britain's remaining colonies and dependencies. The Society's governing body, the Council, is responsible for policy, for the formation of Branches and for the conditions of membership. Although autonomous, the British Red Cross is part of the International Red Cross movement and as such agrees to be bound by its statutes and principles. While the bulk of the Society's fund raising is for its work in the UK, it has a statutory obligation to support the humanitarian work of the whole Red Cross family. International relief is provided in the form of cash, supplies and skilled and professional personnel. Doctors, nurses, physiotherapists, nutritionists and others are recruited on short-term contract, as need demands.

Correspondence should be addressed to:
The British Red Cross Society,
9 Grosvenor Crescent,
London SW1X 7EJ,
UK

CASUALTY SURGEONS ASSOCIATION

Membership of the Casualty Surgeons Association (CSA) is available to doctors whose professional commitment is to accident and emergency medicine and whose interests it will seek to promote and protect. Through its accident and emergency consultants, the CSA will ensure the highest possible standards of primary care to the acutely ill and injured seeking medical aid in the accident and emergency department and the provision of initial care for the less seriously injured whose condition requires hospital facilities. A service will also be provided for those seeking urgent medical advice or care who are unable at the time to make use of general practitioner facilities.

The Casualty Surgeons Association will:

1. Recommend optimum standards of accommodation, facilities, equipment and supporting services and be responsible for establishing and maintaining these standards.
2. Lay down standards for the staffing of accident and emergency departments and ensure that suitably experienced staff are available at all times.
3. Promote and improve the career structure in accident and emergency medicine and ensure that appropriate training and experience is provided for all grades of staff.
4. Co-operate with the Royal Colleges to create a Diploma in Accident and Emergency Medicine of equivalent status to other specialty higher qualifications. A higher examination has been created with the Royal College of Surgeons of Edinburgh as the issuing body, the FRCS (A and E). This was instituted in May 1982.
5. Maintain a programme of postgraduate education.
6. Promote research into all aspects of accident and emergency medicine.
7. Co-operate with other organizations involved in emergency care to produce a national policy on accident and emergency services and to explore the possibility of establishing a single co-ordinating agency which would advise on regional and national major disaster planning.
8. Co-operate in the training of all personnel involved in emergency care and advise on the standardization and provision of equipment within the emergency service.
9. Promote and extend the facilities provided within accident and emergency departments for the training of ambulance personnel.
10. Seek to establish close operational links with professional organizations providing immediate care.
11. Establish a close liaison with general practitioner services to secure the appropriate use of each facility.
12. Improve operational links with community, medical, nursing and social services.
13. Seek to improve liaison with industrial accident services.
14. Promote publicity for accident prevention, the role of the accident and emergency department and the education of the public in the principles of first aid.
15. Maintain close links with other professional organizations so that advances in other specialties may be applied to patients within the accident and emergency department.
16. Protect the professional interests of its members.

    Correspondence should be addressed to:
    The Secretary,
    Casualty Surgeons Association,
    The Royal College of Surgeons,
    35/43 Lincolns Inn Fields,
    London WC2A 3PN,
    UK

CHRISTIAN AID

Christian Aid is the relief and development division of the British Council of Churches and in emergency situations may work under the co-ordination facilities of the World Council of Churches. Assistance is usually provided through the local church organization and usually takes the form of funds related to specific projects. In 1983 Christian Aid made substantial donations to victims of war and disasters, particularly in Lebanon.

Correspondence should be addressed to:
  The Head of Aid Department,
  Christian Aid,
  240/250 Ferndale Road,
  PO Box 1,
  Brixton,
  London SW9 8BH,
  UK

EMERGENCY MEDICINE RESEARCH SOCIETY

The Emergency Medicine Research Society was formed to further research and a common interest in accident and emergency medicine and related topics. The Society holds one or two meetings each year at which original research in accident and emergency medicine is presented and as part of the membership fee the members receive the journal *Archives of Emergency Medicine.* The Society is growing in number and would hope to link with other Societies around the world with similar interests and also to promote collaborative studies in the United Kingdom.

Correspondence should be addressed to:
  Dr K. Little,
  Consultant in A & E Medicine,
  Accident & Emergency Department,
  The Royal Infirmary,
  Edinburgh,
  Scotland EH3 9YW

INTENSIVE CARE SOCIETY

The Intensive Care Society was founded in 1970 and currently has over 450 members including overseas members. Amongst the members are surgeons, anaesthetists, physicians, pathologists and a few non-medical workers who have a major interest in intensive care. The Society exists to facilitate communication and promote high standards of intensive therapy. Council is responsible for organizing Society meetings and advising on intensive care topics. The expanding interests of the Society are now dealt with in part by Sub-Committees on Education and Training, Research, Standards and by a Computer Group. A travelling Fellowship of up to £2000 may be awarded annually.

Correspondence should be addressed to:

Dr D. Ryan,
Consultant Clinical Physiologist,
Freeman Hospital,
Newcastle upon Tyne NE7 7DN,
UK

INTERNATIONAL CIVIL DEFENCE ORGANIZATION

The International Civil Defence Organization (ICDO) is a humanitarian inter-governmental organization whose Constitution of 17th October 1966 has been duly registered with the United Nations Secretariat in New York, in conformity with Article 102 of the Charter. At international level, responsibility for promoting protection and safety measures for persons and property in the face of all kinds of disasters rests with the ICDO, which groups the national authorities in charge of implementing these measures. The ICDO constitutes a forum where professionals working in this field, both in the industrialized and developing countries, can exchange their knowledge and experience with the aim of achieving the highest possible level of readiness with regard to individuals and communities who may be confronted with the simplest of accidents or a major disaster.

The technical co-operation which ICDO has initiated with its Member States, or which it fosters among them at the international and regional level, aims primarily at promoting the establishment, consolidation and growth of national civil protection organizations and at providing assistance in fulfilling their specific tasks such as:

1. Prevention of and intervention in accidents and disasters.
2. Improvement in the population's knowledge about potential hazards.
3. Development of protection and intervention staff and manpower.
4. Co-ordination and development of research on means of protection.
5. Planning and implementation of preparedness plans and safety programme for the population.

The scope of activities of ICDO covers numerous fields:

1. Training of Civil Protection personnel (at all levels).
2. Preparedness and dissemination of basic technical documents and reference material to facilitate the work of the national organizations.
3. Research, collection and registration of literature published throughout the world on the branches assigned to Civil Protection.
4. Promote international collaboration and co-operation in strengthening of EMS and disaster preparedness.

Correspondence should be addressed to:
Dr Milan Bodi,
10–12 Chemin de Surville,
CH-1213 Petit Lancy,
Geneva,
Switzerland

THE TRAUMA FOUNDATION

The Trauma Foundation came into being in June 1971. It arose directly out of recommendations made at an international conference on accident prevention and rehabilitation in Johannesburg in June 1971. The immediate aims of the foundation were to help and encourage existing and developing organizations for research, training and service in the field for prevention and treatment of injuries including the prevention of accidents on the roads, in the home and industry as well as the treatment of war disabled and in the field of the care and rehabilitation of the severely injured, in all parts of the world.

Immediately following this international conference the International Trauma Foundation was established almost simultaneously in different countries, with representatives in many other countries including those of the Third World. The Johannesburg Conference and the establishment of the International Trauma Foundation was made possible by the generous financial support of Mrs May Eden whose continuing generosity and support has made its continued existence possible.

The Registered Office of the Foundation is in the United Kingdom.

In October 1973 the International Trauma Foundation held its first formal meeting in London and this was followed by an inaugural conference in Manchester in June 1975. Many organizations, both in the United Kingdom and overseas were represented at these meetings.

The Trauma Foundation has an office in London staffed by an Administrator and apart from its activities in liaising with all organizations concerned through the medium of its liaison committee, it also acts as a centre at which various organizations and groups can meet. In addition there is a reference library and slide library which is in the process of being built up by the co-operation and help of associated and interested organizations.

The Committee of the Trauma Foundation meets regularly in London and welcomes affiliation from any interested organizations not already on its liaison committee. It in no way serves to duplicate or take over the work of any existing organization but aims to serve as a common meeting ground for many organizations and at intervals to provide a common meeting place for representatives of all those organizations with the aim of furthering knowledge and skills in the care of the injured and hopefully the prevention of those injuries.

Correspondence should be addressed to:
   The Administrator,
   The Trauma Foundation,
   21 West Smithfield,
   London EC1A 9HY,
   UK

LATIN AMERICAN MEDICAL ORGANIZATION FOR DISASTER COUNSELLING AND RESEARCH

The Latin American Medical Organization for Disaster Counselling and Research (OMLAID) is an organization established in San Jose, Costa Rica in

1984. It is affiliated with the College of Physicians and Surgeons of Costa Rica, where its headquarters is located. It is legally registered in Costa Rica and its statutes are in accordance with the Law of Associations number 219 from 8 August, 1939. OMLAID is a private Latin American organization and its members are professionals in the medical science field. The organization specializes in research, advice and training in health matters for natural or man-made disaster situations in the Latin American and Caribbean region. It maintains close ties with similar organizations and will establish regional offices in different countries according to the needs. It is non-profit making and will provide assistance without discrimination to religious, political, philosophical or ethnic groups.

Correspondence should be addressed to:
    Latin American Medical Organization for Disaster Counselling and Research,
    PO Box 548,
    San Jose,
    Costa Rica

LEAGUE OF RED CROSS AND RED CRESCENT SOCIETIES

The League of Red Cross and Red Crescent Societies is the international federation of national Red Cross and Red Crescent Societies. Founded on 5 May, 1919 in Paris, it has 135 member national societies today. The League is an independent, non-governmental, non-political, non-racial and non-sectarian organization. Its object is to inspire, encourage, facilitate and promote at all times all forms of humanitarian activities by its member societies with a view to the prevention and alleviation of human suffering, and thereby to contribute to the maintenance and the promotion of peace in the world.

To achieve this object, the League, among other activities, works as the permanent body of liaison, co-ordination and study between the national societies, giving the societies assistance at their request. It encourages and promotes in every country the establishment and development of an independent and duly recognized national Red Cross or Red Crescent Society. The League acts to bring relief to disaster victims by all available means. It therefore organizes, co-ordinates and directs international relief actions in accordance with the principles and rules adopted by the International Conference of the Red Cross. By the same token, it assists national societies in their disaster relief preparedness, in the organization of their relief actions and in the relief operations themselves.

In addition, the League encourages and co-ordinates national society participation in activities for safeguarding public health and promoting social welfare; and for the exchange of ideas for educating children and young people in humanitarian ideas and the development of friendly relations between young people of all countries. The League assists its members in recruiting adherents to the Red Cross movement and in inculcating the movement's principles and ideals. Last of the League's functions to be mentioned is its role of bringing help to victims of armed conflicts within the framework of its agreed activities as a member of the International Red Cross, in accordance with its agreements with a second component of the International Red Cross, the ICRC International

Committee of the Red Cross. As part of this function, the League assists the ICRC in promoting and developing international humanitarian law, collaborating with that organization in disseminating this law, and of the fundamental principles of the Red Cross, among the national societies.

The League shares with the ICRC the common motto of the Red Cross, *Inter Arma Caritas*, to which it has added a second motto, *Per Humanitatem ad Pacem*, considering that together these reflect the ideas of the movement as a whole.

Correspondence should be addressed to:

League of Red Cross and Red Crescent Societies,
PO Box 276,
CH 1211,
Geneva 19,
Switzerland

MÉDECINS SANS FRONTIÈRES

Médecins sans Frontières provides medical assistance to populations that are victims of war, natural disasters or chronic inadequate medical care. The organization provides all types of health workers and nutritionists who serve from 3–12 months. Volunteers should speak the language of the country to which they are assigned. Médecins sans Frontières will also supply goods. including drugs from the modified WHO list, and other equipment as deemed necessary. The organization was most active in the 1984 Bhopal disaster in India.

Correspondence should be addressed to:

The Executive or Medical Director,
Médecins sans Frontières,
161 Boulevard Lefèvre,
75015 Paris,
France

OXFORD COMMITTEE FOR FAMINE RELIEF

The aims of the Oxford Committee for Famine Relief (OXFAM) are twofold— to promote the development of improved public health standards and to provide relief in disasters. OXFAM provides funding for curative medical services, water supply, sanitation and immunization programmes and, from time to time, will supply personnel, goods and supplies for health services, feeding and water supply. The services are available to virtually any country demonstrating a clear need for assistance.

Correspondence should be addressed to:

The Disaster Unit,
OXFAM,
274 Banbury Road,
Oxford OX2 7DZ,
UK

PAN AMERICAN HEALTH ORGANIZATION

The Pan American Health Organization (PAHO) is the regional office of the World Health Organization for the Americas, and has the same aims and objectives as the World Health Organization. Its membership is drawn from 34 countries in the Americas with Britain, France and the Netherlands as Associate Members. Representatives from each country form the Pan American Sanitary Conference and Directing Council which determines overall policy and administers the Organization. The health care programmes are carried out by the Pan American Sanitary Bureau Director and his staff.

The Organization is devoted to the improvement in public health throughout the Americas which will include adequate nutrition, a clear water supply and sanitation facilities; a comprehensive immunization programme along with epidemiological research and statistics. PAHO helps its member countries in the development and implementation of health care systems and these will include emergency and disaster preparedness and the relief necessary to minimize the effect of such tragedies in line with WHO principles.

The Organization publishes comprehensive reports on its activities including a regular newsletter entitled *Disaster Preparedness in the Americas*. It also produces a most useful directory of the agencies providing health assistance after disasters occurring in Latin America and the Caribbean.

Correspondence should be addressed to:
The Disaster Relief Co-ordinator,
Pan American Health Organization,
525 Twenty Third Street, NW,
Washington DC 20037,
USA

RELIEF INTERNATIONAL

Relief International is an organization providing subsidized assistance to victims of disasters. As with many organizations, the level of provision of help depends on previous fund raising success. The organization can provide personnel and limited material support.

Correspondence should be addressed to:
The Executive Director,
Relief International,
275 Slater Street,
Ottawa,
Ontario K1P 5H9,
Canada

RESUSCITATION COUNCIL (UK)

The Resuscitation Council (UK), formerly the Community Resuscitation Advisory Council, was formed in 1981 with the object of facilitating the educa-tion of the population of the UK in effective methods of resuscitation. The

Council now consists of 15 nominated members who represent the views of the Association of Anaesthetists, BASICS, AEMT, the Intensive Care Society, British Cardiac Society, British Heart Foundation, Casualty Surgeons Association, Trauma Foundation, SURF, World Association of Emergency and Disaster Medicine and the World Federation of Societies of Anaesthesiologists. Close links have also been established with Government organizations and voluntary aid societies.

In the few years since its inception, the Council has formulated its recommendations on advanced resuscitation. Its findings have been published in a series of documents:

1. *The Resuscitation Guide (Basic resuscitation)*—a 5 page pocket size *aide-memoire,* printed on laminated plastic.
2. *Resuscitation for the Citizen (Basic resuscitation)*—a 10 page booklet describing the practice of resuscitation with the aid of simple diagrams and an explanatory text.
3. *ABC of Resuscitation (Basic resuscitation)*—a poster which matches the resuscitation guide.
4. *Cardiopulmonary Resuscitation (Advanced resuscitation)*—a poster for advanced resuscitation.
5. Videofilms on Basic and Advanced Cardiac Life Support.
6. Recommendations for Paediatric Resuscitation.

The Council is examining the results of in-hospital resuscitation in a multicentre study throughout the UK. Work is continuing on recommendations for paediatric resuscitation, trauma resuscitation and the ethics of resuscitation.

Correspondence should be addressed to:

Dr D. Zideman,
Resuscitation Council (UK),
Department of Anaesthetics,
Royal Postgraduate Medical School,
Hammersmith Hospital,
Ducane Road,
London W12 0HS,
UK

RESUSCITATION RESEARCH CENTRE

The Resuscitation Research Centre was initiated by Dr Peter Safar and is supported by the University of Pittsburgh. Its aims are to undertake and promote original research into all aspects of resuscitation, with the ultimate object of preventing unnecessary and premature death and enhancing the quality of life after an episode of cardiorespiratory insufficiency or arrest. To this end many research programmes have been undertaken by Dr Safar and his co-workers. Several projects, including a multinational trial, have been concerned with brain resuscitation after cardiorespiratory arrest and this work is on-going.

Correspondence should be addressed to:

Resuscitation Research Centre,
University of Pittsburgh,
School of Medicine,
3434 Fifth Avenue, 2nd Floor,
Pittsburgh PA 15260,
USA

ROYAL NATIONAL LIFEBOAT INSTITUTION

The Royal National Lifeboat Institution (RNLI) was founded in 1824. It is a registered charity and entirely depends on voluntary contributions for its income. There are 200 RNLI lifeboat stations around the shores of the United Kingdom. The aim of the RNLI is to provide, on call, the permanent day and night lifeboat service necessary to cover known and predicted search and rescue (SAR) requirements out to 30 miles from the coast of the United Kingdom and the Republic of Ireland. Each station has a Station Honorary Medical Adviser (SHMA), who is a member of the British Association for Immediate Care, by virtue of the RNLI medical organization's membership of the Association.
Correspondence should be addressed to:
Royal National Lifeboat Institution,
West Quay Road,
Poole,
Dorset BH15 1NZ,
UK

ST JOHN AMBULANCE

St John Ambulance, formed in 1877 to instruct people in first aid, nursing, hygiene and allied subjects, today operates in 45 countries with 200 000 volunteers and its Cadet branch, a major youth group with 100 000 members, in 33 countries. In Britain the Association trains 150 000 people a year in first aid while the uniformed Brigade is a body of fully-qualified volunteers on duty wherever crowds collect and providing service in the field of community care. The Aeromedical Service repatriated over 500 patients in 1984. In 1985 Her Majesty the Queen presented the Ambulance Air Wing, specializing in transportation of transplant organs, with the prestigious Britannia Trophy. In addition to a comprehensive first aid and nursing manual published in conjunction with St Andrews Ambulance and the British Red Cross, St John Ambulance itself publishes a wide range of manuals on first aid and allied subjects.
Correspondence should be addressed to:
Medical Secretary,
National Headquarters St John Ambulance,
1 Grosvenor Crescent,
London SW1X 7EF,
UK

SALVATION ARMY WORLD SERVICE OFFICE

The Salvation Army World Service Office provides assistance for Salvation Army organizations in over 80 countries in the form of technical help or funds to provide appropriate aid for immediate needs resulting from disasters. The organization can supply physicians, nurses and other health staff as well as cash, goods, medical supplies and equipment.

Correspondence should be addressed to:
  The Director,
  Salvation Army World Service Office,
  1025 Vermont Avenue NW 305,
  Washington DC 20005,
  USA

SAVE THE CHILDREN FUND

The Save the Children Fund is concerned with emergency relief and the long-term welfare of children. There are sister organizations in Australia, New Zealand and Canada. The Fund can supply funds, personnel, goods, medical supplies and equipment for health services and disaster relief. Physicians, nurses, epidemiologists, nutritionists, health teachers and sanitary engineers usually serve for at least a year and should, if possible, speak the language of the country in which they serve.

Correspondence should be addressed to:
  The Senior Medical Officer,
  Save the Children Fund,
  17 Grove Lane,
  London SE5 8SD,
  UK

UNITED NATIONS DISASTER RELIEF ORGANIZATION (UNDRO)

UNDRO is responsible for co-ordinating the disaster relief activities of the United Nations' various specialist agencies.

Correspondence should be addressed to:
  The Office of the UN Disaster Relief Co-ordinator,
  United Nations Building,
  Geneva 19,
  CH 1211,
  Switzerland

WORLD FEDERATION OF SOCIETIES OF ANAESTHESIOLOGISTS

The Cardiopulmonary Resuscitation Committee of the World Federation of Societies of Anaesthesiologists (WFSA) consists of about 10 members elected by the Executive Committee of the WFSA whose task is to promote improved standards of resuscitation amongst the member national societies of the WFSA. The Committee has commissioned two major publications in recent years. *Cardiopulmonary Cerebral Resuscitation* by Peter Safar was published in 1981 by Asmund S. Laerdal of Stavanger, Norway, and is a sequel to his original title *Cardiopulmonary Resuscitation* which appeared in the 1960s. This book has been widely acclaimed and has been distributed worldwide in large numbers due in no small part to the generosity of the Laerdal Corporation. The book has been translated into several languages—French, German, Spanish, Italian, Czechoslovakian, Russian. *Cardiopulmonary Cerebral Resuscitation* is a comprehensive work encompassing both basic and the most advanced life support theories and techniques and is intended as a manual for physicians and paramedical instructors.

The second major publication entitled *Life Supporting Resuscitation and First Aid* was sponsored jointly by the WFSA CPR Committee and the League of Red Cross (and now Red Crescent) Societies. It was prepared by Nancy Caroline and published in 1984 and has been distributed by the League to its member societies. This volume is a manual for instructors of the lay public and is produced in modular form so that the instructor can select the degree of sophistication of training appropriate to the trainees.

Cardiopulmonary Cerebral Resuscitation in the English language, now in its third edition, may be obtained from medical bookshops worldwide or by direct application to the Laerdal Publishing Company in Stavanger or to W. B. Saunders Ltd, in the USA or UK. Other language versions may be obtained from medical bookshops or the local publishers. *Life Supporting Resuscitation and First Aid* may be obtained from national Red Cross Societies.

Further activities of the WFSA CPR Committee include the teaching of resuscitation principles and methods by the WFSA's visiting educational teams. *Correspondence should be addressed to:*

Dr P. J. F. Baskett,
Chairman WFSA CPR Committee,
Department of Anaesthesia,
Frenchay Hospital,
Bristol BS16 1LE,
UK

WORLD ASSOCIATION FOR EMERGENCY AND DISASTER MEDICINE

The World Association for Emergency and Disaster Medicine (formerly the Club of Mainz) was formed in 1976 by a group of individuals led by the late Professor Rudolf Frey and Professor Peter Safar who were interested in fostering improvements and co-operation on an international scale in the field of emergency and disaster medicine. It was intended that the Club of Mainz should be analogous to the Club of Rome and that initially its members should consist of a small number of invited individuals with influence who had considerable experience in the subject and who would be able to advise authorities on a national and international basis. Since 1983, however, the Club has opened its membership to all with an interest in emergency and disaster medicine and applications to join are sought. The membership subscription is currently US $60 per annum and includes the subscription to the Journal. The Club changed its name in 1985 to the World Association for Emergency and Disaster Medicine.

Regular international scientific meetings in Mainz, Monte Carlo, Pittsburgh, Rome, Brighton UK, and Rio de Janeiro over the years have now escalated to World Congress status. The meetings have been open to all with an interest in emergency and disaster medicine. The proceedings of earlier meetings have been published in the Disaster Medicine series, published by Springer Verlag and since 1983 in the Association's own *Journal of Emergency and Disaster Medicine*. Further World Congresses will be held every 2 years.

The Association has formed close links with the League of Red Cross and Red Crescent Societies, the World Health Organization, the United National Disaster Relief Organization and many other national and international bodies. International co-operation has led to projects concerning airport disasters, chemical disasters, earthquakes, volcanoes and terrorism. It is hoped in the future to evaluate international experience and to make authoritative recommendations for improvements in many aspects of emergency and disaster medicine.

Correspondence should be addressed to:
Dr P. J. F. Baskett,
Hon. Secretary,
Department of Anaesthesia,
Frenchay Hospital,
Bristol BS16 1LE,
UK

Editor of the Journal:
Professor R. Adams Cowley MD,
Maryland Institute for Emergency Medicine,
University of Maryland,
22 South Greene Street,
Baltimore, Maryland,
21201 USA

WORLD FEDERATION OF SOCIETIES OF INTENSIVE AND CRITICAL CARE MEDICINE

The World Federation of Societies of Intensive and Critical Care Medicine was established at the Third World Congress on Intensive and Critical Care Medicine, held in Washington DC, in May 1981. It presently consists of 40 societies, including 2 nursing societies, in 38 countries. Its primary aim is to promote the highest standards of intensive care throughout the world. The Federation publishes an *Intensive and Critical Care Digest* which is circulated to over 15500 intensivists in 80 countries around the world. Countries which do not have an intensive or critical care society may join through the Medical Society whose aims are most closely linked with the purpose of the Federation.

Correspondence should be addressed to:
    The Secretary-General,
    WFSICCM,
    National Heart Hospital,
    Westmoreland Street,
    London W1M 8BA,
    UK

WORLD HEALTH ORGANIZATION

The World Health Organization (WHO) provides on-going co-operation with the Health Agencies of its member countries which consist of virtually all the countries of the world. Certain sectors of the world are delegated to regional offices in the execution of its functions, such as the Americas, which are served by the Pan American Health Organization.

The WHO provides guidance on all public health matters and the organization of health care systems and their delivery. In addition, it provides emergency technical assistance in disaster situations threatening the public health of the country. WHO may supply medical equipment according to a prescribed list and may assist in channelling other supplies donated by other sources to the appropriate recipients. Advice is readily available concerning preventive measures, health care provisions and reconstruction after disaster. The WHO publishes regular reports of its aims, objects and activities throughout the world and also publishes booklets relating to specific subjects.

Correspondence should be addressed to:
    The Emergency Relief Operation,
    World Health Organization,
    20 Avenue Appia,
    1211 Geneva 27,
    Switzerland

APPENDIX

APPENDIX

Disaster Profiles of Selected Developing Countries

Country	Indicators — Population annual growth (%)	Indicators — Inf. mort. rate per cap.	Indicators — GNP ($)	Disaster types/ recent history: victims	Vulnerability — Systems problems/assets	Preparedness — Plan/structure	Donor assessment
Burkina-Faso	7·0 million (1984) 1·9%	148/1000	$180	Drought. Famine. Epidemics. Infestations. 1966–1982: 3·9 million	(−) Sanitation. Water. Equipment. Medical care access. Telecommunications. (+) Agriculture. Rail system.	Not clear if plan exists—more like operating procedures. National committee: A permanent famine relief organization. A quasi-military group. Emergency communications network. Other government support groups.	25 major agencies—religious, private, international. Red Cross, Red Crescent and various host groups.
Cape Verde	300000 (1983) 0·9%	78/1000	$320	Persistent poverty. Periodic famine. Emigration. Erratic rainfall. Logistics. *Potential* oil tanker accident. *Potential* air-crash. Hurricanes. 1968–1979: 13 years of drought	(−) Early warning capacity. Search/rescue. Air traffic. Port congestion. Housing. Health personnel. (+) Recognition of preparedness importance/problems.	No known national plan. Response on ad hoc basis via Prime Minister's office. Slow implementation of water conservation programmes. Government recognizes importance of preparedness and mitigation.	Major international, bilateral and religious organizations. 7 US non-profit groups.
Chad	4·8 million (1983) 2·1%	142/1000	$N.A.	Drought. Civil strife/ war. Refugees. Major food shortages. Infestations. 1966–1982: 7 million	(−) Roads. Economy. Equipment. Storage. Diseases. Sanitation. Hospitals. Skill levels. Climate. Ports. Railroads.	Resolution to create full structure. National committee for reconstruction. A working body. Reception, storage and delivery of relief supplies. National disaster relief office: for co-ordination with donors.	International groups. Some French PVOs. 18 US non-profit groups.

APPENDIX

Disaster Profiles of Selected Developing Countries (*continued*)

Country	Indicators		Disaster types/ recent history: victims	Vulnerability Systems problems/assets	Preparedness	
	Population annual growth (%)	Inf. mort. rate per cap. GNP ($)			Plan/structure	Donor assessment
Gambia	700000 (1983) 2·5%	194/1000 $290	Droughts. Epidemics. Power shortages. Civil strife. Infestations. 1968–1981: 1·4 million	(−) Data. Health. Nutrition. Health facilities/staff. Sanitation Agriculture. Transportation. Managerial. Skills. Power. Stockpiles. (+) Member of Sene Gambia Confederation.	Existing plan, but little associated activity. Difficult to assess needs as little known about response capacity.	A number of international, private and religious groups. 15 US non-profit groups.
Ghana	12·4 million 3·1%	86/1000 $360	Droughts. Food shortages. Bush fires. Floods. Refugees. Epidemics. 1968–1985: 5 million	(−) Ports. Communications. Supplies. Environment. Health facilities. Data. Food. Economy. Road. Sanitation. Water. Sewage.	National mobilization programme (part of economic recovery effort). National mobilization committee: Co-ordinates emergency food programmes. Elaborate system, to all parts of economy. Staff/logistical support problems. National repatriation TF (excellent work). Government commitment to disaster planning/preparedness. EWS.	Major donors assisting government. Ghana Red Cross and other host agencies are important. 44 US non-profit groups.

	Population / death rate / GNP / growth	Disaster types and years	Constraints (−) and resources (+)	National plan / organization	Assisting organizations
Mali	7·5 million (1982) 148/1000 $130 2·5%	Regional droughts. Food shortages. Epidemics. 1968–1981: Over 1 million	(−) Diseases. Transportation. Health facilities. Malnutrition. Food. Power. Economy. (+) Storage capacity.	No national plan (1982). Sahel Disaster Relief Organization: Could be restructured for other disasters. Under Ministers of Interior and Defence. Co-ordinating role. Rapid, effective relief efforts.	Wide range of international agencies, bi-lateral religious, and private organizations. 21 US non-profit groups.
Mauritania	1·7 million (1983) 170/1000 $480 2·2%	Chronic drought. Desertification. Malnutrition. Epidemics. Food shortages. Infestations. 1965–1983: 4·5 million	(−) Telecommunications. Transportation. Weather. Urban over-population. Diseases. Squatter settlements. Agricultural research. Health facilities. Health services/ staff. (+) Fishing industry.	National Emergency Action Plan: Focuses on food shortages, health crises, environmental problems. National Committee for Assistance to People Affected by the Droughts: Uses military, key ministers and Red Crescent. Regional Committee. Very focused. Budget inadequate; needs outside help. Part of two regional organizations. Government has begun to tie disaster to development.	Many international private and religious organizations. 11 US non-profit groups.
Niger	6·1 million (1983) 139/1000 $240 3·0%	Infestations. Droughts. Food shortages. Deforestation. Local fires. Local flash floods. Multiplier effects though en-economy; secondary and tertiary disasters. Epidemics. Refugees. 1969–1984: 4·5 million	(−) Health resources. Population growth. Immunization procedures. Agricultural development. Soils. Diseases. Malnutrition. Disaster supplies. Soil conservation. Sanitation. Sewage. Transportation conditions. Urban fuel supplies. Little data analysis. (+) Food production policies. Uranium production. International telecommunications. Road network. Some mining. Good flow of national/ local information.	No national plan. No permanent organization. Ad hoc inter-ministerial committee. Assesses needs and plans for long-term relief. Some good recent government measures: farming and cattle purchasing.	Many international bilateral, and religious groups. Sudan Interior Mission: important role. Over a dozen non-profit groups.

APPENDIX

Disaster Profiles of Selected Developing Countries (*continued*)

Country	*Indicators* Population annual growth (%)	Inf. mort. rate per cap. GNP ($)	Disaster types/ recent history: victims	*Vulnerability* Systems problems/assets	*Preparedness* Plan/structure	Donor assessment
Senegal	6·2 million (1983) 2·6%	140/1000 $440	Civil strife. Epidemics. Droughts. Floods. Storms. Infestations. 1964–1978: 15 million	(−) Disaster supplies. Dependency rate. Health rate. Infrastructure. Safe water. Sanitation. Data. Waterborne and infectious diseases. Communicable diseases and malnutrition. Food importation. Depressed commodity markets. Rainfalls. Soils. (+) Port facilities. Tourism. Long-term economic goals. Roads. Railroads. Senegambia Confederation.	No disaster plan. Disaster relief co-ordinator and disaster relief department in Ministry of Planning and Co-operation. Ad hoc interministerial committee. Distribution and transportation of supplies. UNDRO has offered assistance.	Major international, private and religious organizations. Two dozen US non-profit groups.
Zaire	29·9 million (1983) 2·5%	106/1000 $170	Epidemics. Civil strife. Refugees (permanent). Earthquakes. Volcanic eruptions. Major diseases. 1966–1978: 15 000	(−) Medical services. Agriculture. Relief/rescue. Roads. Airports. Medicines/drug supplies. (+) Ports. Hydroelectric potential. Excellent weather tracking.	No national plan (1975). Economic development and disaster preparedness linked together. Ad hoc national disaster commission (1975). Hierarchy dependent on disaster type. Responses often slow. Satellite connection for weather tracking.	Nearly 60 US non-profit supporters. All major international, private, religious organizations. Major development projects.

	Population	IMR / GNP	Disasters	(−) and (+) factors	National plan / structure	Organizations
Zambia	6·3 million (1983) 2·5%	100/1000 $580	Local droughts. Refugees. Deforestation. Erosion. Air/water pollution. Floods. Accidents. 1964–1978: 34 000	(−) Economy. Politics. Ports. Environmental data. Relief transportation. (+) Health network. Disease controls. Medical staff. Food projects. Industrial development. Roads. Rails. Power. Airport. Communication. Satellite usage.	No clear plan or structure directed (broadly) at disasters. Government and various agencies involved in many development projects which address a range of disaster preparedness/mitigation issues. Use of satellite warning system.	Over 50 countries and US non-profit institutions. Major international, private and religious organizations. Red Cross important. UNHCR help with refugee settlement. No central donor locus.
Djibouti	400 000 (1983) N.A.	High IMR but no figure available. 50% due to food lack in country. GNP per capita not available. One of poorest countries in world.	Floods. Droughts. Refugees. Some earthquakes. 1977–1981: 315 000	(−) Natural resources. Diseases. Public resources. Industry. Weather. Health services. Waterways. Health facilities. Food. Sanitation. Water. Port conjestion. Relief supplies. High unemployment. (+) Thermoelectric plants.	No clear national plan evident, though refugee assistance office appears to have operating procedures. National office of refugee assistance: plans/ implements rehabilitation/ development programmes. Needs substantial outside help. Army, police and most civil servants assist in floods.	Food assistance sporadic; based on availability. CARITAS, Red Cross, UNHCR and WFP assistance are exceptions. CRS also plays an important role.
Ethiopia	40·9 million (1983) 2·7%	122/1000 $120	Drought. Famine. Locusts. Political disorders. Erosion. Refugees. 1965–1981: 4·2 million plus death of millions of cattle.	(−) Population reachability. Logistics. Health services. Security. Data. Malaria. Nutrition. Grain deficits. Labour unrest. Economy: Output stagnation. Resource diversion. Political unrest. (+) Electric power potential. Airport system. Disease prevention. Food/nutrition.	Long-term relief and rehabilitation commission. Problems with availability of data on total areas/populations affected. Red Cross plays an important role in relief. Food and nutrition. Early warning system. No known national plan.	All major organizations involved. Considerable food assistance from FAO. WFP, UNDRO. Red Cross very important. 31 US non-profit groups.

APPENDIX

APPENDIX

Disaster Profiles of Selected Developing Countries (*continued*)

Country	Indicators — Population annual growth (%)	Inf. mort. rate per cap. GNP ($)	Disaster types/ recent history: victims	Vulnerability Systems problems/assets	Preparedness Plan/structure	Donor assessment
Kenya	18·9 million (1983) 4·0%; highest in world	81/1000 $340	Droughts. Floods. Pest infestations. Soil erosion. Deforestation. 1965–1981: Several million (no precise figure available).	(−) High birth rate. Land availability. Cultivation practices. Siltation. (+) Sophisticated government approaches. Family planning. Storage facilities. Airports. Telecommunications. Satellite usage. Geothermal potential. Tourism. Coffee and tea industries.	No national disaster plan. President's office takes care of centralized decision-making. Military plays large role with available equipment. Relief committees at district level. Government does not generally publicize problems.	All major world organizations in Kenya—international, private, and religious. Nearly 100 US non-profit groups.
Somalia	5·1 million (1983) 3·2%	142/1000 $250	Refugees. Critical food shortages. Drought. Some seismicity. Infestations. 1966–1981: Over 5 million	(−) Health facils. Storage capacity. Transportation. Communications. Diseases. Resource strains. Food supplies. Cultivatable land. Firewood supplies. Malnutrition. Disease control implementation. Health services.	No national comprehensive plan. National refugee commission with good planning and implementation: Several dozen refugee camps. Major logistics problems in addressing refugee needs.	Wide range of donors from international, private and religious communities. 23 US non-profit groups.

	Population	Growth	Ratio	GNP	Hazards / Disaster history	(−) / (+)	National plan	Donor organizations
Sudan	20·8 million (1983)		117/1000	$400	Refugees. Deforestation. Erosion. Floods. Water hyacinth. Epidemics. Civil strife. Potential herbicide poisonings. Accidents. Not subject to frequency/intensity of natural disaster as are neighbours. 1965–1980: Over 2 million	(−) Rain excesses. Transportation. Fuel lacks. Agriculture practices. Water. Drainage/irrigation. Refugee strains. Poor sanitation. Malnutrition. Health personnel. Power. Managerial skills. (+) Telecommunications. Government policy on refugees. Health plan.	No national plan. National relief committee. Centralized decision-making. Permanent commission on refugees. Data collection: villages upward. Successful work with refugees.	Major worldwide donor organizations—international, bilateral, private and religious. Donor co-ordination on an ad hoc basis; Sudanese do *not* bring them together.
Tanzania	20·8 million	3·33%	97/1000	$240	Refugees. Infestations. Floods. Civil strife. Food shortages. 1968–1980: Estimated 820000	(−) Rain patterns. Land development. Soils. Population dispersion. Transportation. Communications. Land use. Food supply. Sanitation. Nutrition. Food storage. (+) Food production. Grain reserves. Health services. Industrial expansion. Ports. Airports. Telecommunications. Hydroelectric distribution.	No national disaster plan. Government budgets contingency funds with supplemental appropriations. National milling corporation: Responsible for strategic grain reserves. Data collection sometimes inadequate, though.	Large grouping of religious, international, private agencies. 55 US non-profit groups. Tanzania Red Cross important; attempts to promote preparedness at regional village levels; food relief presence.
Uganda	13·9 million	2·8%	108/1000	$220	Droughts. Civil strife. Refugees. Some earthquake activity. Food shortages. 1961–1981: Over 1 million	(−) Agriculture. Economy. Societal deterioration. Military. Transportation. Food distribution. Medical services. Industrial production. Power system. Telecommunications.	No known plan. National relief and rehabilitation committee; bi-weekly meetings; poor, unreliable data.	Continued donor assistance including 50 US non-profit groups. Years of civil strife. Many operations difficult. Ongoing food programmes.

APPENDIX

Disaster Profiles of Selected Developing Countries (continued)

Country	Indicators — Population annual growth (%)	Inf. mort. rate per cap. GNP ($)	Disaster types/ recent history: victims	Vulnerability — Systems problems/assets	Preparedness — Plan/structure	Donor assessment
Bangladesh	90 million (1981) 2·6%	139/1000 $ N.A.	Cyclones. Storm surges. Floods. Civil strife. Typhoons. Monsoons. 1960–1980: Estimate of 100 million.	(−) Water supply. Infectious diseases. Surface drainage. Costline openness. Flood controls. River bank weaknesses. Pollution. Epidemics. Power and gas systems. Housing. Agriculture. Industry weaknesses.	No national disaster plan; long-term disagreements on authorities. Relief operations: ad hoc. Central committee for floods. Ministry of Relief/ Rehabilitation: policy guidance to agencies and permanent disaster organization: 6 tiers/ EOC/many disputes. Bangladesh cyclone preparedness programme: Joint ventures between Red Cross and MRR. Many infrastructure limitations. Some mitigation efforts. Ongoing disasters disrupt economy. Needs tie to development. Storm warning/floods forecasting systems defined. Good satellite usage.	All major donors (over 120). Red Cross plays important role: large, organized, many resources. World's largest volunteer agency community.
Burma	35 million (1980) 2·3%	56·8/1000 (1979) $140 (Estimated 1977) for (1979)	Flash floods. Cyclones. Fires. Civil strife. 1966–1976: 2·1 million	(−) Health services. Power transmission/distribution/facilities. (+) Economy. Agriculture. Good urban cold storage. Communications. Hydroelectric potential. Energy expansion plans. Disease eradication.	No national disaster plan. Ministry of government and central relief committee: Co-ordination bodies. Limited picture.	Most international donors including 16 US non-profit groups. Selected private organizations.

India	684 million (1981) 2·2%	123·4/1000 $250	Monsoons. Droughts. Deforestation. Floods. Erosion. Cyclones. Desertification. Some earthquake activity. Nuclear and other accidents (chemical: See Bhopal). Epidemics. 1970–1982: Almost 400 million	(−) Communications and transportation links. Dams/power plant/nuclear plant weaknesses. Housing. Irrigation systems. Drinking supplies. (+) Health programmes. Electric power systems.	No national disaster plan. Disaster management: state level. Central government research, surveys, guidance, financial assistance. Multi-disciplinary government teams. Central government role under review. Tamil Nadu State: especially active planning. Extensive mitigation efforts: for droughts, floods, cyclones, earthquakes, diseases, conservation, irrigation, family planning.	Major international, private donors. Extremely large grouping (105) of US non-profits. Host: excellent self-help capability. Government aware of need for long-term efforts. Realizes development programmes contribute to disaster preparedness.
Indonesia	149·4 million (1981) 3·5% (1980)	91/1000 $439	Earthquakes. Floods. Volcanic eruptions. Droughts. Landslides. Tsunamis. Strong winds. Epidemics. 1963–1982: 48 million	(−) Health services. Water. Waterborne diseases. Immunization programmes. Housing. Sewage. Rails. Relief supplies. Urbanization. (+) Economic growth. Agriculture policies. Petroleum. Emergency food storage. Health status. Ports. Roads.	No plan (though drafted in 1977). Operates by executive order. National co-ordination board for disaster relief (for emergencies): policies and co-ordination efforts. Proposed national disaster mnanagement institute. Provincial level disaster relief organizations. Preventive and rehabilitation efforts. District relief organizations.	All major international, private, religious organizations. 69 US non-profit groups. Primary role may be development. Red Cross: major role. Use of military and private equipment and transportation.

APPENDIX

Disaster Profiles of Selected Developing Countries (*continued*)

Country	Indicators — Population annual growth (%)	Indicators — Inf. mort. rate per 1000	Indicators — GNP ($)	Disaster types/ recent history: victims	Vulnerability — Systems problems/assets	Preparedness — Plan/structure	Donor assessment
Nepal	15·3 million (1981) 2·1%	150/1000	$ N.A.	Deforestation. Malaria. Land slides. Floods. Droughts. Earthquakes. 1963–1968: 4·7 million	(−) Economic growth. Agriculture. Population pressures. Surface transportation. Farm lands. Soil conservation. Infrastructure vulnerabilities. Housing. (+) Hydroelectric potential.	No official plan; many proposed; no guidelines. Organizations act independently in relief operations. Nepal Red Cross: operates with unofficial government authority: Own national plan/major role. Central disaster relief operations committee: Formal structure. Several mitigation projects. Development projects can incorporate disaster mitigation.	A number of international, bi-lateral, private groups. Nearly 40 US non-profit groups.
Pakistan	85·6 million (1982) 2·9 million Afghan refugees in addition 3·1%	126/1000	$ N.A. (though economy is growing)	Floods. Deforestation. Land slides. Earthquakes. Droughts. Refugees. Malaria. Chemical toxins. Water contamination. *Potential* pesticide and other chemical poisoning. Infestations. Fires. 1964–1982: Over 19 million	(−) Health sector administration. Road quality. Infrastructure damage. Earthquake zones with major commerce centres. Inadequate storage. Medical capacity. (+) Economy. Industrial growth. Telecommunications network. Rails. Malaria eradication. Extensive integrated irrigation. Emergency medical systems. Natural gas and hydroelectric development.	National disaster plan: co-ordinated with all appropriate ministries. Outlines prevention aspects. Establishes special regulatory bodies. Provincial plans operational. Military. Contingency disaster plans. Red Crescent Society tied to public relief efforts. Disaster/ development NEXUS becoming important. World Meteorological Warning Systems.	All major international, private and religious organizations. Many host organizations. Red Crescent Society plays important role. UNDP serves as liaison for all organizations to government. 40 US non-profit groups.

	Population	Death rate / Income	Disasters	Problems	National planning	Groups
Philippines	48.0 million (1980) 2.5%	66/1000 $885 (1986 estimated)	Typhoons ('Baguios'). Volcanic eruptions. Monsoons. Earthquakes. Epidemics. Fires. Frequent disasters of various types. 1970–1982: 10 million	(−) Housing. Income distribution. Port maintenance. Telecommunications. Sanitation. Sewage disposal. Civil strife. (+) Health services and policy. Housing policy. Long-range planning. Industrial reforms. Roads. Energy resource development and hydroelectric potential.	National guidelines on disaster preparedness; detailed. National disaster co-ordinating council under Minister of Defence, responsible for guidelines allocates disaster priorities. All major government agencies involved. Highly structured/good communications. Co-ordinating councils at many levels. Office of Civil Defence: co-ordinates government and private groups. EOC. 3-phase housing disaster policy. Long-range economic planning.	All major international, private and religious groups. US voluntary agencies play very significant role; nearly 110—one of the largest groupings.
Sri Lanka	15.0 million (1981) 1.8% (1980)	44/1000 $ N.A.	Floods. Droughts. Civil strife. Malaria. Landslides. Some cyclones. 1964–1982: 5.3 million	(−) Vulnerable roads, bridges, ports, crops, livestock. Sporadic warfare. Widespread violence. Water availability. Communications. Data collection/reporting. Health shortages. Transport delivery. Attitudes toward EWS. (+) Health care costs. Disease eradication programmes. Rail and road systems. New radar system.	No comprehensive plan. Proposed plan never enacted (budget problems). Disasters handled by ad hoc co-ordinating committees. National, district and village level committees. Effective response to flooding. Use of Department of Social Services relief instructions. Satellite use: storm warning system (though at times villages do not take warnings seriously).	Many international, private and religious organizations. 22 US non-profit groups.

APPENDIX

Disaster Profiles of Selected Developing Countries (*continued*)

Country	Indicators — Population annual growth (%)	Inf. mort. rate per cap. GNP ($)	Disaster types/ recent history: victims	Vulnerability — Systems problems/assets	Preparedness — Plan/structure	Donor assessment
Turkey	45·0 million (1980) 2·2%	32/1000 $ N.A.	Earthquakes. Epidemics. Accidents (fires, air and train crashes, oil spills). Snows. Floods. 1967–1980: 600 000	(−) Economy. Political environment. Transport systems. Shortages. Forest production. Phone system. Urban slums. Sanitation. (+) Health system. Economic planning. Agriculture policy. Construction standards. Energy development and management.	Disaster legislation. General directorate of natural disasters: establishes EOCs, co-ordinates activities. Well-structured with detailed assignments. Provincial level structures covering all areas. Important Red Crescent (Kizilay) role: large, well-organized and involved in preparedness and relief; close co-ordination with government.	UNDP co-ordinates international relief activities at specific request of *government.* Red Crescent, CARITAS, CRS, WHO. League of Red Cross Societies: major co-operating organizations. Other private and religious agencies also involved, including a dozen US PVOs.
Antigua and Barduda	76.2000 (1981) 1·3%	24/1000 $ N.A.	History of: Hurricanes. Droughts. Earthquakes. No recent damage.	(−) Some communicable diseases. Health personnel. Housing. Drinking water. (+) Eradication programmes. Transport systems. Power. Telecommunications. Literacy rate.	Central disaster committee: composed of all key cabinet, health and security experts. Co-ordinates emergency operations. Relief clearing house. Local and regional councils and committees. Emergency supplies and storage. Regional disaster plan very detailed (PCDPPP).	Red Cross: important role. Host organization plus YWCA, Salvation Army, some religious groups. At least 12 US non-profit organizations.

Barbados	250 000 (1980) 0·5%	27·7/1000 $ N.A.	Subject to: Hurricanes. Floods. Some earthquake activity. No recent history.	(−) Some malnutrition. Housing. Economy. (+) National health service. Safe piped water. Electricity. Sanitation. Roads. Solar power potential. Telecommunications. Literacy rate. Tourism industry.	Complete emergency plan. Central emergency relief committee. Co-ordinating advisory council. Emergency telecommunications centre. Elaborate, detailed system. PCDPPP participation.	Many major private, religious, international organizations.
Belize	146 000 (1981) 1·9%	45/1000 $ N.A.	Hurricanes. 1961–1979: 95 000	(−) Health care delivery/staff. Food sufficiency. Housing. Rails. Power maintenance. High dependency ratio. Potential invasions. (+) Phone system. Water and sewage development.	Hurricane disaster preparedness plan: Annual updates. Central (cabinet level) emergency organization with 12 sub-committees. District emergency organizations. Emergency storage depot. Good array of host resources. Red Cross organizes supply operations. PCDPPP participation.	Many major host inter-national, private and religious groups, including 24 from the US. Red Cross important.
Dominica	84 000 (1980) 1·2% (Affected by emi-gration of working age males)	19·6/1000 $ N.A.	Hurricanes. Droughts and earthquakes limited. 1979: 65 000	(−) Health services/equipment. Health training. Housing. Communicable diseases. Inflation. Road system. Power system vulnerability. (+) Health improvements. Literacy.	National plan directed toward hurricanes: broad procedural application. Central hurricane committee. Many levels of participation. District and local committees. Warning system: simple but good. PCDPPP participation.	Donor profile not clear though at least 14 US non-profit groups. Many international organizational membership.

APPENDIX

Disaster Profiles of Selected Developing Countries (*continued*)

Country	Indicators — Population annual growth (%)	Inf. mort. rate	per cap. GNP ($)	Vulnerability — Disaster types/ recent history: victims	Systems problems/assets	Preparedness — Plan/structure	Donor assessment
Dominican Republic	6·2 million (1981) 3%	78/1000	$1072 (1972)	Hurricanes. Floods. Earthquakes. Deforestation. Erosion. Forest fires. Epidemics. 1963–1983: 2·6 million	(−) Watersheds. land and water resource abused. Population economy. Farming conservation. Health data. Health services. Housing. Agriculture. Irrigation. Fire-fighting capacity. (+) Health staffing. Government change focus. Telecommunications. Road system. Water projects.	National disaster plan. Very detailed assignments: calls upon private resources. 13 annexes covering major need areas. National disaster committee: major government agencies. Civil defence office not adequate to perform fully. Problems of relations between private and government agencies: communications/ authorities. Good emergency communications network. PCDPPP participation.	Red Cross: major role; has own national relief plan; good education programme blood banks/ware-houses. All major inter-national, private, religious groups. Dominican Electric Corporation also has disaster plan. Almost 50 US non-profit groups.
Grenada	108 000 (1980) 2%	15·4/1000	$ N.A.	Hurricanes. Droughts. Earthquakes limited. No historical profile.	(−) Some high infectious disease rates. Unemployment. Roads and bridges. (+) Health system network. Telecommunications. Malaria eradication programme. Tourism industry. Communications.	No plan. Central emergency relief committee: detailed responsibilities for government departments, utilities, voluntary organizations. Well-funded. EOC at Prime Minister's Office. PCDPPP participation.	Member of several international organizations. Donor profile not clear though at least 9 US non-profit groups.

Guyana	800 000 (1982) 1%	44/1000 $690 (1981)	Civil strife. Floods. Power shortages. Fires. People's Temple 'accident'. (1966–1979): 285 000	(−) Drainage. Malaria. Yellow fever. Water. Waste and sewage disposal. Parasitic diseases. Malnutrition. Trained health personnel shortages. Economy. Road system. Power generation. (+) School immunization programmes. Nursing personnel. Government economic plans. Port usage. Hydroelectric potential.	No national plan. Each administration division of government has energy relief plans. Red Cross plays major supply role though has no official assignments. PCDPPP participation.	Many major churches, international and private organizations. 14 US non-profits.
Haiti	6 million (1982) 1 million living abroad % N.A.	115/1000 $270 (1980)	Hurricanes. Floods. Limited earthquakes. Fires. Pesticide hazards. Droughts. Erosion. Fires. Power shortages. 1964–1983: 3·5 million	(−) Poverty. Illiteracy. Transportation. Nutrition. Malnutrition. Housing. Waste disposal. Deforestation. Agriculture practices. Fire services. Political tensions. Corruption (unclear effects of 1986 government overthrow).	Organisation session pré-désastre et de secours (via 1983 legislation). Public Health Department co-ordinates. Very detailed. Not known to be fully operating nor with a comprehensive plan (4/84). Red Cross: major role; excellent. Law calls for committees/intervention teams. PCDPPP participation. Development/disaster focus needed.	Major developmental contributions from many external organizations. Voluntary agencies play significant social/medical services roles. A Haitian association of volunteer agencies. 17 US non-profits.

APPENDIX

Disaster Profiles of Selected Developing Countries (continued)

Country	Indicators — Population annual growth (%)	Indicators — Inf. mort. rate per cap. GNP ($)	Disaster types/ recent history: victims	Vulnerability — Systems problems/assets	Preparedness — Plan/structure	Donor assessment
Jamaica	2·3 million (1980) 1·2%	15/1000 $ N.A.	Heavy rains. Floods. Extended droughts. Hurricanes. Tidal waves. Fires. Erosion. Chemical hazards. Earthquakes (some). Epidemics. Some civil strife. Potential air accidents. 1968–1981: 331 000	(−) Marginal area settlement. Housing, crop, infrastructure weaknesses. Water pressure. Chemical plant waste storage. Water pollution. Mountain roads. Airport safety. Critical electric supplies. Building structures. Phone line vulnerability. (+) Mitigation projects. Research. Health system. Transportation system.	Office of disaster preparedness and emergency relief: Full co-ordination; develops/mobilizes all resources; sophisticated and well-organized. PCDPPP participation. Government/ PVO co-ordination. Good research and risk assessment. National disaster committee. Parish structure plans. Excellent, comprehensive resources.	Government works closely with donors. Donors: powerful/ effective resource. All major inter-national, private and religious groups. Over 40 US non-profit groups.
Montserrat	11 600 (1980) Zero growth	40/1000 $ Fairly high estimates, but no precise figure available.	Hurricanes. (Some) earthquakes. Droughts.	(−) Health information short-ages. Water storage. Public sewage system. Housing quality. (+) Piped water access. Economic growth. Industrial expansion. Erosion policies. Transpor-tation systems. Telecommunica-tions. Access to electric power.	Montserrat emergency organi-zation. Central committee and district committees. Detailed plans. Plan: Government Hurricane Instructions: detailed responsibilities, including Red Cross. Disaster communications system. Food stockpile. PCDPPP participation.	No clear profile: though 5 US non-profits are contributing. Red Cross plays important role.

				Needs	Disaster organization	Donor
St Kitts-Nevis-Anguilla	49 000 (1980) 2%	41/1000 $920 (1980)	Some hurricanes, droughts. Earthquakes (most are minor). No history information.	(−) Skilled labour shortages. Mortality/mobility data. Some infectious diseases. Health care access. Physician supply. Telecommunications capacity. (+) Transportation systems. Government housing programme. Availability of potable water.	Hurricane instruction is national plan. Hurricane relief officer as needed to advise premier. EOC: police. Specialized Government services called upon. Government/private sector co-operation. Member of PCDPPP.	Donor picture not clear. At least 11 US non-profit organizations.
St Lucia	122 000 (1981) 1·5%	32·9/1000 $ N.A.	Hurricanes. Floods. Earthquakes. 1970–1980: Major hurricane damage to crops, infrastructure (telecommunications, ports, roads, bridges, utilities, housing).	(−) Some water shortages. Housing. (+) Economic recovery. Manufacturing and tourism industries. Ports. Power generation. Alternative energy development. Telecommunications. Health facilities.	National disaster plan. Central emergency committee: all cabinet officers. 10 district plans. Emergency communications system.	Important Red Cross supply distribution role. Other donor profiles unclear, though 16 US non-profit groups involved.
St Vincent and the Grenadines	110 000 (1980) 2·1%	59·4/1000 $ N.A.	Hurricanes. Volcanic eruptions. Landslides. 1967–1980: Over 40000	(−) Enteric diseases. Clean water. Water services. Health personnel shortages. Housing. Bridges. (+) Health facilities. Government commitment to private economic development. Recovery from natural disasters. Economic growth. Transportation. Energy source expansion. Telecommunications.	National disaster plan (for hurricanes/volcanic erruptions). Central energy committee: all major government officials, churches, Chamber of Commerce, utilities. Civic associations. Emergency relief organization operations at district level (20 committees). Two disaster eruption commissions. PCDPPP participation.	Private sector clearly involved with government, but no details available. A dozen US non-profit groups involved.

APPENDIX

Disaster Profiles of Selected Developing Countries (*continued*)

Country	Indicators — Population annual growth (%)	Inf. mort. rate per cap.	GNP ($)	Disaster types/ recent history: victims	Vulnerability — Systems problems/assets	Preparedness — Plan/structure	Donor assessment
Trinidad and Tobago	1·2 million (1980) 1·2%	23·9/1000 (1981)	$4800 (1980: fourth highest in hemisphere)	(Some) hurricanes. Floods. Earthquake activity.	(−) Public service facilities expansion rate. Role of agriculture. Some forest exploitation. Auto accident rates. (+) Overall profile. Health status. Medical facility supplies and personnel. Housing. Sewage system. Electricity. Economic growth/diversification. Oil and gas supply. Roads. Power output. Telecommunications. High literacy.	National disaster plan (NERO): Defines government and private responsibilities. Provides co-ordination assistance. National emergency relief organization: implementation. Specific agency/service plans approved yearly. Close Red Cross involvement: own local disaster service.	UNDP. Red Cross. Society of St Vincent De Paul. World Council of Churches, plus 7 US non-profit groups.
Cormoros	408 000 (1982) % N.A.	89/1000	$340 (1982)	Volcanic eruptions. Cyclones. Deforestation. Erosion. Infestations (some). Droughts. Food shortages. Civil strife. Forced repatriation. 1972–1982: 11 incidents; almost 50 000	(−) Cultivation in volcanic areas. Health. Malnutrition. Forest depletion. Storage. Water supplies. Road construction. Port and airport facilities. Economy. Food adequacy. Outside aid dependence.	No known plan or formal structure. Government addressing of erosion, deforestation, road completion would help. Need for better EMS would aid in disaster prevention.	Several donors. Care is major US conduit; 2 other groups involved. Range of international, bi-lateral, private assistance.

	Population (year) growth	Deaths/1000 GNP per capita	Disasters; deaths	Vulnerabilities	National organization/programmes	International assistance
Madagascar	10 million (1984) 2·6%	66/1000 $310 (1983)	Tropical cyclones. Floods. Epidemics. Deforestation. Erosion. Infestations. Civil strife. Landslides. 1964–1984: 3·5 million	Malaria. Communicable diseases. Malnutrition. Weather variations. Growth and development. Increasing imports. Transportation deterioration. Siltation. Safe water. Waste disposal. Drainage. Communication lines. Housing. Agriculture vulnerability.	National organization assistance plan: cyclone emergencies. National relief council: Co-ordinates relief. Executive general staff (under armed services): disaster management operations. Transportation training. Permanent disaster centre. Cyclone warning system. Mitigation-development relationship.	Range of international, bi-lateral, private and religious organizations. 10 US non-profit groups.
Maldives	160000+ (1982) 2·3%	88/1000 $350 (1982)	Little national disaster vulnerability. Some epidemics. Health hazards. 1978: Cholera; 11000 affected	(−) Waterborne and communicable diseases. Medical resource shortages. Roads. Inner-atoll transport. Power and phone systems. Ports. (+) Atoll health centres. Health centre launch system. Natural resource base. Expanding tourism.	Member: regional disaster prevention and preparedness programme. Tropical cyclone committee, SW Indian Ocean. Satellite use: external communications. Members have own disaster plans; are to develop training, information systems, backup procedures. Regional data collection/dissemination.	No clear picture. Co-operative regional involvement. Interactions with WMO, Red Cross Societies, UNDRO, OFDA plus. At least 2 US non-profit groups.
Mauritius	1·0 million (1983) 2·2%	32/1000 $1248 (1984)	Cyclones. Droughts (some). Floods. 1964–1983: 13 cyclones/major crop and infrastructure damage.	(−) Agriculture and infrastructure vulnerabilities. Waterborne disease breakouts. (+) Communications. Roads. Crop Insurance Programme. Free health care. Family planning services. Health facilities. Water and emergency supplies. Harbour.	National cyclone emergency plan: annual review; early preparation. Infrastructure inspections. Preventive maintenance. Comprehensive crop insurance programme. Early warning system. Four main bodies to handle disasters: Central government down to local levels. Good use of Red Cross. Data sharing with Diego Garcia meteorological station. Regional cyclone communication. Participation in Regional Cyclone Committee.	Several international, religious, private donors, including 2 US non-profit groups.

APPENDIX

Disaster Profiles of Selected Developing Countries (*continued*)

Country	Indicators — Population annual growth (%)	Inf. mort. rate per cap.	GNP ($)	Disaster types/ recent history: victims	Vulnerability Systems problems/assets	Preparedness Plan/structure	Donor assessment
Reunion	110 000 (1983) 1·5% (about 5 000/ year emigrate)	N.A.	$ N.A.	Volcanic eruptions. Cyclones. Heavy 1980 cyclone damage.	(−) Lack of natural resources. Underdeveloped industry. Unemployment. Health care system. High food imports. (+) Expanding road system. Telecommunications system adequacy.	National disaster plan (based on plan used by French territories). No clear picture of use or structure.	On-going assistance from France primarily.
Seychelles	68 000 (1983) 2·8%	30/1000	$1800 (1981)	Erosion. Forest fires. No delineated history.	(−) Food sufficiency. *Potential* water shortages. Rainfall variations. (+) Communications facilities. Health care. Transportation system. Tourism industry. Construction industry.	Member of SW Indian Ocean association of cyclone committees. Organizational plan: requires forecasting and warning responsibilities for all members, as well as disaster plans.	Little information except for involvement of 3 US non-profit groups.

Country	Population	Demographics	Disasters	Factors	Disaster plans	Organizations
Chile	10·9 million (1979) 1·7%	54/1000 (1976) $1170 (1977)	Floods. Earthquakes. Droughts. Volcanic eruptions. Avalanches. Civil strife. 1964–1980: 6·5 million	(−) Enteric diseases. Malnutrition pockets. Housing shortages. Limited safe harbours. (+) Health status. Use of military in health delivery. Drugs supplies. Relative economic stability. Land and growth range. Transportation. Power capacity. Telecommunications system.	Elaborate/extensive plans and organization (via legislation). National emergency preparedness office; plans, co-ordinates, executes. Four regional, provincial community emergency committees. Seven plans at various levels. Communications office. Funding may not be adequate. Food stockpile and strategy. Involve voluntary groups.	Major international, host, private and religious organizations, including 4 dozen US non-profits.
Costa Rica	2·4 million (1982) 2·7%	28/1000 $ N.A.	Volcanic eruptions. Floods. Earthquakes. Droughts. Forest fires. 1963–1980: 1·4 million	(−) Some economic downturn. (+) Agriculture and animal husbandry. Transportation system. Health facilities network. Health care. Low disease levels. Electricity. Communications. High literacy.	No formal disaster plan. 1974 National emergency law directs, plans, controls and co-ordinates all disasters. National emergency commission in event of disaster. Cabinet level civil defence organization. No separate storage and distribution facilities for emergencies. Detailed US mission plan to assist government.	All major international, private and religious organizations, including 4 dozen US non-profits.

APPENDIX

Disaster Profiles of Selected Developing Countries (continued)

Country	Indicators Population annual growth (%)	Inf. mort. rate per cap. GNP ($)	Disaster types/ recent history: victims	Vulnerability Systems problems/assets	Preparedness Plan/structure	Donor assessment
Ecuador	8·6 million (1982) 3·4%	60/1000 $N.A.	Floods. Tropical air mass shifts. Intense rainfalls in arrid areas (El Niño') Volcanic eruptions/pyroclastic flows. Landslides. Deforestation. Local droughts. Epidemics. 1964–1983: Estimate of 10 million.	(−) Sanitation. Health conditions. Land settlement problems. Sewage and water systems. Roads and bridges. Agriculture and livestock vulnerability. Housing enforcement. Deforestation projects. Limited emergency communications.	Multi-organizational responsibilities. Ecuadorian civil defence: primary responsibility, but not effective in preparations/ responses. Participates in Pacific Tsunami Warning System. Government ignores hazards/implications. Little hazard identification analysis. Paucity of government data on resources. Haphazard plans. Jurisdictional disputes. No systematic disaster training. Few mitigation efforts.	All major international, private, civilian and religious organizations, including 54 US non-profit groups. Red Cross well organized, effective, great autonomy of operation.
El Salvador	5·1 million (1982) 3·5%	72/1000 (many preventable) $720	Civil strife. Displaced persons. Volcanic activity (some). Earthquakes. Floods. Landslides. Pesticide damage/poisoning. Hurricanes. 1965–1984: 1·5 million	(−) Uneven health service distribution. Some service shortages. Displaced persons. Damage effects (guerilla warfare) on infrastructure. Employment opportunities. Food storage losses. (+) Major port. Rail and road systems. Agrarian reforms. Seismic network. Phone system.	1984 National emergency law: defines national emergency-system. National and local committees. Early warning system. CONADES: autonomous government commission: assistance to displaced persons, warehouse facilities/co-ordinates with volags. EWS. through Red Cross. Green Cross Commandos. Government programmes to improve political/economic situation. Long-range goals.	All major religious, private, international organizations. Red Cross, Green Cross, etc. Three dozen US non-profit groups.

Country	Demographics	Hazards / Losses	Development issues	Emergency plan	Donor organizations
Guatemala	7·1 million (1981) 69/1000 $ N.A. 3%	Pesticide poisoning. Fires. Earthquakes. Floods. Epidemics. Hurricanes. Civil strife. Landslides. 1960–1979: 1·75 million	(−) Safe water supply. Pollution. Gastric diseases. Housing construction standards. Health facilities. Nutrition. Some food shortages. Erosion. Road and bridge maintenance. Emergency supplies. Phone availability. (+) Port capacity and operations. Highway system expansion. Hydroelectric potential.	No formal plan, but well-developed system. National emergency committee with detailed responsibilities. Long-term planning. Volunteer fire system nationwide for emergencies.	At least 70 international, private, host country and religious organizations.
Honduras	3·7 million (1980) 118/1000 $480 3·4%	Hurricanes. Floods. Droughts. Civil strife. Epidemics. Accidents. 1965–1980: 1·2 million	(−) Malnutrition. Sanitation. Medical care access. Health manpower. Electricity availability. Economic growth. Air-port adequacy. Phone system limitations. Power consumption. (+) Hydroelectric potential.	Council for national emergencies: directs, co-ordinates relief, all donor programmes, government agency functions; very detailed. Armed Forces and Red Cross play major roles. National disaster plan: needs improvements. Considerable equipment, but supplies may not be adequate.	Over 80 major international, private and religious organizations with numerous resources.
Nicaragua	2·73 million (1981) 46/1000 (1978) $660 (1979) 3·2%	Earthquakes. Epidemics. Droughts. Volcanic eruptions. Civil strife. Little illumination on history.	(−) Housing. Economy. Civil strife effects. Underemployment. Productivity. Financial markets. Rail system. Electricity access. Telephone system. Water and sanitation. (+) Agrarian reforms. Ten-year health plan. Road network. Hydroelectric development. Storm water disposal. Resettlement measures.	National plan (developed under Somoza government). National emergency commission: limited response capacity. Civil defence plan. National health plan. Red Cross important in relief efforts.	Considerable host dependence on donor resources. All major religious, international, private agencies. 41 known US non-profit organizations. Many in development.

APPENDIX

Disaster Profiles of Selected Developing Countries (*continued*)

Country	Indicators Population annual growth (%)	Inf. mort. rate per cap.	GNP ($)	Disaster types/ recent history: victims	Vulnerability Systems problems/assets	Preparedness Plan/structure	Donor assessment
Peru	17 million 2·9%	101/1000	Estimate $900 (1978)	Earthquakes. Floods. Droughts. Epidemics. Famine. Civil strife. No history profile available.	(−) Illness/death rates. Health care access. Cold facility distribution. Urban migration. Utilities adequacy. Roads. Communications. Economy.	National civil defence system. All phases of disaster operations relief. Substantial military involvement. Elaborate system but not clear profile/effectiveness. No plan indicated: assume operating procedures go with structure. Host disaster team: military.	Extensive donor community, including major international, religious and private organizations. Over 80 US non-profits.
Fiji	620 000 (1979) 2·5%	23/1000 (1978)	$1150	Earthquakes. Hurricanes. Tropical storms. 1973–1975: 113 000	(−) Agricultural industry. Development plans. Road safety. Access to electricity. (+) Health status. Health personnel. Medical school. Road expansion/reconstruction. Pacific refueling stop. Communication centre. Hydroelectric development.	National plan. Emergency services commission (Ministry of Home Affairs): Co-ordinates all levels of plans. Control centres; detailed assignments. Government departments and district levels. Hurricane relief commission: effective performance. Emergency control centre (communications). EWS.	Many international, religious, private groups. Many involved in development work. Red Cross is important. Five US non-profit groups.

	Population / economy	Hazards and disaster history	Constraints (−) and opportunities (+)	National disaster planning	Organizations / aid
Papua New Guinea	3·3 million (1984) 97/1000 $800 (includes expatriates' incomes and added values of selected private enterprises) 2·1%	Volcanic eruptions. Earthquakes. Landslides. Tsunamis. Cyclones/winds. Floods. Frost. (Some) droughts. (Some) accidents. 1970–1985: 224 000	(−) *Potential* aviation and marine accidents. Squatter settlements/marginal areas. Transportation. Infrastructure. Environmental hygiene. Malaria. Lack of services. (+) Aviation link to remote areas. Telecommunications. Long-term resource exploitation/expansion plans.	1984 National disaster management act. National disaster committee. National disaster plan: Comprehensive; planning incorporated into development. National disaster centre. Provincial disaster committees: considerable detail and covering all functions and needs. Government aware of opportunity to integrate mitigation with development. Several electronic warning systems: volcanic eruptions; tsunamis; cyclones; earthquakes.	US aid through nearly 40 donor organizations. Many international, private and religious groups.
Tonga	93 000 (1978) 20·5/1000 (1976) $350 (1976) 1·5% growth	Hurricanes. Floods. Earthquakes. Tsunamis. Volcanic eruptions. Droughts. Epidemics (some have not occurred in many years). No delineated history	(−) Transport and communications limitations. Rescue capacity. Water supply and sanitation. Economic expansion obstacles. Fixed markets. Road deterioration. (+) Clinic/medical service systems. Medical facilities. Power capacity. Upgrading phone system.	No national disaster plan (1980). Central hurricane relief committee. Warning system of limited dimension.	Red Cross: important. Several international, host and religious organizations, including 11 US non-profits.
Western Samoa	154 000 (1978) 40/100 (1976) $350 (1976) 1% (high dependency rate)	Hurricanes. Floods. Earthquakes. Tsunamis. Volcanic eruptions. 1966–1968: 95 000	(−) Increasing heart disease/diabetes. Physician shortage. Under employment. Economic growth limited. Skilled labour. Some agricultural stagnation. (+) High literacy. Health services. Absence of epidemics. Road network. Hydropower. Telecommunications system.	No national plan (1981). Early warning observatory. Seismology station. Participates in international seismic seawave warning system.	Most prominent voluntary organization seems to be the Foundation for the People of the South Pacific. Government is member of many international organizations. At least 14 US non-profits.

Index

479

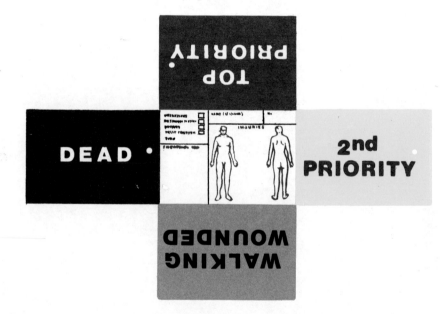

The Perth casualty triage tag.